An Update on Syndemics

An Update on Syndemics

Guest Editors

Nicola Bulled
Merrill Singer

MDPI

Basel • Beijing • Wuhan • Barcelona • Belgrade • Novi Sad • Cluj • Manchester

Guest Editors
Nicola Bulled
Institute for Collaboration on Health, Intervention, and Policy
University of Connecticut
Storrs
USA

Merrill Singer
Department of Anthropology
University of Connecticut
Storrs
USA

Editorial Office
MDPI AG
Grosspeteranlage 5
4052 Basel, Switzerland

This is a reprint of the Special Issue, published open access by the journal *Tropical Medicine and Infectious Disease* (ISSN 2414-6366), freely accessible at: https://www.mdpi.com/journal/tropicalmed/special_issues/2OKIX3T967.

For citation purposes, cite each article independently as indicated on the article page online and as indicated below:

Lastname, A.A.; Lastname, B.B. Article Title. *Journal Name* **Year**, *Volume Number*, Page Range.

ISBN 978-3-7258-4643-6 (Hbk)
ISBN 978-3-7258-4644-3 (PDF)
https://doi.org/10.3390/books978-3-7258-4644-3

Contents

About the Editors

Nicola Bulled

Nicola Bulled is an Assistant Research Professor at the University of Connecticut, affiliated with the Institute for Collaboration on Health, Intervention, and Policy, and a Lecturer at Brown University's School of Public Health. She has over two decades of experience in global and domestic research on syndemic theory, with a particular emphasis on the socio-structural conditions that generate and sustain these co-occurring epidemics. She received a master's in Public Health from Boston University in 2005, a master's degree in Anthropology from the University of Connecticut in 2010, and a Ph.D. degree from the University of Connecticut in 2012. She served as a Fulbright Scholar in Lesotho. She held a Fogarty Foundation/National Institutes of Health Postdoctoral Fellowship at the Center for Global Health, University of Virginia (2013–2015).

Merrill Singer

Merrill Singer was a medical anthropologist and professor emeritus in Anthropology at the University of Connecticut. He was best known for his research on substance abuse, HIV/AIDS, syndemics, health disparities, environmental health, and minority health and his development of two grounding concepts in Medical Anthropology: Critical Medical Anthropology and Syndemics Theory. He received his master's degree in Anthropology from California State University in 1975 and a Ph.D. degree from the University of Utah in 1979. He held a National Institute on Alcohol Abuse and Alcoholism Postdoctoral Fellowship in the Department of Psychiatry, George Washington University (1979–1980) and another at the University of Connecticut School of Medicine from 1982 to 1983. In 2017, he was awarded the Society for Medical Anthropology Career Award.

Tropical Medicine and Infectious Disease

MDPI

Editorial

An Update on Syndemics: Editorial Comments

Nicola Bulled * and Merrill Singer †

Institute for Collaboration on Health, Intervention, and Policy (InCHIP), University of Connecticut, 2006 Hillside Road, Storrs, CT 06269, USA

* Correspondence: nicola.bulled@uconn.edu

† Passed away.

The theory of syndemics hypothesizes that observed clusters of diseases in specific temporal and geographical contexts are the result of harmful socio-environmental conditions resulting in mutually enhancing deleterious consequences. For the past 30 years, the concept has informed an array of health-related disciplines, proving valuable in health research, policy, practice, and education. It has been used to guide recent responses to MPOX [1], COVID-19 [2], and Ebola [3].

For this Special Issue, scholars working in the field were asked to consider novel syndemic attributes of clusters of infectious diseases that result in worse health outcomes than each condition in isolation. While HIV-related syndemics remain the most studied, new disease arrangements have emerged that warrant investigation including those related to novel infectious disease epidemics and re-emerging epidemics, as well as chronic epidemics that, historically, have received limited attention and resources.

In keeping with the three tenets of syndemics, scholars were asked to consider the following: (1) clusters of infectious diseases and other health conditions concentrated in a population; (2) the biological interactions of diseases in a manner that increases infectivity or disease progression beyond that of co-existing/comorbid disease arrangements; and (3) the social, structural, and/or environmental conditions that support the existence of multiple health conditions within a population.

Tenet 1: Clustering of epidemic diseases in a population. Multiple morbidities or comorbidities, the co-occurrence of multiple diseases or health conditions, is well established in the literature. Certain conditions, such as HIV, given its impact on the body's immune response and promoting inflammation, are well recognized as being associated with a host of varied comorbidities including other communicable diseases, chronic non-communicable diseases, and mental health conditions.

While the clustering of health conditions may be seen as serially causal or sequential, with one condition preceding the other, disease interactions are often more dynamic and complex and influenced by the social context. For example, untreated syphilis can facilitate the transmission and acquisition of HIV infection [4]. In turn, HIV increases risk of syphilis acquisition [5] and can alter syphilis manifestations, potentially misleading clinical diagnosis [4]. Co-infection can result in a higher risk of treatment failure, and genital ulcers take longer to heal in patients with HIV than in patients with syphilis alone, increasing the risk of exposure to other sexually transmitted infections [4,5]. These conditions are understood to share "common risk factors", indicating that they cluster among individuals who engage in risk behaviors, hold specific social identities, and experience structural risk factors.

All eight of the articles in this Special Issue highlight the clustering of diseases within a defined population. McCollum et al. [6] present a novel arrangement of Neglected

Tropical Diseases (NTDs) of the skin and mental distress in Liberia. Using a mixed-methods approach to understanding the experiences of individuals with NTDs of the skin, the authors found that disability was significantly associated with higher levels of depression and anxiety, with persons affected experiencing additional financial concerns, stigma, and pain, which all contributed to their mental health conditions. Barret et al. [7] also consider the mental health burden of infectious diseases as they detail syndemics of Lymphatic Filariasis in Malawi. For people affected by Lymphatic Filariasis, absent medical referral pathways, inequalities in healthcare provision or available treatment, and limited knowledge of the condition heightened patients' mental distress. Distress was further exacerbated by stigma and social exclusion, and was shaped by the intersections of gender, poverty, and extreme climate conditions. Collectively, the articles in this Special Issue reveal the value of the syndemics framework in both recognizing previously unexplored comorbidities and considering disease clustering within populations experiencing specific shared social conditions, to focus and mobilize public health and healthcare resources.

Tenet 2: Detailing the interaction of diseases. Disease interaction is a key unique feature of syndemic theory, distinguishing it from the existing frameworks of *comorbidities* and *social determinants of health*. Syndemic theory recognizes that clustered and comorbid diseases interact in a manner that exacerbates the health outcomes of diseases beyond what would be expected from the combination of their independent effects. The name *syn*-demic implies that this interaction is *syn*-ergistic, where the combined effect is greater than the sum of the separate effects.

Presently, the syndemics literature is struggling to address this second tenet. Syndemic theory has been criticized for its inability to clearly articulate and present empirical measures of synergistic interaction [8,9]. The criticism brings to light many questions. How do we present evidence of interaction? What counts as evidence of interaction? Do we have statistical methods or analyses to test hypotheses of interactions of multiple conditions simultaneously?

On the one hand, the criticism suggests that the theory has yet to be evidenced; on the other hand, it raises a larger question about what counts as evidence. Statistically measuring disease interactions does not provide details on the nature of the intricate and complex responses of the body's immune system. Furthermore, current statistical tools only allow us to measure the interaction between two co-existing phenomena, limiting the examination of disease clusters that involve more than two comorbidities. Disease interaction not only still exists but also still matters, irrespective of our ability to measure it [10]. Disease interactions can and have been demonstrated by combining evidence from various forms including literature on disease physiology, epidemiology, cohort studies, clinical trials, and ethnographies or qualitative studies detailing experiences of disease. These assessments present clear evidence supporting syndemic theory.

However, the complexity in fully articulating interaction in syndemic structures is evident in the scoping review of the cardiovascular disease syndemic literature conducted by Quiroz-Mena and colleagues [11] in this Special Issue. The results showed that few studies are adherent to the elements of syndemic theory. The dominant quantitative method to provide empirical evidence supporting disease interaction remains the "sum scores" or cumulative disease approach. The approach assesses whether higher disease concentration is associated with more severe health outcomes; it does not consider the nature of the disease interactions, but does provide evidence of clustering [8,9,12,13].

Tripp et al. [14] present a historical case of the 1918/19 influenza pandemic, using life table analysis to operationalize the syndemic of influenza and pulmonary tuberculosis among impoverished and marginalized adults of reproductive age (20–34 years) in Malta. They show that individuals of reproductive age had a significant increase in pulmonary tuberculosis mortality during the 1918 influenza period, and that those with both infections had a higher probability of mortality than those with only one infection. This does not prove disease interaction, indicating only the accumulation of disease risk. However, there is substantial evidence of biological interaction between the diseases, and the authors point to other studies that have similar findings of higher rates of mortality in individuals infected with both influenza and pulmonary tuberculosis. Tripp et al. complete their presentation of the syndemic of pandemic influenza and pulmonary tuberculosis in Malta by considering the impact of socioeconomic and environmental factors such as the increased cost of living, increased unemployment, political upheaval, temperature, and relative humidity.

Stopka et al. [15] presented a robust empirical analysis of the clustering of serious bacterial infections and Hepatitis C (HCV). Of the participants reporting a past-year hospitalization for a serious bacterial infection, most tested HCV-antibody-positive. To account for disease interaction, the prevalence ratios of past-year serious bacterial infections were calculated with each risk factor in separate models, and the effect of modifications was assessed using multiplicative interaction. No evidence of interaction between HCV and serious bacterial infections was found. Their results indicate that the co-occurrence of HCV and serious bacterial infection is likely mediated by shared risk behaviors. Although no evidence of disease interaction was found in this study population, this is likely due to the small sample size. It is well established that HCV-related liver damage impairs the body's ability to clear bacterial infections, increasing disease susceptibility and severity. This paper indicates how challenging it is to prove disease interaction using present statistical techniques.

Tenet 3: Social vulnerabilities driving disease clusters. Syndemics theory recognizes that disease clusters tend to appear in socially vulnerable populations, indicating that the social, structural, and environmental conditions shared by a population drive disease risk. Furthermore, while epidemics may transcend national borders, driven by various influencing social factors, syndemic diseases take on unique arrangements in different social, political, economic, cultural, and geographic contexts [16,17]. As such, place-based assessments are much needed to develop context-specific solutions.

All of the papers published in this Special Issue attest to the multitude of interacting and intersecting social vulnerabilities that support the existence of clustering disease epidemics within a population. For example, the review by Hernandez Barrios et al. [18] focused on the issue of population vulnerability in the context of the COVID-19 pandemic. Their analysis of 40 articles published between December 2019 and October 2022 found that vulnerability is a systemic issue, with COVID-19 control measures directly increasing vulnerability in some populations. Villacis-Alvarez and colleagues [19] examined gendered and intersecting barriers and facilitators across the range of HIV care before and during the COVID-19 pandemic, which included COVID-19-associated disruptions in services and support structures. This compounded mental health challenges, substance use, violence (including intimate partner violence), internalized and enacted compounded stigma, and discrimination among individuals with HIV.

Bulled [20] contributes to the burgeoning literature on occupational syndemics, detailing the conditions of wine farmworkers in the Western Cape, South Africa. These include dangerous workplace conditions, substandard housing, limited access to healthcare, labor policies that fail to protect workers and worker rights, limited state oversight, and historical legacies of the "dop" (tot) system of payment through alcohol. The occupational and structural factors experienced by farmworkers in the Cape Winelands result in high levels of interacting diseases including HIV, tuberculosis, metabolic syndrome, problem alcohol use, and interpersonal violence.

This confluence of social and structural factors is often difficult to isolate, measure, dissect, and account for causation. Consequently, the elements that drive disease clusters are often disregarded or not fully explored. What is more concerning is that, given new guidance for research studies funded by the US government, future studies may not be allowed to address issues of inequality/inequity, marginalization, and disparity. As such, this third tenet of syndemic theory, which recognizes that those made vulnerable to disease clusters due to historic and present policies, geographies, environments, economies, and culture, may, in the future, be left unexamined. The result will be that either disease burdens ravaging select communities may be unidentified, or significant amounts of resources will be wasted on entire populations to address overlapping disease epidemics that primarily affect communities with unique biological and social characteristics.

The set of papers in this Special Issue adds to the significant body of research and review on syndemics and attests to the value of syndemics theory across health-related disciplines. Future work on syndemics and infectious disease will need to adhere to robust analytic methods for qualitative, quantitative, and mixed-method studies of syndemic interaction and the translation of research into effective intervention. Such research may face increasing challenges based on ideological grounds, a turn of events that will hinder future progress on syndemics and limit its contributions to public health.

Conflicts of Interest: The authors declare no conflict of interest.

References

1. McQuiston, J.; Braden, C.; Bowen, M.; McCollum, A.; McDonald, R.; Carnes, N.; Carter, R.; Christie, A.; Doty, J.; Ellington, S.; et al. The CDC Domestic Mpox Response—United States, 2022–2023. *MMWR Morb. Mortal. Wkly. Rep.* **2023**, *72*, 547–552. [CrossRef] [PubMed]
2. Horton, R. Offline: COVID-19 is not a pandemic. *Lancet* **2020**, *396*, 874. [CrossRef] [PubMed]
3. Delphin, K.; Remco Van De, P.; Thierno Oumar, F.; Alexandre, D.; Willem Van De, P.; Wim Van, D. Guinea's response to syndemic hotspots. *BMJ Global Health* **2021**, *6*, e006550. [CrossRef]
4. Wu, M.Y.; Gong, H.Z.; Hu, K.R.; Zheng, H.Y.; Wan, X.; Li, J. Effect of syphilis infection on HIV acquisition: A systematic review and meta-analysis. *Sex. Transm. Infect.* **2021**, *97*, 525–533. [CrossRef] [PubMed]
5. Ren, M.; Dashwood, T.; Walmsley, S. The Intersection of HIV and Syphilis: Update on the Key Considerations in Testing and Management. *Curr. HIV/AIDS Rep.* **2021**, *18*, 280–288. [CrossRef] [PubMed]
6. McCollum, R.; Barrett, C.; Zawolo, G.; Johnstone, R.; Godwin-Akpan, T.G.; Berrian, H.; Chowdhury, S.; Kollie, J.; Kollie, K.; Rogers, E.; et al. 'The Lost Peace': Evidencing the Syndemic Relationship between Neglected Tropical Diseases and Mental Distress in Liberia. *Trop. Med. Infect. Dis.* **2024**, *9*, 183. [CrossRef] [PubMed]
7. Barrett, C.; Chiphwanya, J.; Matipula, D.E.; Douglass, J.; Kelly-Hope, L.A.; Dean, L. Addressing the Syndemic Relationship between Lymphatic Filariasis and Mental Distress in Malawi: The Potential of Enhanced Self-Care. *Trop. Med. Infect. Dis.* **2024**, *9*, 172. [CrossRef] [PubMed]
8. Tsai, A.C. Syndemics: A theory in search of data or data in search of a theory? *Soc. Sci. Med.* **2018**, *206*, 117–122. [CrossRef] [PubMed]
9. Tsai, A.C.; Burns, B.F. Syndemics of psychosocial problems and HIV risk: A systematic review of empirical tests of the disease interaction concept. *Soc. Sci. Med.* **2015**, *139*, 26–35. [CrossRef] [PubMed]
10. Adams, V. *Metrics: What Counts in Global Health*; Duke University Press: Durham, NC, USA, 2016.
11. Quiroz-Mena, S.; Piñeros-Jimenez, J.G.; Cañon-Montañez, W. Convergence between Cardiometabolic and Infectious Diseases in Adults from a Syndemic Perspective: A Scoping Review. *Trop. Med. Infect. Dis.* **2024**, *9*, 196. [CrossRef] [PubMed]
12. Stall, R.; Coulter, R.W.S.; Friedman, M.R.; Plankey, M.W. Commentary on "Syndemics of psychosocial problems and HIV risk: A systematic review of empirical tests of the disease interaction concept" by A. Tsai and B. Burns. *Soc. Sci. Med.* **2015**, *145*, 129–131. [CrossRef] [PubMed]
13. Starks, T.J.; Millar, B.M.; Eggleston, J.J.; Parsons, J.T. Syndemic Factors Associated with HIV Risk for Gay and Bisexual Men: Comparing Latent Class and Latent Factor Modeling. *AIDS Behav.* **2014**, *18*, 2075–2079. [CrossRef] [PubMed]
14. Tripp, L.; Sawchuk, L.A.; Farrugia, C.J. Assessing the 1918/19 Pandemic Influenza and Respiratory Tuberculosis Interaction in Malta: Operationalizing a Syndemic During a Crisis Event. *Trop. Med. Infect. Dis.* **2025**, *10*, 149. [CrossRef] [PubMed]
15. Stopka, T.J.; Nance, R.M.; Mixson, L.S.; Spencer, H.; Tsui, J.I.; Leahy, J.M.; Pho, M.T.; DeJace, J.; Feinberg, J.; Young, A.M.; et al. Serious Bacterial Infections and Hepatitis C Virus Among People Who Inject Drugs: A Syndemic or Intertwined Epidemics? *Trop. Med. Infect. Dis.* **2025**, *10*, 17. [CrossRef] [PubMed]
16. Singer, M.; Bulled, N.; Leatherman, T. Are there global syndemics? *Med. Anthropol.* **2022**, *41*, 4–18. [CrossRef] [PubMed]

17. Mendenhall, E. The COVID-19 syndemic is not global: Context matters. *Lancet* **2020**, *396*, 1731. [CrossRef] [PubMed]
18. Hernandez Barrios, Y.; Perez Chacon, D.; Molina Gomez, Y.; Gryseels, C.; Verdonck, K.; Peeters Grietens, K.; Nieto-Sanchez, C. Using a Syndemics Perspective to (Re)Conceptualize Vulnerability during the COVID-19 Pandemic: A Scoping Review. *Trop. Med. Infect. Dis.* **2024**, *9*, 189. [CrossRef] [PubMed]
19. Villacis-Alvarez, E.; Sobie, C.; Maier, K.; Lavallee, M.; Daniels, C.; Pashe, H.; Baliddawa, J.; Daniels, N.; Murdock, R.; Russell, R.; et al. Gender and Intersecting Barriers and Facilitators to Access the HIV Cascade of Care in Manitoba, Canada, Before and During the COVID-19 Pandemic: A Qualitative Study. *Trop. Med. Infect. Dis.* **2024**, *9*, 287. [CrossRef] [PubMed]
20. Bulled, N. Occupational Syndemics in Farmworkers in the Cape Winelands, South Africa. *Trop. Med. Infect. Dis.* **2025**, *10*, 179. [CrossRef]

Tropical Medicine and Infectious Disease

MDPI

Review

Convergence between Cardiometabolic and Infectious Diseases in Adults from a Syndemic Perspective: A Scoping Review

Silvia Quiroz-Mena [1,*], Juan Gabriel Piñeros-Jimenez [2] and Wilson Cañon-Montañez [3]

1 Faculty of Health, Technological University of Choco "Diego Luis Cordoba", A.A 292, cra 22 No.18B-10, Quibdó 270001, Colombia
2 National Faculty of Public Health, University of Antioquia, Medellin 050010, Colombia; juan.pineros@udea.edu.co
3 Faculty of Nursing, University of Antioquia, Medellin 050010, Colombia; wilson.canon@udea.edu.co
* Correspondence: silvia.quiroz@udea.edu.co

Abstract: Objective. Synthesize the approaches used to study the convergence between cardiometabolic and infectious diseases in adults from a syndemic perspective based on the scientific evidence available to date worldwide. **Methods**. Scoping review that follows the recommendations of the PRISMA statement. The protocol was registered in INPLASY202150048. The search for studies was carried out in MEDLINE, LILACS, Web of Science and Scopus. **Results**. Since the COVID-19 pandemic, there has been an increase in studies in the field of convergence between cardiometabolic and infectious diseases from a syndemic perspective, but only three studies were classified as true syndemics. There are weaknesses in the adherence to the elements of the syndemic theory, given a low incorporation of population measurements, and until now it has not been possible to find convincing empirical evidence that supports the bio–bio interface. Quantitative methods predominated through models focused on "sum scores". **Conclusions**. Future studies should comprehensively address the elements of syndemics, review discrepancies between additive analyses versus other modeling, and incorporate the influence of large-scale social forces. The lack of these aspects distances studies from the notion of syndemic, bringing them closer to comorbidity or multimorbidity approaches.

Keywords: syndemics; cardiovascular diseases; communicable diseases; public health

1. Introduction

The convergence between cardiometabolic and infectious diseases is not a new issue [1]. Since the 1970s, there have been reports of studies, the results of which show unidirectional relationships, where the infectious agent is an exposure factor that increases the risk or promotes the development of cardiometabolic disease, such as periodontal infection and atherosclerosis [2]. On the other hand, in bidirectional relationships, both diseases can assume the role of exposure and effect. Diabetes mellitus (DM) can lead to a more severe form of tuberculosis (TB) and affect its management, while TB causes impaired glucose tolerance and makes glycemic control difficult in patients with DM [3].

The above is summarized in a pathogen–pathogen view, which has been expanded when trying to understand, where, under what conditions, in whom and how. These convergences occur [1] and add another layer of complexity, going beyond traditional notions of comorbidity and multimorbidity [4]. Syndemic theory, described by medical anthropologist Merrill Singer, offers an opportunity to understand how certain diseases grouped in various social contexts and within specific populations. This theory involves the assessment of two key elements: (i) concentration—grouping of two or more diseases due to the influence of large-scale demographic, social, economic and political factors; and (ii) interaction—these diseases interact through various biological mechanisms (interface bio–bio, such as inflammation) and/or social (bio–social interface, such as stigma). As a result of their interaction, greater adverse health outcomes are generated (excess disease burden and mortality) [5].

One of the challenges has been to achieve coherence between what is stipulated in the theory and the conceptual and methodological approaches used in the analyses [6]. A review of the trends in syndemic research between 2015 and 2019 showed that only 12% of the articles evaluated respond appropriately to the definition of syndemic [7].

There are some reviews on the topic, but these do not focus on the convergence between cardiometabolic and infectious diseases; they do not delve into the types of convergences, methods used and their coherence with theory. In addition, previous reviews include studies before the COVID-19 pandemic, when the rise of the term syndemic became more relevant [7,8]. The appropriation of the elements of syndemic theory must be examined and standardized to guarantee valid results and enhance its usefulness in clinical and public health practice in the face of future pandemics.

The objective of this review is to synthesize the approaches used to study the convergence between cardiometabolic and infectious diseases in adults from a syndemic approach based on the available scientific evidence.

2. Materials and Methods

A scoping review was carried out under the standards established in "PRISMA extension for scoping reviews (PRISMA-ScR)" [9]. The protocol was registered in INPLASY202150048 [10].

Literature searches were carried out in four databases (from inception to October 2023). A combination of English descriptors in MEDLINE, LILACS, Web of Science and Scopus was used using the following search equation: (syndemic OR syndemics) AND (cardiometabolic OR metabolic OR cardiovascular OR noncommunicable diseases OR noncommunicable diseases OR non-infectious Diseases) AND (communicable diseases OR Infectious diseases OR infections OR infection) (Tables S1 and S2).

No language or year of publication restrictions were established. A filter was applied by age (studies over 18 years of age), and in the title and abstract review stage, the following exclusion criteria were used:

- They do not include the two diseases of interest (cardiometabolic and infectious).
- They do not involve convergence between the two types of diseases.
- They are review studies, editorials, case reports, comments or letters to the editor.

From this initial screening process, the studies were selected for full-text review. Subsequently, those studies that did not explicitly refer to a syndemic approach in any section of the article were excluded. The reasons for the non-inclusion of certain documents were listed and discussed by the researchers.

For the extraction and management of data from the definitive studies, a database was created in Microsoft Excel version 16 with the following information: bibliographic database, authors, title, year, country, participants, diseases or syndemic conditions, research design, methods and adverse outcomes.

The data synthesis strategy was qualitative, given the objective of the review, which seeks to describe the different approaches used to evaluate syndemics. For this, the instrument "JBI QARI Data Extraction Form for Interpretive and Critical Research" was used [11]. The synthesis was developed in three steps: (1) extraction of all the findings included in the selected documents; (2) grouping the results into similar themes; and (3) unifying the results into previously defined categories of interest according to the key elements associated with the syndemic theory and in consensus with the research team.

The methodological quality of the studies was assessed using a tool for assessing the quality of diverse studies (QuADS), which allows the assessment of methodological and reporting quality in systematic reviews of mixed or multiple methods studies [12]. Additionally, the "robvis" tool was used to visualize the evaluation of the quality of the studies and the risk of bias [13].

3. Results

The database searches identified 619 publications, of which 56 articles were chosen for full-text selection after reading titles and abstracts. Of this total, 41 did not meet the inclusion criteria, leaving 15 eligible articles. The selection process is summarized in the PRISMA flowchart (Figure 1).

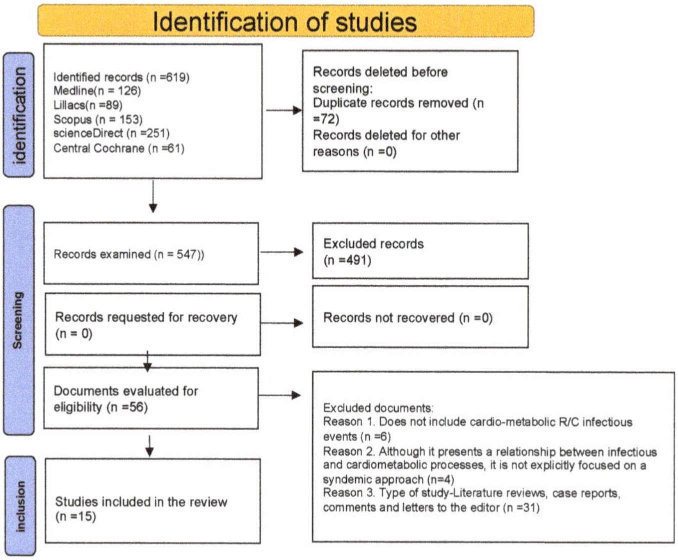

Figure 1. Flowchart—PRISMA [9].

The selected studies were published between 2015 and 2023 [14–28]. The largest number of articles were published following the COVID-19 pandemic (n = 12), and were carried out in the United States (n = 7) and African countries (n = 3). Most of them are quantitative (n = 11) and cross-sectional (n = 12) studies. The number of participants varies in a range from 27 to 12,052 people with specific characteristics defined by age, sex, sexual orientation, ethnic/racial condition, geographic area, socioeconomic status, and index or underlying disease (Table 1).

The syndemic conditions evaluated in the studies incorporate a count of the presence of two or more diseases or health conditions (HIV infection, hypertension, Diabetes mellitus, obesity, depression or anxiety), risk factors (stress or psychoactive substance consumption) and social determinants (low educational level, unemployment, violence, sexual abuse and child abuse). Some authors called the sum of these factors the syndemic burden. The main outcomes reported are linked to impairments in the progression, control and management of an index disease; lower quality of life; higher risks of complications; and death (Table 1).

The quality assessment, considering the QuADS tool, showed that all studies are based on a theoretical framework (syndemic theory); moreover, it also declared the objectives, described the collection procedures and provided recruitment data, but only 53% of the studies evaluated had a high methodological quality (n = 8). Problems related to the coherence between the methodological framework and the objectives were evident, as well as the lack of evidence on the participation of research stakeholders in its design and execution (Figure 2).

Table 1. Characteristics of the included studies.

Author(s), Year	Country	Study Design	Participant Characteristics (n = Sample Size)	Syndemic Conditions Evaluated	Adverse Outcomes	Main Results
Chicheto et al., 2023 **[14].**	USA	Quantitative–Cohort	Women with HIV (n = 3282) between 1987 and 2017 from urban and rural areas	Excessive drinking + smoking + depressive symptoms hypertension + diabetes in people with HIV	Mortality	Clustering of two or more conditions affected nearly one in five Women with HIV and was associated with higher mortality.
Costa et al., 2023 **[15].**	Brazil	Quantitative–Cross-sectional	Adults between 18 and 19 years old (n = 2515)	Socioeconomic inequalities + obesity + insulin resistance	Burden of chronic oral diseases (caries and periodontitis)	They found a syndemic framework linking obesity and the Insulin Resistance Phenotype with the Chronic Oral Disease Burden. Socioeconomic Inequalities were associated with a higher Chronic Oral Disease Burden.
Wildman et al., 2022 **[16].**	England	Qualitative–Cross-sectional	Patients with noncommunicable diseases—NCDs (n = 29)	Social circumstances + cardiovascular diseases + diabetes, depression + anxiety during the COVID-19 pandemic	Lower quality of life	The public health response to the pandemic increased the work required to manage conditions in those most vulnerable to harm from COVID-19. Mental distress was amplified by fear of infection and social distancing requirements that removed usual sources of support. Poor housing, low incomes and the need to earn a living further amplified the work of managing daily life and put mental health at risk.

Table 1. *Cont.*

Author(s), Year	Country	Study Design	Participant Characteristics (n = Sample Size)	Syndemic Conditions Evaluated	Adverse Outcomes	Main Results
Perelman, 2022 [17].	Portugal	Quantitative–Cross-sectional	Adults between 25 and 79 years old (n = 12,052)	Asthma, chronic bronchitis, CVD and cerebrovascular diseases, diabetes, HT, chronic kidney disease (CKD) and obesity	COVID-19 mortality	High socioeconomic inequalities were evident for all eight diseases assessed and were associated with COVID-19 mortality.
Mendenhall, 2022 [18].	South Africa	Mixed–Cross-sectional	Adults from neighborhoods of an urban settlement (n = 783)	Stress + multimorbidity (HT + diabetes + hyperlipidemia + chronic pain + HIV)	Lower quality of life	The quality of life impacts of multimorbidity were conditioned by participants' illness experiences. The strongest finding reveals a robust interaction between a locally designed stress scale and multimorbidity. Stress was associated with medical complications, financial difficulties, family discord and an unsettled future.
Rizk & Shaya, 2022 [19].	USA	Quantitative–Ecological	Counties (n = 160)	Burden of NCDs (HT, DM, obesity and COPD) + socioeconomic inequalities measured in four factors (education, employment, poverty and household income)	Lower vaccination rates and worse outcomes from COVID-19	Counties with higher rates of noncommunicable diseases (COPD, obesity, diabetes and hypertension) and socioeconomic disparities had lower COVID-19 vaccination coverage.

Table 1. *Cont.*

Author(s), Year	Country	Study Design	Participant Characteristics (n = Sample Size)	Syndemic Conditions Evaluated	Adverse Outcomes	Main Results
Rodríguez et al., 2021 **[20]**.	USA	Quantitative–Cross-sectional	Adults with and without HIV (n = 503)	Low education + child abuse + depressive symptoms + HIV status + obesity	Atherosclerotic plaque and elevated blood pressure	A high prevalence of Cardiovascular disease risk measured by carotid atherosclerotic plaque, and elevated systolic and diastolic blood pressure, was identified. There was also a high prevalence of syndemic conditions. Each syndemic condition was associated with increased odds of cardiovascular disease risk, resulting in high risk for detection of atherosclerosis and elevations in blood pressure when multiple syndemic conditions were present.
Chicheto et al., 2021 **[21]**.	USA	Quantitative–Longitudinal	Veterans with and without HIV (5621)	Alcohol consumption + smoking + depressive symptoms + HIV status	CVD incidence	Having at least two of the syndemic conditions (smoking, Unhealthy alcohol use, depressive symptoms) was common among veterans. Having two or more of these conditions was associated with increased risk for incident cardiovascular disease, regardless of HIV status, even after adjusting for comorbidities and traditional risk factors.

Table 1. *Cont.*

Author(s), Year	Country	Study Design	Participant Characteristics (n = Sample Size)	Syndemic Conditions Evaluated	Adverse Outcomes	Main Results
Cuschieri & Grech, 2021 **[22]**.	Malta	Quantitative–Cross-sectional	Adults with a history of COVID-19 (n = 3947)	Multimorbidity (DM + overweight/obesity + CVD dyslipidemia)	Mortality from COVID-19 and years of life lost	Half the study population had a single noncommunicable disease while a third had multimorbidity. Of these, 6.55% were estimated to be at risk of COVID-19 and requiring hospitalization admission. COVID-19 Years of life lost over 12 months was 5228.54 years. The presence of a single chronic disease or multimorbidity from a young age, as identified in this study, is a public health concern.
Chung et al., 2021 **[23]**.	Hong Kong	Quantitative–Cross-sectional	Adults with a history of COVID-19 (n = 3074)	Socioeconomic position + multimorbidity (cardiovascular, kidney, nervous system, digestive diseases, diabetes, cancer and HIV)	COVID-19 severity	Despite an independent adverse impact of multimorbidity on COVID-19 severity, it varied across the socioeconomic ladder, with no significant risk among those living in the wealthiest places. Socioeconomic position interacted with multimorbidity to determine COVID-19 severity with a mitigated risk among the socioeconomically advantaged.

Table 1. *Cont.*

Author(s), Year	Country	Study Design	Participant Characteristics (n = Sample Size)	Syndemic Conditions Evaluated	Adverse Outcomes	Main Results
Zefp et al., 2020 **[24]**.	USA	Quantitative–Cross-sectional	Older men living with HIV who have sex with men (MSM) (n = 281)	Symptoms of depression, symptoms of post-traumatic stress disorder, past physical or sexual abuse, intimate partner violence, stimulant use and excessive alcohol consumption	Worse adherence to treatment in MSM with HIV	The findings suggest that syndemic conditions may impact medication adherence in older MSM living with HIV.
Jones et al., 2020 **[25]**.	USA	Quantitative–Cross-sectional	Women with HIV (n = 131)	Low education + obesity + cigarette smoking + depressive symptoms	HIV status, increased blood pressure and inflammation	Syndemic factors may play a role in HIV health status, thereby contributing to an increased risk of transmission. Additionally, the accumulation of syndemic burden may increase the risk of hypertension.
Byg et al., 2016 **[26]**.	USA	Quantitative–Cross-sectional	MSM with HIV (n = 88)	Diabetes + HIV	Glycemic control	One-third had inadequate glycemic control, which was correlated with other markers of disease (hypertension and depression) and independently associated with substance use, high triglycerides and unsuppressed HIV viral load.

Table 1. *Cont.*

Author(s), Year	Country	Study Design	Participant Characteristics (n = Sample Size)	Syndemic Conditions Evaluated	Adverse Outcomes	Main Results
Mendehall et al., 2015 **[27]**.	Kenya	Mixed–Cross-sectional	Patients from a public hospital (n = 100)	Stress + diabetes + infections	Syndemic suffering	Diabetes accompanies a complex web of social, mental and physical suffering among participants. The study indicates that infection intercepts the stress–diabetes interface among low-income residents. Women revealed more social problems, psychological distress and physical morbidities.
Mendenhall & Norris, 2015 **[28]**.	USA	Qualitative–Cross-sectional	Black women (n = 27)	Diabetes + HIV	Syndemic suffering	Women conceive syndemic social and health problems as mutually exacerbating, co-constructions of suffering in everyday life. They communicated the factors in their lives that caused stress; they prioritized social problems as opposed to medical ones. They showed how reconstructing families and raising grandchildren after losing children to AIDS was not only socially challenging but also affected how they ate and accepted and managed their diabetes.

HIV: Human Immunodeficiency Virus. NCD: Noncommunicable diseases. MSM: Men who have sex with men.

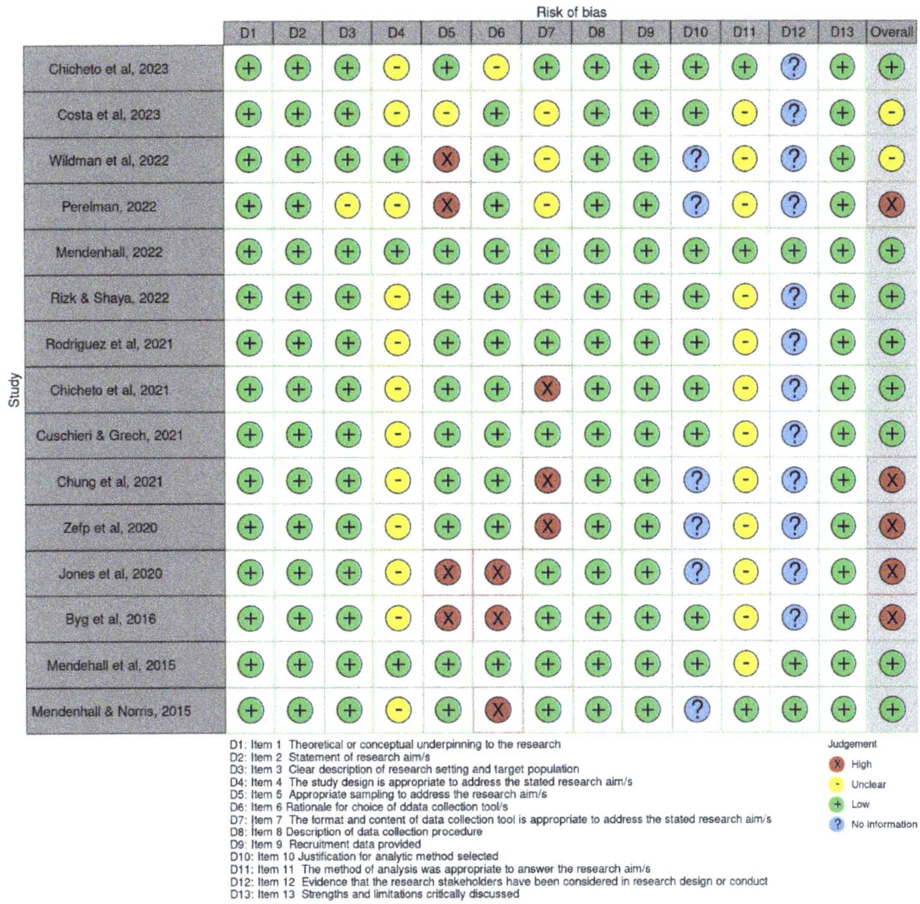

Figure 2. Results of the application of the quality assessment tool for studies with diverse methods (Quality assessment with diverse studies—QuADS).

3.1. Level of Measurement and Application of the Key Elements of Syndemic Theory

Most studies focus on the individual level (n = 9). The element of concentration, defined as the coexistence of two or more diseases in defined temporal and geographic contexts due to detrimental social conditions, was evaluated in only eight studies. Bio–social interaction is the most evaluated element (n = 13), while the bio–bio interface is only addressed in four studies (Table 2).

Considering what was stipulated by Singer, Bulled and Ostrach in their text "Whither syndemics?: Trends in syndemics research, a review 2015–2019", two initial categories were defined to classify the evaluated studies. Firstly, those studies that included both the population and individual level and the two key elements of the theory were classified as "syndemics", that is, they analyze the spatiotemporal grouping and the true interactions of the evaluated cardiometabolic and infectious diseases or the health burdens within a specific population. Furthermore, they incorporate how the bio–bio interactions of these health burdens result in worse diseases, and shared social or structural factors within populations further exacerbate biological conditions creating true synergy rather than simply co-occurrence of disease Within this category, only three studies were included (Table 2).

Table 2. Description of the application of the key elements of syndemic theory.

Studies	Measurement Level		Key Elements			Classification	
	Population	Individual	Concentration	Bio–Social Interaction	Bio–Bio Interaction	Syndemic [1]	Syndemic Potential [2]
Chicheto et al., 2023 [14].	No	Yes	No	Yes	No	-	✓
Costa et al., 2023 [15].	Yes	Yes	Yes	Yes	Yes	✓	-
Wildman et al., 2022 [16].	No	Yes	No	Yes	No	-	✓
Perelman, 2022 [17].	No	Yes	Yes	No	No	-	✓
Mendenhall et al., 2022 [18].	Yes	Yes	Yes	Yes	Yes	✓	-
Rizk & Shaya, 2022 [19].	Yes	No	Yes	Yes	No	-	✓
Rodríguez et al., 2021 [20].	No	Yes	No	Yes	No	-	✓
Chicheto et al., 2021 [21].	No	Yes	No	Yes	No	-	✓
Cuschieri & Grech, 2021 [22].	Yes	Yes	No	No	No	-	-
Chung et al., 2021 [23].	Yes	Yes	Yes	Yes	No	-	✓
Zefp et al., 2020 [24].	No	Yes	No	Yes	No	-	✓
Jones et al., 2020 [25].	No	Yes	No	Yes	Yes	-	✓
Byg et al., 2016 [26].	No	Yes	Yes	Yes	No	-	✓
Mendehall et al., 2015 [27].	Yes	Yes	Yes	Yes	Yes	✓	-
Mendehall et al., 2015 [28].	No	Yes	Yes	Yes	No	-	✓

[1] Syndemics: Studies with interactions that involve the clustering of at least two diseases or conditions within a specific population. Bio–bio interactions of these health burdens result in worse health outcomes and evidence the influence of shared social factors within populations that further exacerbate biological conditions creating a true synergy rather than simply co-occurrence of disease or the addition of various social and health factors [7,8].
[2] Potential syndemics: studies that do not fully develop the bio–bio and bio–social interaction.

Secondly, those studies that only focused on the individual level and did not fully develop the key elements of the theory, especially the bio–bio interaction or the mechanisms by which the cardiometabolic and infectious diseases are evaluated, were classified as "potential syndemics". And social conditions interacted to exacerbate harmful health outcomes (n = 11) (Table 2).

3.2. *Consistencies between the Underlying Conceptual Model, the Methodologies Used and the Postulates of the Syndemic Theory*

Two conceptual models were represented based on the objectives set and the arguments described in the different studies. The first model presented groups-3 studies and attempts to represent in a unified manner approaches focused on evaluating the syndemic as the effect of the sum of a series of conditions related to cardiometabolic and infectious diseases on negative health outcomes, such as increased risk, complications and death in population groups with specific characteristics and/or a defined index disease.

The second conceptual model presented groups-8 studies and involves not only the aspects described in the first model, but also incorporates the influence of social factors, reinforcing the bio–social interface. This model also incorporates the understanding of biological mechanisms related to the bio–bio interface (Figure 3). It should be noted that in the quantitative studies evaluated, the independent effect of each social factor included is measured.

The conceptual models represented incorporate a variety of both quantitative and qualitative methodologies. It is highlighted that the element of disease concentration was evaluated mainly with traditional epidemiological methods, specifically, estimation of measures of occurrence of the diseases and conditions of interest. These tend to be stratified by demographic and socioeconomic variables.

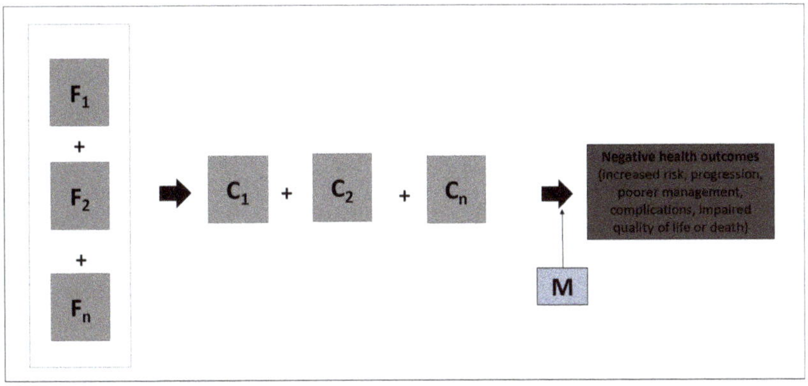

Figure 3. Conceptual model for addressing syndemics between cardiometabolic and infectious diseases according to the reviewed studies. F: Effect of social factors. C: Conditions (diseases and risk factors). M: Mediating factors (physiological or mental).

The interaction element was evaluated using bivariate and multivariate inferential techniques, including interaction terms in some cases. A dominant modeling focused on "sum scores" is evident. Qualitative studies address the elements of the theory through in-depth interviews, ethnographies and life stories. Mixed studies, which incorporate the variety of techniques described, were evident.

4. Discussion

This scoping review synthesized the approaches used to study the convergence between cardiometabolic and infectious diseases in adults from a syndemic perspective for the scientific evidence available to date. The COVID-19 pandemic showed complex and unexpected interactions among the diseases evaluated here, environmental factors and socioeconomic disparities, which makes the use of the syndemic theory important [16]. The results of this review become an opportunity to better understand this problem in order to address current and future pandemics.

The first finding of this review indicates that most studies focus only on the individual level. Strictly speaking, this finding is worrying, because if the origin of the term "syndemic" is reviewed, it is necessary to include the population level, for the term is derived from the Greek word "synergos", which means two or more agents working together to create an effect greater than the sum of each one working alone. And we deduce that it refers to population, as it has been used in basic epidemiological concepts: epidemic, pandemic and endemic [5].

Additionally, falling into the individualistic fallacy, as proposed by Tsai, leads the syndemic area to lose opportunities to incorporate multilevel approaches, which allow us to understand how epidemics interact both at the level of populations and individuals, using as many ecological study designs as possible: cohort, case-control and cross-sectional studies. This author has incorporated important reflections on this aspect and has recently criticized how studies that ignore interactions with ecological influences to focus exclusively on the interaction of factors at the individual level can reach erroneous conclusions [29].

Other authors highlight that empirical evidence on syndemics require a greater understanding of the ways in which health conditions and social adversity interact in marginalized populations to further weaken these groups [30]. Emily Mendenhall, one of the great proponents of the theory, mentioned that "The COVID-19 syndemic is not global: context matters" because what drives the virus to move and interact with biological and social factors differs among countries and regions [31].

The second finding was linked to low adherence to the elements of the theory. Only three studies were classified as true syndemics since they incorporated both the individual and population levels and addressed aspects related to the concentration and interaction of diseases [15,18,27]. This has been reported in studies on the use of this theory before 2019 [7,8]. It has been mentioned that the confusion surrounding the non-application of these elements could be due to the fact that researchers are referring to conceptualizations from Singer's early work. For this reason, we insist on the relevance of recognizing the developments that have been made over the years to articulate the elements in a complete and adequate manner [32].

So far, the empirical evidence supporting the bio–bio interface proposed in the theory is insufficient. Other systematic reviews have shown that most studies, especially epidemiological ones, have attempted to document the existence of syndemics only using the "sum score" specification, and it constitutes the dominant modeling in quantitative studies [29,33,34].

Since 1979, the concept of "interaction" has had a long and controversial history in the epidemiological literature. Renowned authors such as Rothman [35] and VanderWeele [36] have made contributions to direct the analysis of this element, providing foundations for its theoretical distinction and the implementation of formal tests to analyze the interaction within statistical models, ranging from interaction in additive models to the introduction of multiplicative terms [6].

The third finding shows that there is no single conceptual model to represent the syndemic between cardiometabolic and infectious diseases and that it depends on the nature of the interactions that are proposed. However, the studies evaluated have common characteristics in terms of their objectives and approaches, which allowed them to be grouped into two large types of conceptual models. The resulting models do not differ substantially from others proposed in previous literature reviews for other types of syndemics, where the interaction of factors, diseases and conditions in specific population groups is linked. For example, Tsai and Burns [37] in 2015 conducted a systematic literature review on syndemics of psychosocial problems and HIV risk, and as a result of the study, they constructed simple syndemic models in which two conditions (depression and substance abuse) coexist, and they are determined by the poverty and interact synergistically to increase HIV risk [37].

The fourth finding indicates a marked predominance of the positivist paradigm and the use of quantitative methods to address the syndemic between cardiometabolic and infectious diseases. However, it recognizes a strong incursion of qualitative methods, which are part of the anthropological roots of the theory and have been widely applied with other types of syndemics, especially those related to HIV and risk behaviors. The inclusion of mixed methods and longitudinal studies is highlighted as a response to the challenges posed in previous literature reviews [7,8]. In this order, expanding the spectrum of methods and understanding the type of syndemic addressed here has become an urgent need among researchers in this field.

Consistent with the results of this review, Tsai [29] indicates that future studies should aim to gain ground in the validation of the theory, and therefore, six aspects are suggested: (i) the clear exposure of the possible discrepancies that may arise among the additive analyses (score sum) versus those that test synergistic interactions from another type of modeling; (ii) the need to understand the complexity of large-scale social forces or structural determinants of health that influence the convergence of multiple diseases results; (iii) the use and triangulation of data from multiple sources; (iv) the assessment of the temporal effect of health risks following approaches such as the life course; (v) the comprehensive understanding of the effect of clinical and public health interventions for the management of these diseases; and (vi) the incorporation of studies at the population level and contextual effects, given that syndemics have been explicitly theorized as multilevel phenomena, as Singer highlights "the interaction between diseases occurs at both the population and individual levels" [6].

Not explicitly modeling social forces distances the field from political, economic and cultural explanations; downplays the first element of the theory (concentration); and brings it closer to notions of comorbidity or multimorbidity.

Finally, identifying and addressing syndemics globally contributes to the fulfilment of the United Nations 2030 Agenda for Sustainable Development Goals (SDGs) by adopting an integrative, collaborative and multi-sectoral perspective, which is in line with current approaches such as "One Health". Both approaches are based on the recognition that health problems are often interconnected and cannot be addressed in isolation [38]. By considering the broader social, environmental and animal health contexts, the One Health approach can help identify and address the underlying factors that contribute to syndemics.

Limitations

The results of this review must be interpreted with caution due to some limitations. First, the search strategy was restricted to studies reported in the English language, which could have overlooked other aspects reported in other studies in a non-English language. Second, it is likely that our review will have missed relevant articles that do not mention another type of convergence in their title, abstract or key words. On the same hand, we may not have captured all conceptual linkages with regard to common definitions within syndemics.

5. Conclusions

Syndemics appear to have played an important role in human history and are likely to continue to influence the global burden of disease today [5]. Understanding the syndemic between cardiometabolic and infectious diseases is an urgent issue, not only for facing the great challenges raised by COVID-19, but also for being able to cope with future pandemics and the emerging and re-emerging of public health threats.

With this scoping review, it would be expected that future empirical studies on syndemics would include both the individual and population levels within their approaches and would be natural candidates for the application of multilevel models. The findings of this review show the lack of adherence to the key elements of the syndemic theory. Therefore, the need also arises for future research to appropriate and incorporate the concentration of diseases and interaction as foundations when it comes to evaluating syndemics.

Linked to the above, it is necessary to include methodologies consistent with the elements of the theory. A recommendation that comes from this review and other studies is the use of mixed methodologies, the combination of different sources of information and exploration of data analysis methods. Additionally, the use of longitudinal studies that can more fully capture the complex interconnections among syndemic conditions is highlighted.

It is recommended that future studies achieve greater coherence among the objective, the theoretical framework (syndemics) and the methodology. This aspect is crucial to ensure logical research that increases the validity of the findings and reduces bias.

With respect to health interventions, multicomponent or comprehensive ones are suggested, yet more evidence is required, one that documents multiple pathways and encourages their use through advocacy for program implementers or policymakers. The study of syndemics involves drawing on various disciplines, including epidemiology and anthropology. This often means collaboration among researchers with different academic and professional backgrounds from different areas.

Clinical care and public health must consider the complexity of syndemics. They cannot be limited only to the understanding of comorbidities and the clinical management of convergent diseases [30]. Mastering the interaction of multiple diseases requires a change in interventions, to adequately manage not only infectious diseases but also the increasing burden of cardiometabolic diseases through a "one health" approach [2].

Supplementary Materials: The following supporting information can be downloaded at: https://www.mdpi.com/article/10.3390/tropicalmed9090196/s1, Table S1: Syndemics between cardiometabolic and infectious diseases in adults; Table S2: Specific searches.

Author Contributions: All authors conceived of the presented idea. S.Q.-M. collected the data and designed the analysis. J.G.P.-J. and W.C.-M. verified the analytical methods and supervised the findings of this work. All authors discussed the results and contributed to the final manuscript. All authors have read and agreed to the published version of the manuscript.

Funding: Ministry of Science, Technology and Innovation—Minciencias (Doctoral Scholarship Agreement no. 20230017-11-20).

Institutional Review Board Statement: Not applicable.

Informed Consent Statement: Not applicable.

Data Availability Statement: The raw data supporting the conclusions of this article will be made available by the authors on request.

Conflicts of Interest: The authors declare no conflicts of interest.

References

1. Nicholson, A.; Negussie, Y.; Mundaca, C.; Ayano, O. *The Convergence of Infectious Diseases and Noncommunicable Diseases;* Ogawa, V.A., Shah, C.M., Negussie, Y., Nicholson, A., Eds.; National Academies Press: Washington, DC, USA, 2019. [CrossRef]
2. Beck, J.; Garcia, R.; Heiss, G.; Vokonas, P.S.; Offenbacher, S. Periodontal disease and cardiovascular disease. *J. Periodontol.* **1996**, *67* (Suppl. S10), 1123–1137. [PubMed]
3. Yorke, E.; Atiase, Y.; Akpalu, J.; Sarfo-Kantanka, O.; Boima, V.; Dey, I.D. The Bidirectional Relationship between Tuberculosis and Diabetes. *Tuberc. Res. Treat.* **2017**, 1702578. [CrossRef] [PubMed]
4. Valderas, J.M.; Starfield, B.; Sibbald, B.; Salisbury, C.; Roland, M. Defining comorbidity: Implications for understanding health and health services. *Ann. Fam. Med.* **2009**, *7*, 357–363. [CrossRef]
5. Singer, M. *Introduction to Syndemics: A Critical Systems Approach to Public and Community Health;* John Wiley & Sons: Hoboken, NJ, USA, 2009; 301p.
6. Quiroz Mena, S.; Cañon Montañez, W. Teoría sindémica como un enfoque para explicar la interacción entre problemas de salud pública. *Sci. Med.* **2021**, *31*, e38309. [CrossRef]
7. Singer, M.; Bulled, N.; Ostrach, B. Whither syndemics?: Trends in syndemics research, a review 2015–2019. *Glob. Public Health* **2020**, *15*, 943–955. [CrossRef]
8. Mendenhall, E.; Singer, M. What constitutes a syndemic? Methods, contexts, and framing from 2019. *Curr. Opin. HIV AIDS* **2020**, *15*, 213–217. [CrossRef] [PubMed]
9. Tricco, A.C.; Lillie, E.; Zarin, W.; O'Brien, K.K.; Colquhoun, H.; Levac, D.; Moher, D.; Peters, M.D.J.; Horsley, T.; Weeks, L.; et al. PRISMA extension for scoping reviews. (PRISMA-ScR): Checklist and explanation. *Ann. Intern. Med.* **2018**, *169*, 467–473. [CrossRef]
10. Quiroz, S.P.; Piñeros, J.G.; Cañon-Montañez, W. Syndemics between cardiometabolic and infectious diseases in adults: A scoping review protocol. *Inplasy Protoc.* **2021**, *5*, 48. [CrossRef]
11. Lockwood, C.; Porrit, K.; Munn, Z.; Rittenmeyer, L.; Salmond, S.; Bjerrum, M.; Loveday, H.; Carrier, J.; Stannard, D. Chapter 2: Systematic reviews of qualitative evidence. In *Joanna Briggs Institute Reviewer's Manual;* Aromataris, E., Munn, Z., Eds.; The Joanna Briggs Institute: Adelaide, Australia, 2017.
12. Harrison, R.; Jones, B.; Gardner, P.; Lawton, R. Quality assessment with diverse studies (QuADS): An appraisal tool for methodological and reporting quality in systematic reviews of mixed- or multi-method studies. *BMC Health Serv. Res.* **2021**, *21*, 144. [CrossRef]
13. McGuinness, L.A.; Higgins, J.P.T. Risk-of-bias VISualization (robvis): An R package and Shiny web app for visualizing risk-of-bias assessments. *Res. Syn. Meth.* **2021**, *12*, 55–61. [CrossRef]
14. Chichetto, N.E.; Gebru, N.M.; Plankey, M.W.; Tindle, H.A.; Koethe, J.R.; Hanna, D.B.; Shoptaw, S.; Jones, D.L.; Lazar, J.M.; Kizer, J.R.; et al. Syndemic trajectories of heavy drinking, smoking, and depressive symptoms are associated with mortality in women living with HIV in the United States from 1994 to 2017. *Drug Alcohol. Depend.* **2023**, *249*, 110838. [CrossRef]
15. Costa, L.L.C.; Nascimento, G.G.; Leite, F.R.M.; Alves-Costa, S.; Barbosa, J.M.A.; Alves, C.M.C.; Thomaz, E.B.A.F.; Batista, R.F.L.; Ribeiro, C.C.C. Obesity, Insulin Resistance, Caries, and Periodontitis: Syndemic Framework. *Nutrients* **2023**, *15*, 3512. [CrossRef]
16. Wildman, J.M.; Morris, S.; Pollard, T.; Gibson, K.; Moffatt, S. "I wouldn't survive it, as simple as that": Syndemic vulnerability among people living with chronic non-communicable disease during the COVID-19 pandemic. *SSM Qual. Res. Health* **2022**, *2*, 100032. [CrossRef] [PubMed]
17. Perelman, J. Pandemia Sindémica em Portugal: Desigualdade Social nos Fatores de Risco Associados à Mortalidade por COVID-19 [Syndemic Pandemic in Portugal: Social Inequality in Risk Factors Associated With COVID-19 Mortality]. *Acta Med. Port.* **2022**, *35*, 433–449. [CrossRef] [PubMed]
18. Mendenhall, E.; Kim, A.W.; Panasci, A.; Cele, L.; Mpondo, F.; Bosire, E.N.; Norris, S.A.; Tsai, A.C. A mixed-methods, population-based study of a syndemic in Soweto, South Africa. *Nat. Hum. Behav.* **2022**, *6*, 64–73. [CrossRef] [PubMed]

19. Rizk, J.G.; Shaya, F.T. County-Level COVID-19 Vaccination Rates, Non-Communicable Diseases, and Socioeconomic Inequities: Applying Syndemic Theory to Vaccines. *J. Health Care Poor Underserved* **2022**, *33*, 1736–1746. [CrossRef]
20. Rodriguez, V.J.; Chahine, A.; Parrish, M.S.; Alcaide, M.L.; Lee, T.K.; Hurwitz, B.; Sawhney, M.; Weiss, S.M.; Jones, D.L.; Kumar, M. The contribution of syndemic conditions to cardiovascular disease risk. *AIDS Care* **2021**, *33*, 585–593. [CrossRef] [PubMed]
21. Chichetto, N.E.; Kundu, S.; Freiberg, M.S.; Koethe, J.R.; Butt, A.A.; Crystal, S.; So-Armah, K.A.; Cook, R.L.; Braithwaite, R.S.; Justice, A.C.; et al. Association of Syndemic Unhealthy Alcohol Use, Smoking, and Depressive Symptoms on Incident Cardiovascular Disease among Veterans With and Without HIV-Infection. *AIDS Behav.* **2021**, *25*, 2852–2862. [CrossRef]
22. Cuschieri, S.; Grech, S. Insight into the Occurrence of Common Non-communicable Diseases at a Population Level and the Potential Impact During the Coronavirus Pandemic—A Need for a Syndemic Healthcare Approach? *SN Compr. Clin. Med.* **2021**, *3*, 2393–2400. [CrossRef]
23. Chung, G.K.; Chan, S.M.; Chan, Y.H.; Yip, T.C.; Ma, H.M.; Wong, G.L.; Chung, R.Y.; Wong, H.; Wong, S.Y.; Yeoh, E.K.; et al. Differential Impacts of Multimorbidity on COVID-19 Severity across the Socioeconomic Ladder in Hong Kong: A Syndemic Perspective. *Int. J. Environ. Res. Public Health* **2021**, *18*, 8168. [CrossRef]
24. Zepf, R.; Greene, M.; Hessol, N.A.; Johnson, M.O.; Santos, G.M.; John, M.D.; Dawson-Rose, C. Syndemic conditions and medication adherence in older men living with HIV who have sex with men. *AIDS Care* **2020**, *32*, 1610–1616. [CrossRef]
25. Jones, D.L.; Rodriguez, V.J.; Alcaide, M.L.; Carrico, A.; Fischl, M.A.; Chichetto, N.E.; Rodriguez, C.J.; Welsch, M.A.; Farah-Abraham, R.; Adimora, A.A.; et al. Syndemic burden and systemic inflammation, HIV health status, and blood pressure among women with unsuppressed HIV viral loads among women living with HIV. *AIDS* **2020**, *34*, 1959–1963. [CrossRef] [PubMed]
26. Byg, B.; Bazzi, A.R.; Funk, D.; James, B.; Potter, J. The Utility of a Syndemic Framework in Understanding Chronic Disease Management Among HIV-Infected and Type 2 Diabetic Men Who Have Sex with Men. *J. Community Health* **2016**, *41*, 1204–1211. [CrossRef]
27. Mendenhall, E.; Omondi, G.B.; Bosire, E.; Isaiah, G.; Musau, A.; Ndetei, D.; Mutiso, V. Stress, diabetes, and infection: Syndemic suffering at an urban Kenyan hospital. *Soc. Sci. Med.* **2015**, *146*, 11–20. [CrossRef] [PubMed]
28. Mendenhall, E.; Norris, S.A. When HIV is ordinary and diabetes new: Remaking suffering in a South African township. *Glob. Public Health* **2015**, *10*, 449–462. [CrossRef] [PubMed]
29. Tsai, A.C. Syndemics: A theory in search of data or data in search of a theory? *Soc. Sci. Med.* **2018**, *206*, 117–122. [CrossRef] [PubMed]
30. Weaver, L.J.; Kaiser, B.N. Syndemics theory must take local context seriously: An example of measures for poverty, mental health, and food insecurity. *Soc. Sci. Med.* **2022**, *295*, 113304. [CrossRef]
31. Mendenhall, E. The COVID-19 syndemic is not global: Context matters. *Lancet* **2020**, *396*, 1731. [CrossRef]
32. Pirrone, I.; Dieleman, M.; Reis, R.; Pell, C. Syndemic contexts: Findings from a review of research on non-communicable diseases and interviews with experts. *Glob. Health Action* **2021**, *14*, 1927332. [CrossRef]
33. Stall, R.; Coulter, R.W.S.; Friedman, M.R.; Plankey, M.W. Commentary on "Syndemics of psychosocial problems and HIV risk: A systematic review of empirical tests of the disease interaction concept". by A. Tsai and B. Burns. *Soc. Sci. Med.* **2015**, *145*, 129–131. [CrossRef]
34. Logie, C.H.; Coelho, M.; Kohrt, B.; Tsai, A.C.; Mendenhall, E. Context, COVID-19 and comorbidities: Exploring emergent directions in syndemics and HIV research. *Curr. Opin. HIV AIDS* **2022**, *17*, 46–54. [CrossRef]
35. Rothman, K.J. Synergy and antagonism in cause-effect relationships. *Am. J. Epidemiol.* **1974**, *99*, 385–388. [CrossRef] [PubMed]
36. VanderWeele, T.J. Sufficient cause interactions and statistical interactions. *Epidemiology* **2009**, *20*, 6–13. [CrossRef] [PubMed]
37. Tsai, A.C.; Burns, B.F. Syndemics of psychosocial problems and HIV risk: A systematic review of empirical tests of the disease interaction concept. *Soc. Sci. Med.* **2015**, *139*, 26–35. [CrossRef] [PubMed]
38. Sinclair, J.R. Importance of a One Health approach in advancing global health security and the Sustainable Development Goals. *Rev. Sci. Tech.* **2019**, *38*, 145–154. [CrossRef]

Tropical Medicine and Infectious Disease

MDPI

Article

'The Lost Peace': Evidencing the Syndemic Relationship between Neglected Tropical Diseases and Mental Distress in Liberia

Rosalind McCollum [1,*,†], Carrie Barrett [1,*,†], Georgina Zawolo [2,*,†], Rachel Johnstone [1], Tiawanlyn G. Godwin-Akpan [3], Hannah Berrian [2], Shahreen Chowdhury [1], Jerry Kollie [2], Karsor Kollie [4], Emerson Rogers [4], Colleen Parker [2], Maneesh Phillip [5], Lucas Sempe [6], Maaike Seekles [1], John Solunta Smith [2], Wede Seekey [2], Anna Wickenden [1,5], Zeela Zaizay [7], Sally Theobald [1] and Laura Dean [1]

1. Department of International Public Health, Liverpool School of Tropical Medicine, Liverpool L3 5QA, UK
2. Pacific Institute for Research and Evaluation, University of Liberia, Monrovia 1000, Liberia
3. Programs Department, American Leprosy Mission, 27 Jungle Road, East Legon, Accra GA-374-5385, Ghana
4. Department of Health Services, Ministry of Health-Liberia, Congo Town Back Road, Monrovia 1000, Liberia
5. International Programs Department, Effect Hope, 200-90 Allstate Pkwy, Markham, ON L3R 6H3, Canada
6. The Institute for Global Health and Development Division, Queen Margaret University, Edinburgh EH21 6UU, UK
7. Action Transforming Lives, Congo Town Backroad, Monrovia 1000, Liberia

* Correspondence: rosalind.mccollum@lstmed.ac.uk (R.M.); carrie.barrett@lstmed.ac.uk (C.B.); gzawolo2009@gmail.com (G.Z.)

† These authors contributed equally to this work.

Abstract: Neglected Tropical Diseases (NTDs) are a group of chronic infectious diseases of poverty affecting over one billion people globally. Intersections of NTDs, disability, and mental ill-health are increasingly evidenced but are rarely studied from a mixed-methods perspective. Here, we advance syndemic understandings by further assessing and contextualising the syndemic relationship between NTDs (particularly their associated disability) and mental distress in Liberia. Participatory qualitative methods, including body mapping (56 participants), social mapping (28 participants), and in-depth interviews (12) provided space for persons affected by NTDs to narrate their experiences. Simultaneously, 201 surveys explored experiences of common mental health conditions among persons affected by skin NTDs. An intersectionality approach was applied within the analysis for both qualitative and quantitative methods informed by Meyer's minority stress model, adapted for NTDs. Qualitative data was analysed thematically and gender-disaggregated, univariable and multivariable analyses were applied to survey data for the outcome measures depression (PHQ-9) and anxiety (GAD-7). Disability was associated with higher levels of depression and anxiety ($p < 0.001$). An interaction between disability and being a women increased incidence risk ratio of depression ($p < 0.001$). In alignment with qualitative findings, persons affected experienced additional generalised (financial concerns), external (experience of stigma) and internal (experience of pain and physical symptoms) minority stressors, to varying degrees, which contributed towards their mental distress, and mental health conditions. These findings were used to co-develop a syndemic-informed person-centred health system response to address the suffering associated with NTDs and mental distress, including a focus on strengthening relationships between formal and informal community health actors and the broader health system.

Keywords: syndemics; neglected tropical diseases; Liberia; mental health; depression; anxiety; disability

1. Introduction

Neglected Tropical Diseases (NTDs) are a group of chronic infectious diseases of poverty that affect more than one billion people, primarily from low- and middle-income countries (LMICs) [1,2]. NTDs, particularly those that affect the skin, lymphatic filariasis

(LF), leprosy, Buruli ulcer, Yaws and onchocerciasis, present significant pain and physical disfigurement; stigma and discrimination are also common experiences [3]. LF and onchocerciasis are vector borne diseases caused by filarial nematodes, LF presents most commonly as hydrocoele and lymphoedema, and onchocerciasis can cause disfiguring skin conditions and blindness [4]. An estimated 36 million people are living with LF symptoms, and 14.6 million people living with skin disease and 1.15 million with blindness as a result of onchocerciasis [5–7]. Yaws is caused by a bacterium and characterised by papillomas (noncancerous lumps) and ulcers, with over 80,000 new cases reported each year [8]. Leprosy affects the skin and the peripheral nerves and Buruli ulcer leads to ulceration and skin loss, both are caused by a different species of mycobacterium, and transmission routes are not fully understood [9–11]. Over 200,000 new leprosy cases are reported each year within 120 countries [9].

Mental distress and mental health conditions (depression and anxiety) amongst people affected by NTDs are significantly higher than in the general population [3,12–19]. The link between NTDs and common mental health conditions (depression, anxiety and suicidal ideation) is increasingly documented through epidemiological clustering studies [16,20–26]. A recent review evidences three multi-directional pathways that are shaping epidemiological clustering, namely: (1) people experiencing mental distress or mental health conditions are more at risk to NTDs, and people with NTDs are more at risk to mental distress; (2) people with NTDs experience increased levels of stigma and discrimination leading to higher levels of mental distress; and (3) people with mental health conditions experience high levels of stigma and discrimination heightening vulnerability to NTDs due to delayed care seeking and the poverty-disability nexus [15]. Stigma is often identified as a catalyst of such epidemiological clustering, yet limited research in the field of mental health, stigma and NTDs has taken an equity lens, guided by gendered and intersectionality theory, to understand the drivers of these burdens [3,27]. Thus, understanding broader meso and macro social and structural inequalities driving these multi-directional pathways becomes essential to ensure appropriate person-centred responses for people affected by NTDs and mental health conditions [3,15]. The application of syndemic theory, that considers the biosocial relationships that drive 'synergistically related' epidemics, becomes critical and essential in shaping these understandings [28].

Person-centred responses to NTDs and mental health conditions require a re-orientation of health systems, so that holistic understandings of health (i.e., those that extend beyond the biomedical) are championed. Adjusting care models in this way requires a prioritisation of primary health care interventions that are co-produced with persons affected by NTDs and communities who become active change agents promoting good health and wellbeing throughout the life-course [26,27]. Yet, evidence on 'what works' to address the synergistically related epidemics of NTDs and mental (ill-) health is sparse, and where intervention(s) do exist they have largely been top-down with limited integration within national health systems [29]. Further contextualising the syndemic relationship between NTDs and mental distress, including moving beyond stigma, to think about additional underlying social and structural inequities, becomes imperative to support evidence based, demand driven systems reform. People affected by NTDs and mental health conditions are critical assets in this process, and co-production should be a central value in promoting positive shifts toward normative frameworks of person-centred care [17,27].

1.1. The Context of Liberia

Liberia has experienced protracted drivers of fragility in the past 3 decades, including civil wars (1989–1996, 1999–2003), Ebola virus disease (EVD) epidemic (2013–2016) and the COVID-19 pandemic [30]. Liberia's unique political history, shaped by the post-slavery, post-colonial experience, where disunity between 'settlers' (freed American slaves) and indigenous peoples contributed to protracted unrest and fragility [31]. Subsequent economic mismanagement shapes the ongoing high levels of poverty (with 50.9% of Liberians living below the national poverty line [32]); low levels of education and a weakened health system [31]. These factors contribute to a reliance on traditional medicine by many Liberians. The health system was further devastated by the deaths of 192 health workers responding to the EVD epidemic [33]. These macro-level determinants predispose people to the chronic effects of NTDs and mental distress [31]. Consequently, experiences of mental ill-health are common, although evidence is limited [30], estimates indicate 40% of the population meeting the criteria for major depressive disorder (albeit based on data from 2008) [34]. Infectious diseases of poverty, including NTDs, are frequently diagnosed late, coupled with poor management of NTDs due to limited systems capacity, causes increased morbidity and mortality [3]. Dean (2022), characterise the relationship between mental distress and NTDs (particularly their associated chronic morbidity/disability e.g., lymphoedema) in Liberia as a syndemic driven by three key factors: (1) ongoing structural violence in Liberia pre-disposes people and communities to the chronic effects of NTDs as well as other generalised stressors (e.g., poverty); (2) people affected by NTDs and or mental health conditions face additional stressors, largely related to stigma and discrimination; and (3) the impact of general stressors, and NTD/mental health related stressors synergistically interact with identity based characteristics, including gender and age to shape individual experiences of syndemic suffering [3]. However, within the analysis presented by Dean (2022), an epidemiological evidence gap remains due to the lack of quantitative studies considering the epidemiological clustering of mental health conditions and NTDs in this context. The syndemic is theorised through the application and adaptation of Mendenhall's (2017) model of syndemic approaches to health, with stigma highlighted as a critical catalyst through the adaptation and application of Meyer's (2003) minority stress model [28,35].

Within this study, we draw on mixed-methods approaches to further contextualise the syndemic relationship between NTDs (and their associated disability) and mental distress (depression, anxiety) in Liberia. The biological interaction between the NTDs of focus and mental health conditions has not been explicitly explored, with the exception of onchocerciasis which is increasingly linked to neurodevelopment disorders [36]. Whilst no research has specially looked at the biological relationship between NTDs and mental distress, some research has highlighted the vicious cycle of stress-induced inflammatory events related to other skin conditions, potentially leading to worsening of symptoms [37]. Physical pain, disability stage, and duration of illness leads to poor mental health outcomes among persons affected by NTDs; poor mental health delays health seeking, negatively impacting physical health; NTD related medications may impair mood and cause anxiety, agitation or psychosis; and some NTDs directly affect the brain, leading to mental and neurological consequences [3,13,16,17]. Although, this hasn't been investigated extensively for NTDs, by advancing the Consequently, within this study, we focus on the social and structural mechanisms through which NTDs and mental health conditions synergistically interact and exacerbate health inequalities, as a stigma syndemic. However, we do recognise that further study of the biological interactions between NTDs and mental distress is needed to advance the syndemic argument [38].

This study was completed to support the development of person-centred approaches to skin NTDs, including the integration of mental health services in Liberia, through the REDRESS programme. REDRESS is a five-year, multi-disciplinary research consortium established at the request of the Ministry of Health, Liberia to identify effective strategies to detect, refer, treat and support people living with NTDs that are acceptable, affordable and sustainable especially amongst the most vulnerable [39]. REDRESSS' underpinning methodology is participatory action research to support the co-designing and testing of innovative health systems interventions. In line with participatory health research values and principles [40], this study prioritises the views and experiences of people affected by NTDs, including them as co-researchers within study design, delivery and analysis.

1.2. Contextual Framework: Meyer's Minority Stress Model

Meyer's minority stress theory argues that minority individuals experience psychosocial stress as a consequence of stigma and discrimination that is experienced as direct result of a minority identity [35]. Minority stress theory was originally documented and theorised in relation to the experiences of sexual minorities, largely in the United States [35]. However, Dean (2022) have adapted this model in relation to NTDs in Liberia based on narrative accounts of people affected [3]. In their adaptation and application of Meyer's model, Dean (2022) (see Figure 1) hypothesise that the disadvantage associated with being diagnosed with an NTD presents a minority status. This minority status is thought to exacerbate 'general stressors' for the majority of individuals and communities in Liberia which exist as a consequence of ongoing structural violence due to the post conflict environment, coupled with additional periods of fragility, as a consequence of multiple disease outbreaks (including Ebola, COVID-19). External and internal minority stressors associated with being affected by an NTD then become added stressors that can contribute to poorer, synergistically related health outcomes, specifically, mental distress (depression, anxiety, suicidal ideation) and morbidity/disability. Intersecting axes of inequity, such as gender, age and geography (minority identities) are described as having an interactional relationship with these stressors shaping embodiment/internalisation of oppression and nuanced experiences of the syndemic.

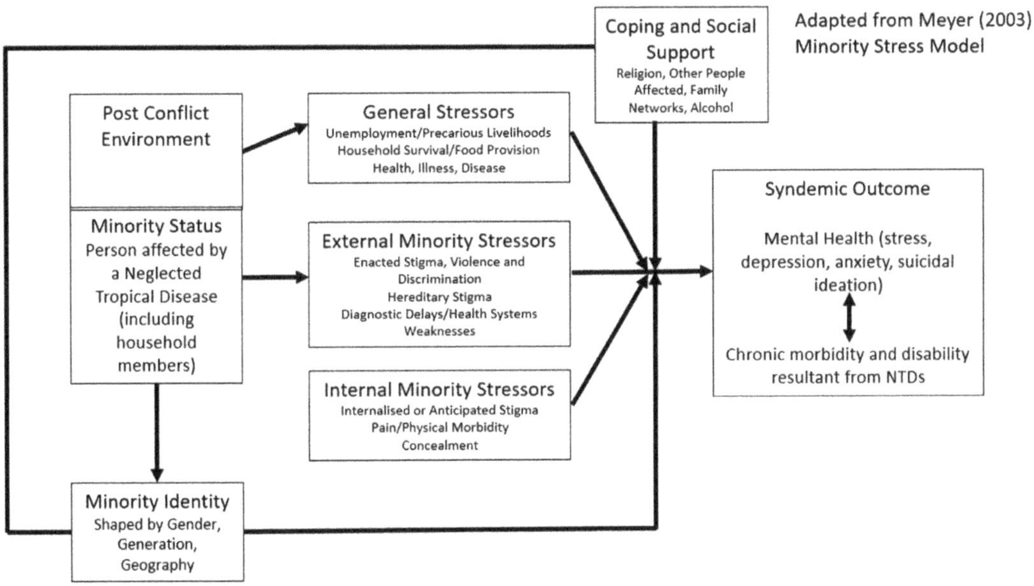

Figure 1. Minority stress model for NTDs and mental distress, reprinted with permission from Dean (2022) [3] which is an adapted from Meyer (2003) [35].

2. Methodology

2.1. Study Context and Sites

We used mixed-method approaches to further interrogate the syndemic relationship between skin NTDs of priority (yaws, Buruli ulcer, LF, onchocerciasis, leprosy) and mental distress (anxiety, depression and suicidal ideation) for persons affected in Liberia. Participatory, qualitative and quantitative data was collected from persons affected by skin NTDs. Drawing on participatory health research principles [40], we involved co-researchers as part of the research team, including community health workers and affected people. Co-researchers received training in research methods, safeguarding and ethics, and took part in data collection, analysis and validation.

The REDRESS study was implemented within three counties in Liberia: Grand Gedeh, Lofa and Margabi (subsequently referred to as the 'REDRESS counties'). These counties were purposively selected in collaboration with the Ministry of Health, Liberia to ensure maximum variation in: (1) the service delivery context of the integrated case management of skin NTDs; (2) endemicity (for all skin NTDs of focus); (3) geography (peri-urban and rural); and (4) socio-demographics (e.g., ethnicity, literacy).

2.2. Survey Data Collection

We completed a cross-sectional survey in the three 'REDRESS counties' (Grand Gedeh, Lofa, Margabi) and one comparator (for the main REDRESS evaluation) county Grand Kru between October 2022 and January 2023 to ascertain the mental health status of adults (>18 years) affected by one of the five endemic skin-NTDs. Grand Kru was purposively selected as a comparator due to similarities in disease endemicity, geography and health service delivery to the 'REDRESS counties'. This cross-sectional survey was part of the wider REDRESS study to evaluate subsequent interventions. Consequently, the sample size of 75 men and 75 women was derived to observe changes in depression scores (PHQ-9) pre- and post-REDRESS interventions and comparisons between gender.

All survey data was collected using REDCAP software (version 13.7.6) and uploaded via electronic tablets (Samsung Galaxy Tab A7 Lite, Monrovia, Liberia). Data were downloaded as a CSV file and imported onto R programme (version 4.3.1) for descriptive and statistical analysis.

2.3. Survey Information

Participants were identified by co-researchers from facility registers, in partnership with trained community health assistants and verified (as living with an NTD) by county health NTD focal persons. Survey questions focused on the participants socio-demographics (gender, age, education level, county), disease (NTD), common mental health conditions (depression and anxiety), stigma and disability scores. Education level was self-reported and described in three categories: no education (i.e., never attended school); attending primary education (i.e., elementary (Grades 1–6)); and attended above primary level education (Grades 7+).

Outcome Measures

Depression and anxiety were assessed using the 9-item Patient Health Questionnaire (PHQ-9) and Generalised Anxiety Disorder 7-item (GAD-7) questionnaire, respectively [41,42]. Stigma was assessed using the Stigma Assessment and Reduction of Impact (SARI) scale and disability was assessed using the World Health Organization (WHO) Disability Assessment Schedule 2.0 (WHODAS 2.0) [43,44]. A Likert scoring system was used to collect questionnaire answers which ranged from 0–27 for depression (PHQ-9), 0–21 for anxiety (GAD-7), 0–100 for stigma (SARI) and 0–4 for disability (WHODAS). The PHQ-9 tool has widely defined cut-off score categories, no depression (0–4), mild depression (5–9), moderate depression (10–14), moderately severe depression (15–19) and severe depression (20–27), previously used in Liberia [45,46]. Similarly, GAD-7 categorised no anxiety (0–5), mild anxiety (5–9), moderate anxiety (10–14), severe anxiety (15–21). There are no validated cut-off scores for the stigma SARI score and degrees of disability and so this score was used as a count variable. WHODAS score for disability defined as categories, no disability (0), mild disability (1), moderate disability (2), severe disability (3) and extreme disability (4) [47].

2.4. Qualitative Data Collection

A mixture of qualitative (in depth interviews (12) and participatory methods (body mapping (56 participants), social mapping (28 participants)) were used in order to help understand the experiences, meanings and views of persons affected (Pope and Mays 1995). Qualitative data collection took place across five counties in Liberia, the three 'REDRESS counties', plus an additional two purposively selected counties (Bong and Nimba) between June 2021 and July 2022. Bong and Nimba were purposively selected due to the high prevalence of endemic skin NTDs. Participants for the in depth interviews (IDIs), body mapping, and social mapping were purposively selected from facility records to support maximum variation in gender, age and disease condition.

In depth interviews explored more about individual experiences with their condition, including both physical and mental wellbeing, seeking care, health beliefs, stigma, and participation within community life. Body mapping was either completed during a group discussion (Grand Gedeh, Lofa, and Margibi) (8 groups) or on a one-to-one basis (Bong and Nimba) (21 participants). Participants were invited to draw a map of themselves and to add to this symbols and images relating to their experiences with their condition, including mental and physical wellbeing. Social mapping was conducted in a group setting and participants were invited to draw out their community identifying key locations for social gatherings within the community, e.g., church or mosque, water pump. This map was then used as a prompt for discussion about their participation within the community. All interviews were audio recorded, transcribed verbatim and stored to SharePoint. A selection of approximately 10% were randomly selected, with the transcript cross-checked against the audio for quality assurance purposes.

2.5. Data Analysis

All data analysis was guided by the main dimensions within Meyer's (2003) minority stress model: general stressors, external minority stressors, internal minority stressors, coping and social support (Meyer 2003). We also considered minority identity by drawing on intersectionality theory to consider how experiences are mediated by social and structural processes to create unique experiences for individuals based on their personal characteristics through the application of intra-categorical analysis (e.g., how are the experiences of men and women living with NTDs aligned/different) [48,49].

2.5.1. Qualitative—Data Analysis

For the qualitative data, thematic framework analysis was carried out to help classify and organise the data according to the main themes, concepts and categories emerging from the data [50]. Categories, guided by the model, were deductively identified, although space was provided to identify emerging issues inductively to ensure an iterative approach to analysis. As a research team (including co-researchers) we familiarised ourselves with the data in the transcripts before then jointly discussing the main themes within the transcripts which were subsequently developed into the coding framework. The coding framework was applied to data using Nvivo 12 to help manage data as part of analysis. After coding of the data, charts were developed, with narratives developed which included comparisons drawn based on gender, county and disease condition.

2.5.2. Quantitative—Data Analysis

For the survey data, two sets of analysis were conducted each with two arms and guided by Meyer's minority stress model and emerging issues identified within the qualitative data: (1) gender-disaggregated descriptive analysis with (i) socio-demographics and (ii) mental health (depression, anxiety and suicide ideation (iii), stigma and disability; (2) risk factor analysis: (i) univariable and (ii) multivariable analysis. Univariable analysis was performed on candidate risk factors: gender, age, diagnosed NTD, county and education level, stigma and disability. Relative-risk ratios (RRs), 95% confidence intervals (CIs) were plotted, and p-values were calculated and reported for all candidate risk factors. The internal reliability of the PHQ-9 and GAD-7 was derived the Cronbach's α calculation.

Gender-disaggregated descriptive analysis was used to understand differences between genders. The overall prevalence and 95% CI for depression, suicide ideation, anxiety, stigma and disability, reported and t-tests were performed. Chi-squared tests were performed to understand the relationship between gender and categories (i.e., mild, moderate, severe etc) for depression, anxiety and disability.

Multi-variable analysis was conducted to understand key risk factors interactions and associations with depression and anxiety and a model selection process was performed. Gender-disaggregated and univariable analysis identified candidate risk factors to be carried forward to multi-variable modelling stage, by screening for statistical significance (p-value < 0.05). Multi-variable models were performed, firstly including all identified candidate risk factors and secondly investigating candidate risk factor interactions. Multi-variable modelling and quantitative findings identified key risk factors associated with depression and anxiety which informed the final models reported in this paper, which included with and without interactions between identified key risk factors. Stigma was excluded from final models due to missing data entries, and anxiety was excluded due to the co-occurrence of depression and anxiety [51,52].

2.6. Ethical Considerations

All researchers and co-researchers took part in training about safeguarding and considerations of power dynamics prior to data collection. The study received ethical approvals from the Liverpool School of Tropical Medicine Research Ethic Committee, United Kingdom (Protocol ID 20-040) and University of Liberia Pacific Institute for Research and Evaluation (UL-PIRE)'s Institutional Review Board, Liberia (Protocol ID 20-09-233) in March and April 2020, respectively. All participants were provided with information about the study and interview. Written informed consent was obtained from all participants.

2.7. Findings

A total of 201 participants were included in the survey (Table S1), across Grand Gedeh (N= 41 [20.4%]), Lofa (N = 72 [35.8]), Margibi (N = 34 [16.9%]) and Grand Kru (N = 53 [26.4%]). More than two-thirds of the participants were male (N = 125 [62.2%]) and the remaining female (N = 76 [37.8%]), with the total average age 46 years (range from 18 to 87) standard deviation (SD) of 16.0). Participants presented with five skin-NTDs; Buruli ulcer (N = 70 [34.8%]), LF-related hydrocoele (N = 49 [24.4%]), LF-related lymphoedema (N = 54 [26.9%]), leprosy (N = 21 [10.5%]), Yaws (N = 6 [3.0]), onchocerciasis (N = 1 [0.5%]). The majority of participants did attend primary education or above, with (N = 79 [39.3%]) attending higher than primary education, (N = 44 [21.9%]) only attending primary school education and (N = 77 [38.3%]) not attending education.

A total of 96 participants took part in qualitative and or participatory data collection activities (Table S2).

2.8. Syndemic Outcomes

Our mixed-methods evidence is indicative of a syndemic relationship between NTDs and mental health, specifically depression, anxiety and suicidal ideation in Liberia, as described in Table 1. Of 201 participants surveyed, 47.8% (95% CI 40.7 to 54.9) reported moderate depressive symptoms or above (PHQ-9 $\geq$ 10). For anxiety, 30.8% (95% CI 24.5 to 54.9) reported moderate or severe symptoms (GAD-7 $\geq$ 10). The internal reliability for both the PHQ-9 and GAD-7 was assessed as excellent, with Cronbach's α of 0.9 and 0.88, respectively.

Comparison of gender means for depression ($t(164) = 3.92$, $p < 0.001$) and anxiety ($t(164) = 3.94$, $p < 0.001$), showed statically significantly higher scores in women in comparison to males. Additionally, women had statistically significantly higher disability scores ($t(158) = 3.64$, $p < 0.001$). Of the 201 baseline surveys, 128 had available stigma SARI scores, used for statistical analysis. No statistically significant difference was found between gender in overall stigma, experienced (enacted) and anticipated stigma SARI scores, and internalised stigma domain scores ($t(90.9) = 2.54$, $p = 0.013$) were statistically significantly higher amongst women.

Table 1. Gender-disaggregated analysis and illustrative qualitative evidence.

	Total, N (%)	Women, N (%)	Men, N (%)	Comparison	Illustrative Qualitative Evidence
Total	201 (100)	76 (37.8)	125 (62.1)		
Depression					
PHQ-9 mean SD	9.4 (6.1)	11.5 (5.8)	8.2 (6.0)	(t(164) = 3.92, p < 0.001) *	*"Very bad, I couldn't sleep at all and I couldn't eat because I only drank water for about one month, two weeks, I only live on water."* ***Bodymapping with male participant, Grand Gedeh*** *"I was feeling bad and crying and don't know what to do."* ***Bodymapping with male participant, Grand Gedeh***
Depression Clinical Scores					
With depression (PHQ-9 ≥ 10)	96 (47.8)	46 (60.5)	50 (40.0)		
None (0–4)	49 (24.4)	10 (13.2)	39 (31.2)	X^2 = 37.831, df = 4, p < 0.001 *	
Mild (5–9)	56 (27.9)	20 (26.3)	36 (28.8)		
Moderate (10–14)	56 (27.9)	23 (30.3)	33 (26.4)		
Moderately severe (15–19)	28 (13.9)	16 (21.1)	12 (9.6)		
Severe (20–27)	12 (6.0)	7 (9.2)	5 (4.0)		
Self-harm/Suicidality	96 (47.8)	50 (65.8)	46 (36.8)	(t(173) = 2.68, p = 0.008) *	*"I was feeling bad myself and even [at] that time I was having bad plan about myself for me to kill myself because I was feeling too bad. So, I say let me just die one time. It's not good living here inside."* ***Bodymapping with male participant with Leprosy, Nimba***
Anxiety					
GAD-7 mean, SD	7.1 (4.9)	8.6 (5.0)	6.1 (4.6)	(t(164) = 3.94, p < 0.001) *	*"Sometimes I can be thinking because if I sit down sometimes, I can be thinking too much, especially this sickness business."* ***Social mapping with male participant, Margibi*** *"You know as a patient sometime when you sick, you can be discouraged. Sometime in the night sleep all you can't sleep."* ***IDI with male participant with hydroocele, aged 34, Lofa***
Anxiety Clinical Scores					
Moderate anxiety or above (GAD-7 ≥ 10)	62 (30.8)	34 (44.7)	28 (22.4)		
None (0–4)	74 (36.8)	21 (27.6)	53 (42.4)	X^2 = 11.462, df = 3, p = 0.009 *	
Mild (5–9)	65 (32.3)	21 (27.6)	44 (35.2)		
Moderate (10–14)	48 (23.9)	27 (35.5)	21 (16.8)		
Severe (>15)	14 (7.0)	7 (9.2)	7 (5.6)		
Stigma					
Total SARI mean, SD	22.6 (14.5)	25.8 (15.8)	20.5 (13.3)	(t(93.5) = 1.97, p = 0.051)	
SARI experienced mean, SD	7.5 (5.9)	8.6 (6.3)	6.9 (5.6)	(t(139) = 1.87, p = 0.064)	*"When it is on you most people don't like to get around you; your friends themselves, some of them don't like to be around you. So, I have been experiencing all those ones them, since this sickness got on me."* ***IDI with male participant with hydrocoele, aged 73, Grand Gedeh***
SARI internalised mean, SD	5.7 (4.2)	6.8 (4.6)	4.9 (3.7)	(t(90.9) = 2.54, p = 0.013) *	*"The water was just coming out, myself, I used to be ashamed to go among my friend then. The water used to be so stink."* ***Bodymapping with male participant with Buruli ulcer, aged 47, Lofa***
SARI anticipated mean, SD	4.1 (3.5)	4.7 (3.7)	3.6 (3.3)	(t(101) = 1.67, p = 0.097)	*"Because whenever I walked, they see my foot they start to laugh at me, so it makes me shy to go anywhere."* ***Social mapping with male participant, Grand Gedeh***

Table 1. *Cont.*

	Total, N (%)	Women, N (%)	Men, N (%)	Comparison	Illustrative Qualitative Evidence
Disability					
WHODAS mean SD	9.4 (6.1)	11.5 (5.8)	8.2 (6.0)	(t(158) = 3.64, $p < 0.001$) *	*"I can't stand on my feet so because of that I am not able to walk to go sit down to the town hall."* ***Social mapping with female participant, Lofa*** *"Yes, as for me, because of my foot business I cannot even go to the market."* ***Social mapping with male participant, Grand Gedeh***
Disability Category Scores					
No disability	18 (8.9)	3 (3.9)	15 (12.0)	$X^2 = 10.752$, df = 3, $p = 0.013$ *	
Mild	102 (50.7)	33 (43.4)	69 (55.2)		
Moderate	60 (29.9)	30 (39.5)	30 (24.0)		
Severe	16 (8.0)	9 (11.8)	7 (5.6)		

* Statistically significant $p < 0.05$ in paired *t*-test (t) and independence chi squared test (X^2).

Qualitatively, irrespective of age or gender, respondents described feelings related to their mental wellbeing as 'feeling bad', 'thinking too much', 'feeling low', 'very bad' or 'very sad and crying'. Anxiety was indicated within one body map as small lines inside the head (Figure 2a), with sadness and loneliness indicated with tears or crying (Figure 2b).

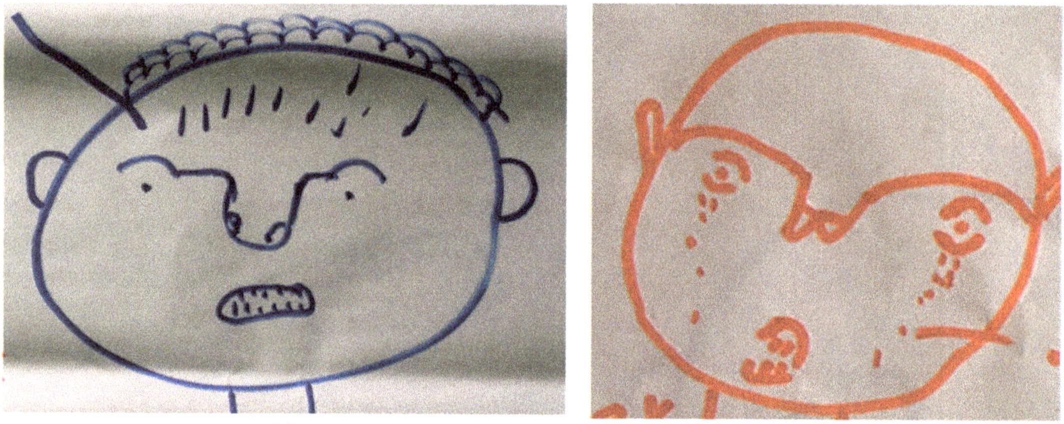

(**a**) (**b**)

Figure 2. (**a**) Bodymap with male participants, Margibi. (**b**) Bodymap with male participant with BU, Lofa.

Women more frequently described feeling hopeless about their situation. A minority of respondents described thoughts of self-harm or suicidal ideation, as also apparent within the quantitative data with 47.8% (n = 96) of participants identifying as having thoughts of self-harm or suicide within the last two weeks. Suicidal ideation was also described qualitatively. A male participant, living with lymphoedema further articulated the connection between their mental and physical wellbeing, highlighting the detrimental impact of stress on them physically.

> *"Sometime[s] when I go to bed, I can't sleep. I will be worrying, thinking, thinking, thinking, until I understand. So, people just advise me now I need not to worry now... So, I need not to be worrying too much. Because the more I worry, that the more my body will be draining."* ***Bodymapping male person affected by lymphoedema, 46 years old, Margibi***

2.9. Risk Factor Analysis

For depression, Figure 3 shows estimated RRs, 95% CIs and *p*-values for univariable generalised linear regression Poisson analysis with all candidate risk factors. Participants that were female (RR 1.41 [95% CI 1.29 to 1.54]) were associated with higher depression scores in comparison to men. Participants above the age of 60 years (RR 1.26 [95% CI 1.12 to 1.42]) were associated with higher levels of depression in comparison to 18–39 and 40–50 years olds. Participants who received no education were associated with higher depression in comparison to those that attended primary education (RR 0.80 [95% CI 0.71 to 0.90]) and those that attended higher than elementary (RR 0.79 [95% CI 0.71 to 0.87]). Participants presenting with leprosy, (RR 1.44 [95% CI 1.26 to 1.65]), Buruli ulcer (RR 1.45 [95% CI 1.21 to 1.73]) and LF-related lymphoedema (RR 1.90 [95% CI 1.67 to 2.17]) were associated with higher depression scores in comparison to LF-related hydrocoele. Participants with a mild anxiety (RR 2.74 [95% CI 2.38 to 3.16]), moderate anxiety (RR 3.99 [95% CI 3.47 to 4.58]), severe anxiety (RR 5.05 [95% CI 4.26 to 5.99]), were associated with higher levels of depression in comparison to no anxiety. Participants with a mild disability (RR 2.20 [95% CI 1.69 to 2.87]), moderate anxiety (RR 4.15 [95% CI 3.19 to 5.41]), or severe anxiety (RR 4.75 [95% CI 3.57 to 6.31]), were associated with higher levels of depression in comparison to no disability.

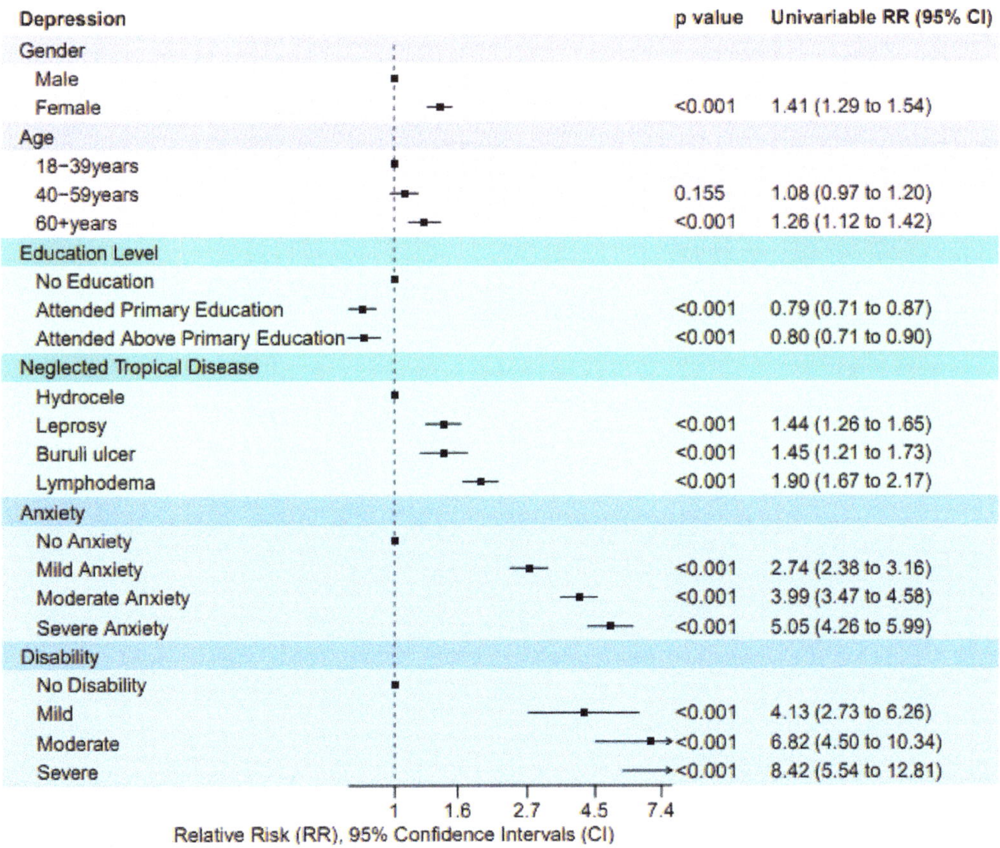

Figure 3. Relative-risk Ratios (RR) and 95% CIs for depression derived from univariable generalised linear regression Poisson models. RR above 1 (dotted line) shows a greater association with depression and RR below 1 means a lesser association in comparison to the first item listed for each variable.

For anxiety, Figure 4 shows estimated RRs, 95% CIs and p-values for univariable generalised linear regression Poisson analysis with all candidate risk factors. Participants that were female (RR 1.40 [95% CI 1.26 to 1.55]) were associated with higher anxiety scores in comparison to men. Participants above the age of 60 years (RR 1.29 [95% CI 1.13 to 1.49]) were associated with higher levels of anxiety scores in comparison to 18–39 and 40–69 years old. Participants that received no education were associated with higher levels of anxiety in comparison to those that attended elementary (RR 0.77 [95% CI 0.67 to 0.88]) and those that attended higher than elementary (RR 0.79 [95% CI 0.70 to 0.88]). Participants presenting with leprosy, (RR 1.47 [95% CI 1.26 to 1.71]), Buruli ulcer (RR 1.38 [95% CI 1.12 to 1.70]) and LF-related lymphoedema (RR 1.89 [95% CI 1.62 to 2.20]) were associated with higher anxiety scores in comparison to LF-related hydrocoele. Participants with a mild disability (RR 2.12 [95% CI 1.56 to 2.88]), moderate anxiety (RR 4.02 [95% CI 2.96 to 5.46]), severe anxiety (RR 5.91 [95% CI 4.28 to 8.15]), were associated with higher levels of anxiety in comparison to no disability.

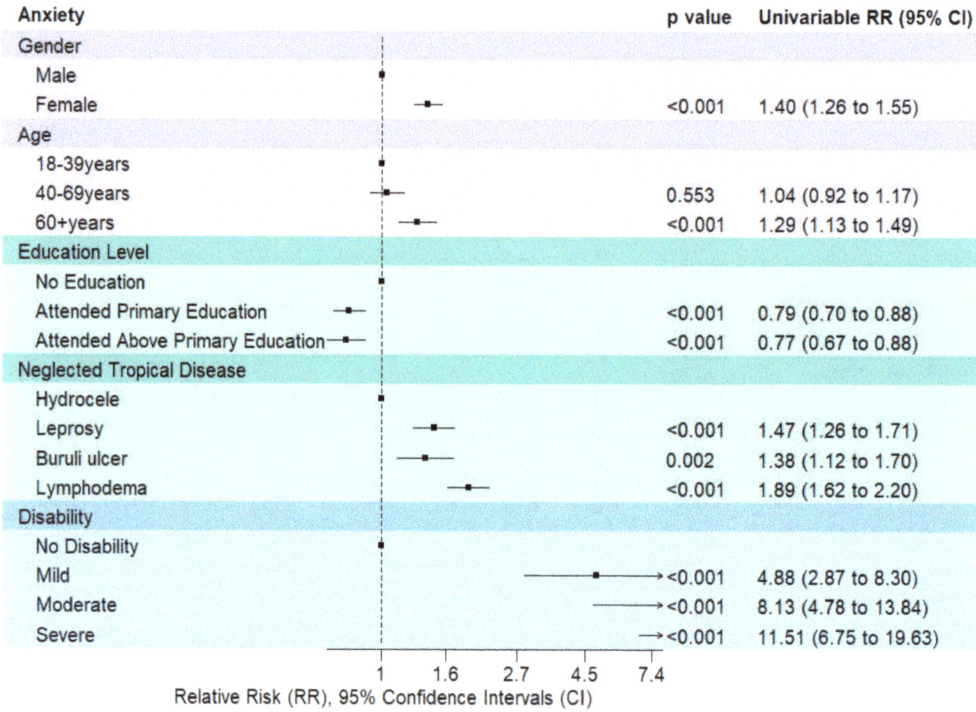

Figure 4. Relative-risk Ratios (RR) and 95% CIs for anxiety derived from univariable generalised linear regression Poisson models. RR above 1 (dotted line) shows a greater association with anxiety and RR below 1 means a lesser association in comparison to the first item listed for each variable.

Key risk factors, gender and disability were identified respectively from gender-disaggregated data analysis (Table 1), univariable risk factor analysis (Figures 1 and 3), multi-variable analysis, previous studies, and qualitative findings. Four multivariable models were performed, two models for each outcome variable: depression and anxiety, model 1 displayed no interaction between gender and disability, and model 2 an interaction, as described in Table 2. Across all models, we identified that higher disability scores were associated with an increased incidence risk ratio of high depression and anxiety scores, see Table 2.

Table 2. Multivariable generalised linear regression Poisson models for depression and anxiety. Presenting an interaction (model 2) and no interaction (model 1) between gender and disability.

	Depression Model 1			Depression Model 2			Anxiety Model 1			Anxiety Model 2		
Characteristic	**IRR [1]**	**95% CI [1]**	***p*-Value**	**IRR [1]**	**95% CI [1]**	***p*-Value**	**IRR [1]**	**95% CI [1]**	***p*-Value**	**IRR [1]**	**95% CI [1]**	***p*-Value**
Gender												
Male	—	—		—	—		—	—		—	—	
Female	1.15	1.05, 1.27	0.003	2.00	1.51, 2.66	<0.001	1.11	0.99, 1.23	0.067	1.40	1.0, 1.97	0.052
Disability	1.03	1.03, 1.04	<0.001	1.04	1.04, 1.05	<0.001	1.04	1.04, 1.05	<0.001	1.04	1.04, 1.05	<0.001
Gender * Disability												
Female * Disability				0.98	0.97, 0.99	<0.001				0.99	0.98, 1.00	0.2
Log-likelihood		−669			−661			−555			−554	
AIC		1344			1330			1116			1116	

[1] IRR = Incidence Rate Ratio, CI = Confidence Interval, * = interaction.

We found that the incidence risk ratio for depression in females was higher in comparison to men, which was statistically significant across both depression models. For persons affected by NTDs, being a male and having no/mild disability moderated the negative effects of depression, as shown in Figure 5. The interaction between gender and disability in anxiety model 2 and being female in anxiety model 1 were not statistically significantly associated with a higher incidence risk ratio of anxiety. This shows for anxiety, disability has the greatest contribution to incidence risk ratio.

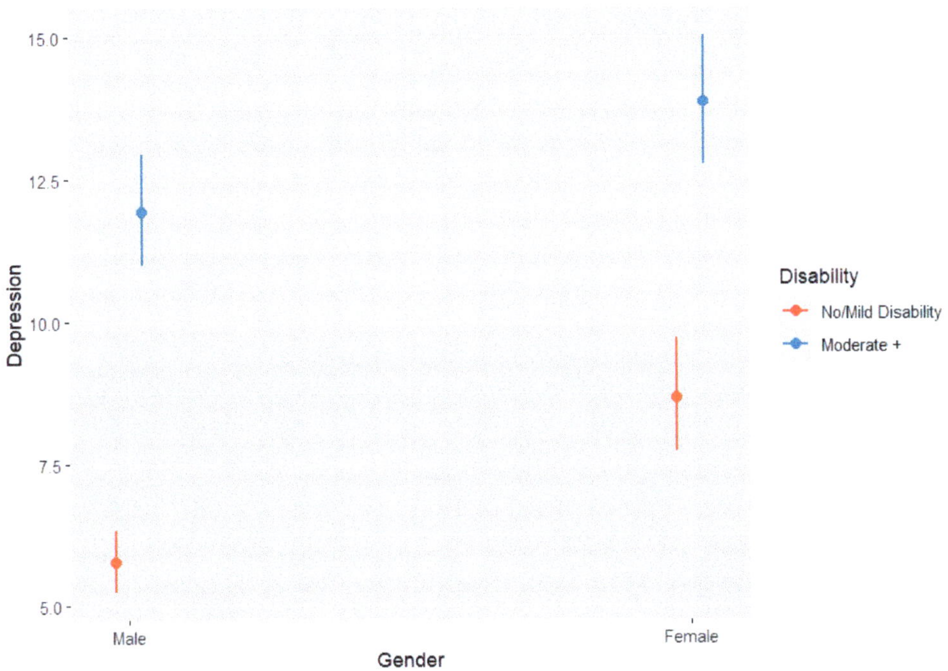

Figure 5. Interaction effect between gender and disability for depression.

In the subsequent sections, we present further qualitative evidence linked to the differing domains of Meyer's Minority Stress Model (2003), as adapted by Dean (2022) (see Figure 1), to consider the biosocial factors shaping this syndemic outcome.

2.10. General Stressors

Our evidence shows the impact of general stressors for people affected by skin NTDs in Liberia. Specifically, they emphasise the influence of income losses and challenges with health seeking, largely due to accessibility related issues.

2.11. Loss of Income Due to Physical Consequences of Their Condition

Physical limitations associated with skin NTDs were linked to financial difficulties due to loss of work, with some participants becoming dependent on relatives or begging as a means of survival. The perception of inappropriate appearance due to physical symptoms also posed challenges to livelihood activities with one person affected by leprosy describing being unable to wear shoes due to ulcers on his feet which created a barrier to office work. Some participants also described stigma (see below) leading to some people refusing to engage with them in selling or employment. Self-care, as a key strategy to managing skin NTDs, was described by some persons affected as important, however the time taken to do these activities was often outweighed by a need to provide for family members and go out to "look for my daily bread." IDI with Male person affected by leprosy, aged 26 years, Lofa county.

> *"...here most of my friends, some encourage me to work with them. [To] do letter work, pen and paperwork, but then, the problem that I have now, I can't wear shoes."* ***IDI with male person affected by leprosy, aged 26 years, Lofa***

> *"...I learned the tailoring, I learned the tie and dye I can do some work, but only this my hand I do it with and this my hand can't permit me."* ***Bodymapping with female person affected by leprosy, Bong***

Both men and women described these negative livelihood impacts. However, adult men (aged 25–49 years) more commonly described both the economic consequences of their condition, as well as the negative impact of this on their own wellbeing. They frequently described feeling 'bad', worried, discouraged or anxious at being unable to go out and work to provide for their families. Some elderly participants described changing what they ate to cheaper alternatives due to lack of money.

> *"I said the place I am now I am still feeling bad! I feeling bad of it, yes! Young man like me and this foot just get on me [pain in foot from NTD], I can't be in peace, yes. I am still feeling bad about it and I am just asking God how we will be free from it."* ***Bodymapping with male person affected, Grand Gedeh***

2.12. Health Seeking Challenges from Both Formal and Informal Providers

Accessing appropriate healthcare was identified as a challenge, driven by three key factors: (1) high costs associated with travel and lost work; (2) fear of medical procedures (e.g., amputation) within biomedical facilities; and (3) loss of confidence in the health system, largely due to irregular or absent medicine supply. These challenges often led to treatment cessation, as well as creating complex care pathways. For example, some have sought care from an informal provider followed by biomedical care, others vice versa, and some seeking care from both simultaneously. Several participants with lymphoedema described having had their foot *"cut open"* by a herbalist/traditional healer. Other traditional practices such as providing something to drink leading to patients experiencing vomiting and diarrhoea, feeling "helpless" as a result. This resulted in negative impact for the person affected, who felt like the herbalist was "trying to destroy them".

"Somebody [traditional healer] cutting human being flesh putting it down and say that's medicine . . . He wanted to destroy me, so that's the bad care people there." **IDI with female person affected by lymphoedema, aged over 49, Margibi**

"They say they don't have the drugs there in the hospital. So, when we go there, they can only prescribe drugs and give it to us. Then we go buy the drugs in the other clinics. So, what is the use of [me] going there still?" **IDI with male person affected by Buruli ulcer, aged 69, Grand Gedeh**

Chaotic and complex care seeking pathways were largely responsible for people affected having 'lost-peace', 'thinking too much' and experiencing anxiety. This was particularly common for male participants around the time of their diagnosis, due to their limited knowledge about what to expect, including what treatment would be needed. Where participants had been on such complex care seeking journeys but were still searching for a cure, a sense of hopelessness and resignation was often articulated.

"You know as a patient sometime when you sick, you can be discouraged. Sometime in the night you can't sleep." **IDI with male person affected by leprosy, aged 34, Lofa**

"Starting from this year I have gone nowhere yet because I am tired now. I am just spending money and no result so, I am just tired sitting down now and waiting for God's time." **IDI with Female person affected by Buruli ulcer, aged over 49, Margibi**

2.13. External Minority Stressors: Experienced Stigma

Experienced stigma was commonly described by participants across counties, ages and genders and was largely attributed to: community members' perception that the condition is transmissible by physical contact/proximity; smell coming from wounds; belief systems including superstition and witchcraft. Experienced stigma was described by participants with all conditions; persons affected by leprosy described it most frequently and extensively. One of the most frequent forms described by people with leprosy and lymphoedema was name calling, such as *"the old man that gets leprosy"* IDI with a female person affected by leprosy, aged 98, Grand Gedeh or *"rotten man"* IDI with a male person affected by lymphoedema, aged 25–49 years, Margibi. Other forms of stigma described include verbal abuse, mocking, being the subject of gossip within the community, having people spitting due to bad smell from an ulcer and having been driven away or isolated by others, including being carried to spend time in the 'sick bush'.

"I even left the place. I left them because of the stigma" Social mapping with male participants, Lofa

Participants often described 'feeling bad' or ashamed in response. The sense of isolation was described more frequently by female participants, with male participants describing continued support from their wife (although they had also experienced loss of friendships). However, one male participant described having experienced rejection from his family, which provoked an angry response.

"... when you find yourself like this when you were not like that, family turned their back, friends turned their back... When you are well, you are for people. People will like you, they will come around you, you will do things together, but this type of condition now nobody can come to your rescue." **Bodymapping with female person affected by Lymphoedema, aged 50, Margibi**

"I am angry with my family... They cannot [do not] visit me, they cannot [do not] keep time with me... So, I am very angry of that. From there, when I sit down on my own when I think about my condition, I always cry, 'what I do to my family they do not look at me, what I do to them they do not look at me.'" **Bodymapping with male person affected by Buruli ulcer, aged 47, Margibi**

Some participants also described experiencing discrimination from health workers if they showed any evidence of previously having sought care from an informal provider. One older female participant with lymphoedema gave a compelling story of a health worker refusing to treat her, shouting at her and ordering her to leave the facility. This stigmatising response led her to feel confused, adding additional stress for her when she was already feeling unwell.

> *"They [name of hospital] didn't even touch me! Later, when the Doctor came, he said "they touched this foot oh, because I can see chalk on it" so he didn't even touch me. He didn't feel the skin like this, he didn't touch me; they just walked in group and went...and myself too I am sick and feeling bad and then I go somebody said "your carry her on that side, we don't have place for her!" they were just shouting."* ***IDI with female person affected by lymphoedema, aged over 49, Margibi***

2.14. Internal Minority Stressors

2.14.1. Physical Symptoms

Participants described a wide range of symptoms related to their condition, including pain, swollen and/or itchy limb, ulcer/ sore, leaking ulcer, smell from ulcer, loss of sensation. These symptoms were frequently linked with a sense of shame and self-isolation by participants, particularly the foul-smelling exudate described by many participants with Buruli ulcer. The pain in particular impacted mental wellbeing among persons affected, contributing towards sleeplessness, loss of appetite and sadness. Bodymapping participants frequently showed pain, using red to indicate the severity of their pain linked to swelling and ulcers (Figure 6a,b). Other less commonly described symptoms include rash, loss of appetite, irritation from flies and several women described having lost their eyebrows, which they found distressing.

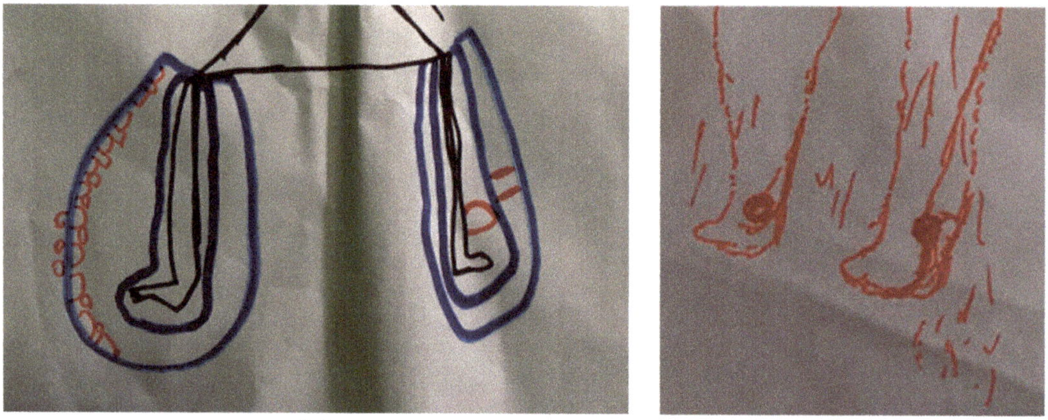

(a) (b)

Figure 6. (**a**) Bodymap with male participant with Buruli ulcer, 69 years old, Lofa (**left**). (**b**) Bodymap with female participants, Margibi (**right**).

2.14.2. Internalised or Anticipated Stigma

People affected experienced shame related to physical symptoms, leading them to isolate themselves from others in the community, avoid social gatherings, with a reluctance to name or disclose their health condition, and describing themselves as 'rotten'. It was common for participants to describe altering their clothing in order to try and hide their condition. These feelings were often described more intensely by younger participants.

"Like for [me], [I] felt bad because looking at [my] age, [I am] very young and then, [I] get that kind of condition, [I] felt bad. Seeing [my] friends walking good, normal, and [I] have that condition, [I] felt very bad." ***Bodymapping with female person affected by lymphoedema, aged 30, Lofa***

2.14.3. Coping and Social Support

Support from family, friends and faith in God were all described as forming essential coping strategies among persons affected. Participants regularly described placing their faith in God for healing, at times this was in response to having been abandoned by others. Faith was also described as playing a part in some people affected accepting their condition as being the will of God.

"for me, I never lose hope because God is there, I never disappointed because the lord is always there for me." ***Social mapping with male participants, Margibi***

"I [am] sick, I not have nobody to help me only God. My children...they not big...Ain't got no husband." ***Bodymapping with female person affected by lymphoedema, aged 50, Margibi***

Having someone to talk to was widely discussed as an important source of encouragement and companionship with a positive influence on overall wellbeing. For some, this role was played by the health worker, while for others if was a family member or friend. For those who were older, this support often came from children. In contrast among youth, aged 18–25 years, support was often came from their parents. Where support was present, this was highly encouraging for persons affected.

"Yes, my family really catered to me in my sickness and they never gave me any word to make me feel bad, they make me always happy, and my community people, too, they did the same." ***Social mapping with male persons affected, Margibi***

The support included practical support such as helping to bring them to the health facility or to a traditional healer, as well as providing encouragement and emotional support. Where participants were married, gender was a clear mediator in shaping experience, with men often describing being supported by a spouse, whereas women frequently described being abandoned or alone. Male participants who received caring support from their spouse recognised the impact on their spouse.

"When you find yourself like this when you were not like that, family turned their back, friends turned their back...When you are well, you are for people. People will like you, they will come around you, your will do things together, but this type of condition now nobody can come to your rescue." ***Bodymapping with female person affected by lymphoedema, aged 50, Margibi***

"Lying down whole day and whole night, crying, the woman [wife] will come haul the clothes from under my foot and put different one there. She goes wash, hang it and put different one there. Five minutes, she comes again take that one, put different one there. Go wash it." ***Bodymapping with male person affected by Buruli ulcer, aged 41, Lofa***

Some participants felt that their friends continued to support them, after the diagnosis, although this was not universal and even those who generally felt supported by friends often still described instances of having been stigmatised by others in their community.

"...some of my friends actually we move together, we do things together. Yes, they make me feel like them. they make me happy. They make me laugh. We all joke together, we do things together, we live happy life, but criticize. Some they stigma, some they talked about it, some even if you go around them, they take you different." ***IDI with male person affected by leprosy, aged 26, Lofa***

"That's just God, for me God love me and people been helping me, people know me, better people." ***IDI with female person affected by lymphoedema, aged over 49, Margibi***

3. Discussion

To our knowledge, this is the first study to presents mixed-methods approaches to evidence the syndemic relationship between NTDs and mental distress, specifically mental health conditions (depression and anxiety). Our study provides needed empirical evidence for the syndemic of concern, within the context of structural violence in Liberia, a post-conflict setting, with high levels of poverty, gendered social norms, stigma and weak health infrastructure [3]. This study used an adapted Meyers (2003) minority stress model, as is evidenced within other skin-NTD work [53–55], to present quantitative findings together with qualitative and participatory findings. Quantitative and qualitative findings informed analysis approaches to strengthen understanding in intersectionality for individual identities, stressors and syndemic outcomes mental health and disability (Figure 1). We utilised mixed-methods evidence in this under-researched area to support the collaborative design of holistic person-centred approaches to end syndemic suffering. The findings presented in this study were used to support intervention development workshops linked to the REDRESS programme, with findings presented in collaborative design workshops to shape recommendations for intervention design. Specifically, we illuminate the need for early case detection to prevent NTD-related disability and mental distress, as well as social and structural interventions to improve the health and wellbeing of those affected. Box 1 presents some of the recommendations for intervention areas identified following the presentation of these study results and that went on to be piloted within the REDRESS programme (results forthcoming).

Box 1. Co-designed interventions developed in response to findings.

- Delivery of awareness about NTDs and mental health in marketplaces and on the radio, led by community advisory boards that constitute of multiple community stakeholders.
- Establish peer support groups or networks for persons affected by skin NTDs to provide opportunities for experience sharing and mutual support, with seed funding to support financial sustainability.
- Support community health workers and informal providers to recognise the signs and symptoms of NTDs and mental distress, including tackling myths and misconceptions to support early identification and referral.
- Support health–workers through the provision of training and resource materials to diagnose NTDs and provide support for mental distress, including enhancing communication skills and supporting stigma reduction.
- Integrate screening tools for depression (PHQ9) and anxiety (GAD7) at point of NTD diagnosis.
- Provide mhGAP training for selected health workers at facility level, highlighting mental health and NTD links.

3.1. The Syndemic Spiral

Our findings align with those previously presented by Dean (2022) which emphasise that the post-conflict environment, minority status and minority identity of persons affected by NTDs interact with and exacerbate a person's experience of generalised stressors. Their experience of external minority stressors, experienced through enacted stigma, and internal minority stressors, including physical symptoms and anticipated symptoms interact in a potentially 'vicious spiral' contributing to ever worsening physical and mental wellbeing. These effects can be buffered (or exacerbated) through the presence (or absence) of a strong health system, robust support from family and friends and holistic, non-stigmatising care from trained and trusted faith and traditional healers (Figure 7).

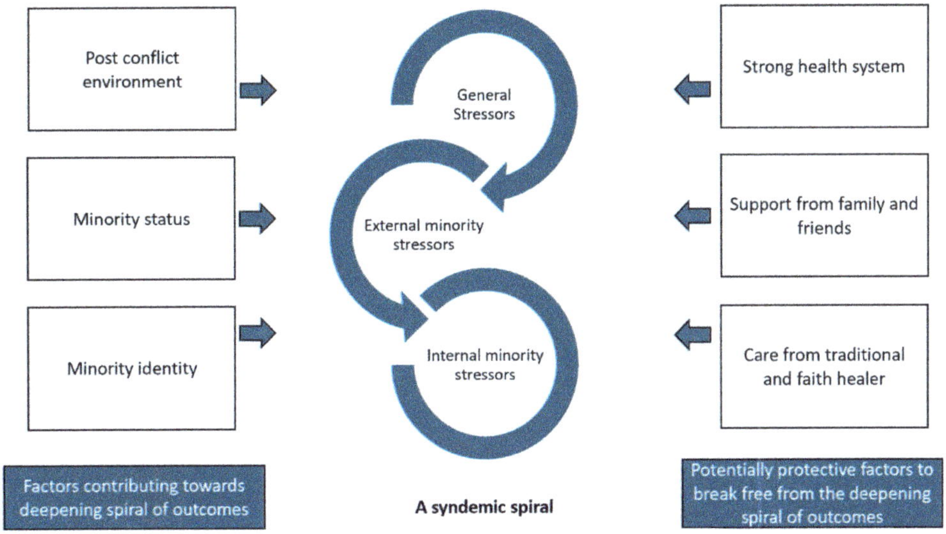

Figure 7. The Syndemic Spiral of NTDs and Mental Distress in Liberia.

3.2. General Stressors

In our study, we found one of the main general stressors described by persons affected was their experience of financial insecurities in consequence of their frequent loss of work due to the physical impacts of their condition. Similar to results from Nigeria where a contextually adapted collaborative care model for persons affected by skin-NTDs was developed for implementation in the primary care system [56]. Thus, the provision of economic support to persons affected is a key potential strategy to address the 'syndemic spiral'. This could include the promotion of income generation activities for persons with disabilities, such as socio-economic rehabilitation, i.e., training in skills, educational opportunities and enhancing entrepreneurship [57–59]. Understanding the best and most sustainable ways to provide this economic support is likely to rely on linkages across sectors to ensure a person-centred response [17].

Alongside the financial insecurities, challenges related to health seeking via both formal and informal providers stemmed from pursuit of a 'cure', widely described in the literature, related to underlying health beliefs about causation of the condition, as well as health system limitations [60]. This oscillation between providers and inability to understand the cause of their condition has previously been described as distressing for persons affected [3,31]. Given the reliance of persons affected by NTDs on informal providers (both traditional and faith healers), as well as the holistic nature of care provided for persons affected by these informal providers in Liberia [61], there is opportunity to engage with traditional and faith healers, providing them training and mentorship to identify and refer persons affected, while supporting them to provide basic psychosocial support and referral (Box 1). Fear of biomedical care and frequent drug stock-outs created a loss of confidence in seeking care from the formal health system, as previously documented [62]. Thus, a strong supply chain has been described as a cornerstone for integrated case management [62].

3.3. External Minority Stressors

Enacted stigma was widely described by participants in the form of name calling, mocking, verbal abuse, being driven away by others, including being carried to the 'sick bush' [out of the community into the forest] which has previously been described in other studies among persons with NTDs in Liberia [63]. Quantitative findings emphasise the association between stigma with depression and anxiety. The experience of stigma by persons affected by skin NTDs has been widely described in the literature across multiple contexts and settings [64–66]. In our study, the experience of stigma was linked and often catalytic of mental distress, related to a sense of shame, isolation and loneliness from having been rejected. Social stigma related to disease has been identified as a key promotor of syndemic interactions and overall suffering [67], previously identified in the stigma syndemic of mental distress and LF/NTDs (Malawi and Liberia respectively) [3,57]. Stigma can further complicate recognition, treatment and prevention of disease [67]. Links between stigma, mental health and NTDs are well documented [15,64]. Challenging stigma through the work of peer support groups, and training of local community leaders and change agents such as traditional and faith healers were recommended as necessary strategies to respond to some of these findings (Box 1). Peer support groups have been shown to improve wellbeing and self-esteem amongst persons affected by skin-NTDs, as well as can encourage adherence to self-care [68]. Wider community stigma reduction interventions such as community awareness campaigns, stepping stones, and community conversations, have been implemented in other settings and relevant to other infectious diseases to support more holistic responses to the stigma experienced (HIV in South Africa and NTD podoconiosis in Ethiopia) [69].

3.4. Internal Minority Stressors

Physical symptoms caused participants' considerable distress as described in the qualitative findings, and from the quantitative findings, greater degrees of disability were associated with higher levels of depression and anxiety. Experience of pain relating to Buruli ulcer and lymphoedema has previously been widely described [70,71], with up to 95% of persons affected by Buruli ulcer describing pain in one study from Ghana [71]. Alongside pain, symptoms of anxiety contributed to further physical symptoms, such as the inability to sleep and loss of appetite. The interlinking of symptoms between NTDs and mental health, creates a vicious cycle which can self-perpetuate with pain contributing to sleeplessness, contributing to anxiety and depression, contributing to reduced appetite, potentially contributing to worsening of physical symptoms related to poor nutrition.

Other physical symptoms such as foul-smelling exudate and leaking wounds among persons affected by Buruli ulcer contributed to feelings of shame and internalised and/or anticipated stigma among persons affected, leading them to isolate themselves from others within their community. In this study, surveys showed women to have statistically higher internalised stigma scores in comparison to men. The enacted, anticipated and internalised stigma experienced by persons affected by Buruli ulcer and lymphoedema is in keeping with findings from a systematic review exploring social stigma towards NTDs [64].

3.5. The Equity Implications of NTD and Mental Health Syndemic Relationship

The existing structural and social inequities resulting from the macro-forces shaping Liberia's complex history and present situation (including war, high poverty and low educational levels), mean the people affected by skin NTDs are frequently already among those most marginalised within communities at the onset of their symptoms. Experiencing the added generalised (financial concerns), external (experience of stigma) and internal (experience of pain and physical symptoms) minority stressors which persons affected in our study describe (to varying extents) contributes towards mental distress and the development of mental health conditions. Related to this, persons affected by NTDs and mental health conditions experience a loss of power, and restriction in participation in the life of their community and/or family, emphasised in a recent review of mental health, stigma and NTDs [15]. At times, this may be self-imposed due to anticipated stigma, or imposed by the community, through enacted stigma, shaped by fear of infection, discrimination and ableism norms. By adopting an intersectionality approach within our analysis [72], we can see that the experiences of persons affected are not homogenous, rather, there are many variations shaped by the unique circumstances of power, privilege and identity experienced in the life of each individual that shape the underlying pathways toward syndemic suffering. We found gender, age, (dis)ability and socio-economic status to be important 'axes of privilege, power and inequity' [73] shaping this path.

3.6. Addressing Gender Inequities

This work further evidences the need to address gender-based inequalities and disparities within NTD and mental health programmes [74]. This gendered impact of NTDs creates a disproportionate burden on women and girls, largely due to gender roles and responsibilities, increased experience of stigma, discrimination and lack of spousal support; resulting in social and financial losses for women [75]. This disproportionate effect of the social consequences of NTDs for women, may explain the higher co-occurrence of depression and anxiety among women, in our study. Meanwhile, men of working age in our study described greater distress relating to their loss of ability to work due to their condition, and their inability to fulfil the traditionally male breadwinner role. This may have been shaped by the existing "hypermasculinity" norms previously described within Liberia [76] but warrants further exploration in subsequent work. Younger persons affected experienced distress at the changes they experienced in their life circumstances (loss of educational and work opportunities, and of 'good health'), which they considered to be unfair at their stage of life [57]. Transforming the social, environmental and political factors which contribute towards the interactions between health conditions is needed to reduce the burden of ill health associated with NTDs and mental distress for all [3].

3.7. Limitations and Trustworthiness

This study benefited from mixed-method approaches where qualitative findings helped to interpret and add meaning to quantitative results. Some of the qualitative data were collected at different time points and in different counties; however, the findings were consistent, adding an additional layer of triangulation to the data. The role of co-researchers (including community health workers and a persons affected) as part of the research cycle, including data collection and co-analysis, provided opportunity to strengthen the trustworthiness of this work. The absence of a control group measuring depression and anxiety of the general population, does not allow us to make comparisons to overall population in Liberia, and quantitative prevalence studies are somewhat limited in Liberia [30]. The missing data entries from SARI stigma scores should be acknowledged when interpretating quantitative stigma findings presented in this paper. There is limited evidence on the validity, cultural interpretability and the use of the PHQ-9 and GAD-7 in Liberia, which may introduce measurement bias, and possibly underestimate the prevalence of mental health outcomes in this survey study group.

4. Conclusions

We find strong evidence which adds to our understanding of the syndemic relationship between NTDs, and mental distress (anxiety and depression) within the context of structural violence in Liberia, in response to generalised, external minority and internal minority stressors. Persons affected by NTDs currently rely upon two main coping mechanisms, centred around support from their faith in God, and emotional, financial and social support from family and/ or friends. NTD programmes should strengthen these naturally occurring coping strategies, by providing training for faith healers, family and friends to provide basic psychosocial support, as well as strengthening multi-sectoral collaboration to support persons affected with opportunities for suitable income-generation activities.

Supplementary Materials: The following supporting information can be downloaded at: https://www.mdpi.com/article/10.3390/tropicalmed9080183/s1, Table S1: Means (SD) for each continuous outcome measure and proportion (N) for binary outcome by group for each socio-demographic characteristic. Table S2: Participant characteristics for qualitative and participatory research methods.

Author Contributions: Conceptualization, R.M., C.B., G.Z., M.S., T.G.G.-A., R.J. and L.D.; methodology, R.M., C.B., G.Z., R.J., M.S., L.S. and L.D.; formal analysis, R.M., C.B., G.Z., R.J., H.B., S.C., J.K., C.P., J.S.S., W.S., Z.Z. and L.D.; investigation, R.M., C.B., G.Z., R.J., H.B., S.C., J.K., C.P., J.S.S., L.S., M.S., W.S., Z.Z., S.T. and L.D.; resources, K.K., E.R., C.P., S.T. and L.D.; data curation, R.M., G.Z., R.J., L.S. and C.B.; writing—original draft preparation, R.M., C.B., G.Z. and L.D.; writing—review and editing All; supervision, R.M., Z.Z., K.K., S.C., M.S., E.R., S.T. and L.D.; project administration, R.M., Z.Z., S.T. and L.D.; funding acquisition, L.D., S.T., A.W., M.P. and K.K. All authors have read and agreed to the published version of the manuscript.

Funding: This work was supported and funded by the National Institute for Health Research (NIHR), [REDRESS: Reducing the Burden of Severe Stigmatising Skin Diseases through equitable person-centred approaches to health systems strengthening (project reference NIHR200129)/Research and Innovation for Global Health Transformation]. The views expressed are those of the author(s) and not necessarily those of the NIHR or the Department of Health and Social Care.

Institutional Review Board Statement: The study was conducted in accordance with the Declaration of Helsinki, and approved by the Institutional Review Board (or Ethics Committee) of Liverpool School of Tropical Medicine Research Ethic Committee, United Kingdom (protocol ID 20-040) and University of Liberia Pacific Institute for Research and Evaluation UL-PIRE's Institutional Review Board, Liberia (protocol ID 20-09-233).

Informed Consent Statement: Informed consent was obtained from all subjects involved in the study.

Data Availability Statement: All data generated and analyzed during this study are included in this manuscript. Raw qualitative data are not available and will not be publicly shared, as this would compromise the anonymity and protection of our study participants.

Acknowledgments: The authors wish to thank the co-researchers (Satta S. Kollie, Emmanuel G. Zaizay, Jallah Kessellie, Kebeh Lavala, Christopher Morris, Hagar Kruah, Robert G Jaffa, Harrison Wenjor), community health workers, programme coordinators and managers, county health workers, and county officials and participants who made this study possible. We would like to thank the participants who took the time to engage with us as part of this study and for their sharing honest, challenging and personal experiences.

Conflicts of Interest: The authors declare no conflicts of interest.

References

1. Hotez, P.J.; Damania, A.; Naghavi, M. Blue Marble Health and the Global Burden of Disease Study 2013. *PLoS Neglected Trop. Dis.* **2016**, *10*, e0004744. [CrossRef]
2. Singer, M.; Bulled, N. Interlocked Infections: The Health Burdens of Syndemics of Neglected Tropical Diseases. *Ann. Anthropol. Pract.* **2012**, *36*, 328–345. [CrossRef]
3. Dean, L.; Theobald, S.; Nallo, G.; Bettee, A.; Kollie, K.; Tolhurst, R. A Syndemic Born of War: Combining Intersectionality and Structural Violence to Explore the Biosocial Interactions of Neglected Tropical Diseases, Disability and Mental Distress in Liberia. *PLoS Glob. Public Health* **2022**, *2*, e0000551. [CrossRef] [PubMed]
4. Ashford, R.W. Parasitic Diseases 5th Edition. *Parasitology* **2006**, *132*, 449–455. [CrossRef]
5. World Health Organization. Lymphatic Filariasis. 2023. Available online: https://www.who.int/news-room/fact-sheets/detail/lymphatic-filariasis (accessed on 1 June 2023).
6. Ramaiah, K.D.; Ottesen, E.A. Progress and Impact of 13 Years of the Global Programme to Eliminate Lymphatic Filariasis on Reducing the Burden of Filarial Disease. *PLoS Negl. Trop. Dis.* **2014**, *8*, e3319. [CrossRef] [PubMed]
7. Global Burden of Disease. Keys Facts. 2018. Available online: https://www.who.int/news-room/fact-sheets/detail/onchocerciasis (accessed on 1 July 2024).
8. World Health Organization. Yaws (Endemic Treponematoses). 2024. Available online: https://www.who.int/health-topics/yaws#tab=tab_1 (accessed on 1 June 2024).
9. World Health Organization. Leprosy. 2023. Available online: https://www.who.int/news-room/fact-sheets/detail/leprosy (accessed on 1 May 2024).
10. Huang, G.K.L.; Johnson, P. *Chapter 28—Buruli Ulcer (Atypical Mycobacteria). Emerging Infectious Diseases*; Ergönül, Ö., Can, F., Madoff, L., Akova, M., Eds.; Academic Press: Amsterdam, The Netherlands, 2014; pp. 373–383.
11. Ploemacher, T.; Faber, W.R.; Menke, H.; Rutten, V.; Pieters, T. Reservoirs and transmission routes of leprosy: A systematic review. *PLoS Negl. Trop. Dis.* **2020**, *14*, e0008276. [CrossRef]

12. Abdulmalik, J.; Nwefoh, E.; Obindo, J.; Dakwak, S.; Ayobola, M.; Umaru, J.; Samuel, E.; Ogoshi, C.; Eaton, J. Emotional Difficulties and Experiences of Stigma among Persons with Lymphatic Filariasis in Plateau State, Nigeria. *Health Hum. Rights* **2018**, *20*, 27–40.
13. Bailey, F.; Eaton, J.; Jidda, M.; van Brakel, W.H.; Addiss, D.G.; Molyneux, D.H. Neglected Tropical Diseases and Mental Health: Progress, Partnerships, and Integration. *Trends Parasitol.* **2019**, *35*, 23–31. [CrossRef]
14. Bailey, F.; Mondragon-Shem, K.; Haines, L.R.; Olabi, A.; Alorfi, A.; Ruiz-Postigo, J.A.; Alvar, J.; Hotez, P.; Adams, E.R.; Vélez, I.D.; et al. Cutaneous Leishmaniasis and Co-Morbid Major Depressive Disorder: A Systematic Review with Burden Estimates. *PLoS Neglected Trop. Dis.* **2019**, *13*, e0007092. [CrossRef]
15. Koschorke, M.; Al-Haboubi, Y.; Tseng, P.-C.; Semrau, M.; Eaton, J. Mental Health, Stigma, and Neglected Tropical Diseases: A Review and Systematic Mapping of the Evidence. *Front. Trop. Dis.* **2022**, *3*, 808955. [CrossRef]
16. Obindo, J.; Abdulmalik, J.; Nwefoh, E.; Agbir, M.; Nwoga, C.; Armiya, A.; Davou, F.; Maigida, K.; Otache, E.; Ebiloma, A.; et al. Prevalence of Depression and Associated Clinical and Socio-Demographic Factors in People Living with Lymphatic Filariasis in Plateau State, Nigeria. *PLoS Neglected Trop. Dis.* **2017**, *11*, e0005567. [CrossRef] [PubMed]
17. World Health Organization. *Mental Health of People with Neglected Tropical Diseases: Towards a Person-Centred Approach*; World Health Organization: Geneva, Switzerland, 2020.
18. Semrau, M.; Davey, G.; Bayisenge, U.; Deribe, K. High Levels of Depressive Symptoms among People with Lower Limb Lymphoedema in Rwanda: A Cross-Sectional Study. *Trans. R Soc. Trop. Med. Hyg.* **2020**, *114*, 974–982. [CrossRef] [PubMed]
19. Ton, T.G.; Mackenzie, C.; Molyneux, D.H. The Burden of Mental Health in Lymphatic Filariasis. *Infect. Dis. Poverty* **2015**, *4*, 34. [CrossRef] [PubMed]
20. Suma, T.K.; Shenoy, R.K.; Kumaraswami, V. A Qualitative Study of the Perceptions, Practices and Socio-Psychological Suffering Related to Chronic Brugian Filariasis in Kerala, Southern India. *Ann. Trop. Med. Parasitol.* **2003**, *97*, 839–845. [CrossRef] [PubMed]
21. Richard, S.A.; Mathieu, E.; Addiss, D.G.; Sodahlon, Y.K. A Survey of Treatment Practices and Burden of Lymphoedema in Togo. *Trans. R. Soc. Trop. Med. Hyg.* **2007**, *101*, 391–397. [CrossRef] [PubMed]
22. Kanda, K. The Quality of Life among Lymphedema Patients Due to Lymphatic Filariasis in Three Rural Towns in Haiti. Ph.D. Thesis, University of South Florida, Tampa, FL, USA, 2004.
23. Wijesinghe, R.S.; Wickremasinghe, A.R.; Ekanayake, S.; Perera, M.S.A. Physical Disability and Psychosocial Impact Due to Chronic Filarial Lymphoedema in Sri Lanka. *Filaria J.* **2007**, *6*, 4. [CrossRef] [PubMed]
24. Molyneux, D.H. Mental Health and Neglected Tropical Diseases—The Neglected Dimension of Burden: Identifying the Challenges and Understanding the Burden. *Int. Health* **2023**, *15* (Suppl. 3), iii3–iii6. [CrossRef]
25. Thapa, D.K.; Dahal, H.R.; Chaulagain, D.R.; Karki, A.; Sharma, N.; Baral, B.; Nepal, C.; Paudel, P.; Thapa, J. Stigma, Depression and Quality of Life among People Affected by Neglected Tropical Diseases in Nepal. *Int. Health* **2023**, *15* (Suppl. 3), iii79–iii86. [CrossRef]
26. Seekles, M.L.; Kadima, J.K.; Ding, Y.; Bulambo, C.B.; Kim, J.J.; Kukola, J.K.; Omumbu, P.O.L.; Mulamba, R.M.; Nganda, M.; Ngenyibungi, S.M.; et al. Mental Health, Stigma and the Quality of Life of People Affected by Neglected Tropical Diseases of the Skin in Kasai Province, Democratic Republic of the Congo: A Sex-Disaggregated Analysis. *Int. Health* **2023**, *15* (Suppl. 3), iii28–iii36. [CrossRef]
27. Dean, L.; Eaton, J. People, Power and Participation: Strategic Directions for Integrated Person-Centred Care for Ntds and Mental Health. *Int. Health* **2024**, *16* (Suppl. 1), i1–i4. [CrossRef]
28. Mendenhall, E.; Kohrt, B.A.; Norris, S.A.; Ndetei, D.; Prabhakaran, D. Non-Communicable Disease Syndemics: Poverty, Depression, and Diabetes among Low-Income Populations. *Lancet* **2017**, *389*, 951–963. [CrossRef]
29. Litt, E.; Baker, M.C.; Molyneux, D. Neglected Tropical Diseases and Mental Health: A Perspective on Comorbidity. *Trends Parasitol.* **2012**, *28*, 195–201. [CrossRef] [PubMed]
30. Hook, K.; Ando, K.; Ghebrehiwet, S.; Harris, B.; Ojediran, B.; Syeda, H.; Henderson, D.; Borba, C. Current State of the Literature on Mental Health in Liberia: A Systematic Review. *S. Afr. J. Psychiatr.* **2020**, *26*, 1502. [CrossRef] [PubMed]
31. Dean, L.; Tolhurst, R.; Nallo, G.; Kollie, K.; Bettee, A.; Theobald, S. Neglected Tropical Disease as a 'Biographical Disruption': Listening to the Narratives of Affected Persons to Develop Integrated People Centred Care in Liberia. *PLoS Neglected Trop. Dis.* **2019**, *13*, e0007710. [CrossRef]
32. The World Bank. 2023. Available online: https://www.worldbank.org/en/about/annual-report#:~:text=and%20Central%20Asia-,World%20Bank%20Fiscal%20Year%20Commitments,$1.1%20billion%20in%20IDA%20commitments. (accessed on 19 July 2024).
33. Nyenswah, T.G.; Kateh, F.; Bawo, L.; Massaquoi, M.; Gbanyan, M.; Fallah, M.; Nagbe, T.K.; Karsor, K.K.; Wesseh, S.; Sieh, S.; et al. Ebola and Its Control in Liberia, 2014–2015. *Emerg. Infect. Dis.* **2016**, *22*, 169–177. [CrossRef] [PubMed]
34. Johnson, K.; Asher, J.; Rosborough, S.; Raja, A.; Panjabi, R.; Beadling, C.; Lawry, L. Association of Combatant Status and Sexual Violence with Health and Mental Health Outcomes in Postconflict Liberia. *JAMA* **2008**, *300*, 676–690. [CrossRef] [PubMed]
35. Meyer, I.H. Prejudice, Social Stress, and Mental Health in Lesbian, Gay, and Bisexual Populations: Conceptual Issues and Research Evidence. *Psychol. Bull.* **2003**, *129*, 674. [CrossRef] [PubMed]
36. Hotterbeekx, A.; Namale Ssonko, V.; Oyet, W.; Lakwo, T.; Idro, R. Neurological manifestations in Onchocerca volvulus infection: A review. *Brain Res Bull.* **2019**, *145*, 39–44. [CrossRef] [PubMed] [PubMed Central]
37. Chen, Y.; Lyga, J. Brain-skin connection: Stress, inflammation and skin aging. *Inflamm Allergy Drug Targets* **2014**, *13*, 177–190. [CrossRef] [PubMed] [PubMed Central]

38. Singer, M.; Clair, S.J.M. Syndemics and public health: Reconceptualizing disease in bio-social context. *Med. Anthropol. Q.* **2003**, *17*, 423–441. [CrossRef] [PubMed]
39. REDRESS Liberia. Strengthening People-Centred Health Systems for People Affected by Severe Stigmatising Skin Diseases in Liberia. Available online: https://www.redressliberia.org/ (accessed on 1 May 2024).
40. Ozano, K.; Dean, L.; Adekeye, O.; Bettee, A.K.; Dixon, R.; Gideon, N.U.; Gwani, N.; Isiyaku, S.; Kollie, K.; Lar, L.; et al. Guiding Principles for Quality, Ethical Standards and Ongoing Learning in Implementation Research: Multicountry learnings from Participatory Action Research to Strengthen Health Systems. *Health Policy Plan.* **2020**, *35* (Suppl. 2), ii137–ii149. [CrossRef]
41. Kroenke, K.; Spitzer, R.L.; Williams, J.B.W. The Phq-9: Validity of a Brief Depression Severity Measure. *J. Gen. Intern. Med.* **2001**, *16*, 606–613. [CrossRef] [PubMed]
42. Spitzer, R.L.; Kroenke, K.; Williams, J.B.; Löwe, B. A Brief Measure for Assessing Generalized Anxiety Disorder: The Gad-7. *Arch. Intern. Med.* **2006**, *166*, 1092–1097. [CrossRef]
43. Dadun, D.; Peters, R.; Van Brakel, W.; Lusli, M.; Damayanti, R.; Bunders, J.; Irwanto, I. Cultural Validation of a New Instrument to Measure Leprosy-Related Stigma: The Sari Stigma Scale. *Lepr. Rev.* **2017**, *88*, 23–42. [CrossRef] [PubMed]
44. World Health Organization. Who Disability Assessment Schedule 2.0. Available online: https://www.who.int/classifications/icf/whodasii/en/ (accessed on 1 July 2024).
45. Secor, A.; Macauley, R.; Stan, L.; Kagone, M.; Sidikiba, S.; Sow, S.; Aronovich, D.; Litvin, K.; Davis, N.; Alva, S.; et al. Mental Health among Ebola Survivors in Liberia, Sierra Leone and Guinea: Results from a Cross-Sectional Study. *BMJ Open* **2020**, *10*, e035217. [CrossRef] [PubMed]
46. Fabian, K.E.; Fannoh, J.; Washington, G.G.; Weetol, W.B.G.; Nyachienga, B.; Cyrus, G.; Hallowanger, J.N.; Beste, J.; Augusto, O.; Wagenaar, B.H. Psychometric Properties of Two Mental Health Screening Tools in Southeast Liberia: The Liberian Distress Screener and Patient Health Questionnaire. *Transcult. Psychiatry* **2022**, *59*, 425–437. [CrossRef] [PubMed]
47. American Psychiatric Association. Online Assessment Measures. Available online: https://www.psychiatry.org/File%20Library/Psychiatrists/Practice/DSM/APA_DSM5_WHODAS-2-Self-Administered.pdf (accessed on 6 November 2021).
48. Christensen, A.-D.; Jensen, S.Q. Doing Intersectional Analysis: Methodological Implications for Qualitative Research. *NORA-Nordic J. Fem. Gend. Res.* **2012**, *20*, 109–125. [CrossRef]
49. McCall, L. The Complexity of Intersectionality. *Signs* **2005**, *30*, 1771–1800. [CrossRef]
50. Ritchie, J.B.; Lewis, J.; Nicholls, C.M.; Ormston, R. *Qualitative Research Practice: A Guide for Social Science Students and Researchers*; SAGE Publications Ltd.: New York, NY, USA, 2013.
51. Kessler, R.C.; Birnbaum, H.G.; Shahly, V.; Bromet, E.; Hwang, I.; McLaughlin, K.A.; Sampson, N.; Andrade, L.H.; de Girolamo, G.; Demyttenaere, K.; et al. Age differences in the prevalence and co-morbidity of DSM-IV major depressive episodes: Results from the WHO World Mental Health Survey Initiative. *Depress. Anxiety* **2010**, *27*, 351–364. [CrossRef]
52. Kessler, R.C.; Berglund, P.; Demler, O.; Jin, R.; Merikangas, K.R.; Walters, E.E. Lifetime prevalence and age-of-onset distributions of DSM-IV disorders in the National Comorbidity Survey Replication. *Arch Gen Psychiatry* **2005**, *62*, 593–602. [CrossRef] [PubMed]
53. Bartlett, J.; Deribe, K.; Tamiru, A.; Amberbir, T.; Medhin, G.; Malik, M.; Hanlon, C.; Davey, G. Depression and Disability in People with Podoconiosis: A Comparative Cross-Sectional Study in Rural Northern Ethiopia. *Int. Health* **2015**, *8*, 124–131. [CrossRef] [PubMed]
54. Ali, O.; Mengiste, A.; Semrau, M.; Tesfaye, A.; Fekadu, A.; Davey, G. The Impact of Podoconiosis, Lymphatic Filariasis, and Leprosy on Disability and Mental Well-Being: A Systematic Review. *PLoS Negl. Trop. Dis.* **2021**, *15*, e0009492. [CrossRef] [PubMed]
55. Ali, O.; Deribe, K.; Semrau, M.; Mengiste, A.; Kinfe, M.; Tesfaye, A.; Bremner, S.; Davey, G.; Fekadu, A. A Cross-Sectional Study to Evaluate Depression and Quality of Life among Patients with Lymphoedema Due to Podoconiosis, Lymphatic Filariasis and Leprosy. *Trans. R. Soc. Trop. Med. Hyg.* **2020**, *114*, 983–994. [CrossRef] [PubMed]
56. Eaton, J.; Afolaranmi, T.; Tsaku, P.; Nwefoh, E.; Ode, P.; Baird, T.; Sunday, P.; Obindo, T. Integration of Services for Neglected Tropical Diseases and Mental Health in Nigeria: Development of a Practical Model Informed by International Recommendations, Contextual Factors and Service-User Perspectives. *Int. Health* **2023**, *15* (Suppl. 3), iii47–iii58. [CrossRef]
57. Barrett, C.; Chiphwanya, J.; Matipula, D.E.; Douglass, J.; Kelly-Hope, L.; Dean, L. Addressing the Syndemic Relationship between Lymphatic Filariasis and Mental Distress in Malawi: The Potential of Enhanced Self-Care. *Trop. Med. Int. Health* **2024**, *9*, 172. [CrossRef]
58. Ebenso, B.; Fashona, A.; Ayuba, M.; Idah, M.; Adeyemi, G.; S.-Fada, S. Impact of socio-economic rehabilitation on leprosy stigma in northern Nigeria: Findings of a retrospective study. *Asia Pac. Disabil. Rehabil. J.* **2007**, *18*, 98–119.
59. Alamsyah, T.; Usman, S.; Yusuf, M.; Elvin, S.D. Effectiveness of Traditional Healers in Program to Control Leprosy in Nagan Raya District in Aceh. *Dermatol. Res. Pract.* **2018**, *2018*, 3176762. [CrossRef] [PubMed]
60. McCollum, R.; Berrian, H.; Theobald, S.; Zaizay, Z.; Kollie, K.; Dean, L. Barriers and Enablers to Health-Seeking for People Affected by Severe Stigmatising Skin Diseases (Sssds): A Scoping Review. *Soc. Sci.* **2022**, *11*, 332. [CrossRef]
61. Berrian, H.; Dean, L.; Chowdhury, S.; Zaizay, Z.; Theobald, S.; Seekey, W.; Jerry, K.; Smith, J.S.; Parker, C.; Rogers, E.; et al. The Role of Informal Health Providers in the Management of Neglected Tropical Diseases: A Participatory Investigation. 2024, submitted for publication.

62. Kollie, K.K.; Jenkins, J.; Theobald, S.; Nallo, G.; Kpadeh, O.; Jones, L.; Borbor, D.; Phillip, M.; Wickenden, A.; Kollie, J.T.; et al. Unpacking the Impact of Integrating the Neglected Tropical Disease Supply Chain into the National Supply Chain System: Illustrative Evidence from Liberia. *Parasitology* **2023**, *150*, 1052–1062. [CrossRef]
63. Dean, L. *Narratives of Neglect*; University of Liverpool: Liverpool, UK, 2019.
64. Hofstraat, K.; van Brakel, W.H. Social Stigma Towards Neglected Tropical Diseases: A Systematic Review. *Int. Health* **2016**, *8* (Suppl. 1), i53–i70. [CrossRef] [PubMed]
65. Hotez, P.J. Stigma: The Stealth Weapon of the Ntd. *PLoS Negl. Trop. Dis.* **2008**, *2*, e230. [CrossRef]
66. Kuper, H. Disability, Mental Health, Stigma and Discrimination and Neglected Tropical Diseases. *Trans. R. Soc. Trop. Med. Hyg.* **2020**, 115. [CrossRef] [PubMed]
67. Ostrach, B.; Lerman, G.S.; Singer, M. *Stigma Syndemics: New Directions in Biosocial Health*; Lexington Books: Lanham, MD, USA, 2017.
68. Chowdhury, S.; Adekeye, O.; McRae, A.; Olorunfemi, T.; Dubukumah, L.; Makinde, O.; Ozokede, E.; Ewemade, J.; Abdulkadir, S.; Ayuba, R.; et al. A holistic approach to well-being and 939 neglected tropical diseases: Evaluating the impact of community-led support groups in Nigeria using community-based partic- 940 ipatory research. *Int. Health* **2023**, *15* (Suppl. 1), i87–i99. [CrossRef] [PubMed]
69. Jewkes, R.; Nduna, M.; Levin, J.; Jama, N.; Dunkle, K.; Puren, A.; Duvvury, N. Impact of stepping stones on incidence of HIV and HSV-2 and sexual behaviour in rural South Africa: Cluster randomised controlled trial. *BMJ* **2008**, *337*, a506. [CrossRef] [PubMed]
70. Akogun, O.B.; Akogun, M.K.; Apake, E.; Kale, O.O. Rapid Community Identification, Pain and Distress Associated with Lymphoedema and Adenolymphangitis Due to Lymphatic Filariasis in Resource-Limited Communities of North-Eastern Nigeria. *Acta Trop.* **2011**, *120*, S62–S68. [CrossRef] [PubMed]
71. Woolley, R.J.; Velink, A.; Phillips, R.O.; Thompson, W.A.; Abass, K.M.; van der Werf, T.S.; de Zeeuw, J.; Stienstra, Y. Experiences of Pain and Expectations for Its Treatment among Former Buruli ulcer Patients. *Am. J. Trop. Med. Hyg.* **2016**, *95*, 1011–1015. [CrossRef]
72. Hankivsky, O. Intersectionality. 2014, 64, p. 101. Available online: https://bccampus.ca/wp-content/uploads/2020/07/Hankivsky-Intersectionality101-2014.pdf (accessed on 19 July 2024).
73. Theobald, S.; MacPherson, E.E.; Dean, L.; Jacobson, J.; Ducker, C.; Gyapong, M.; Hawkins, K.; Elphick-Pooley, T.; Mackenzie, C.; Kelly-Hope, L.A.; et al. 20 Years of Gender Mainstreaming in Health: Lessons and Reflections for the Neglected Tropical Diseases Community. *BMJ Glob. Health* **2017**, *2*, e000512. [CrossRef] [PubMed]
74. Shomuyiwa, D.O.; George, N.S.; Sunday, B.A.; Omotayo, F.O.; Mwaba, M.; David, S.C.; Nabiryo, M.; Yangaza, Y. Addressing Neglected Tropical Diseases in Africa: A Gender Perspective. *Health Sci. Rep.* **2023**, *6*, e1726. [CrossRef]
75. Ochola, E.A.; Elliott, S.J.; Karanja, D.M.S. The Impact of Neglected Tropical Diseases (Ntds) on Women's Health and Wellbeing in Sub-Saharan Africa (Ssa): A Case Study of Kenya. *Int. J. Env. Res. Public Health* **2021**, *18*, 2180. [CrossRef]
76. World Health Organization. *Culture and Mental Health in Liberia: A Primer*; World Health Organization: Geneva, Switzerland, 2017.

Tropical Medicine and Infectious Disease

MDPI

Article

Addressing the Syndemic Relationship between Lymphatic Filariasis and Mental Distress in Malawi: The Potential of Enhanced Self-Care

Carrie Barrett [1,*], John Chiphwanya [2], Dorothy E. Matipula [2], Janet Douglass [3], Louise A. Kelly-Hope [1,4] and Laura Dean [1]

[1] Centre for Neglected Tropical Disease, Department of Tropical Disease Biology, Liverpool School of Tropical Medicine, Pembroke Place, Liverpool L3 5QA, UK

[2] National Lymphatic Filariasis Elimination Programme, Ministry of Health, P.O. Box 30377, Lilongwe 3, Malawi

[3] College of Public Health, Medical and Veterinary Sciences, James Cook University, Townsville, 1 James Cook Drive, Douglas, QLD 4811, Australia

[4] Department of Livestock and One Health, Institute of Infection, Veterinary and Ecological Sciences, University of Liverpool, 146 Brownlow Hill, Liverpool L3 5RF, UK

* Correspondence: carrie.barrett@lstmed.ac.uk

Abstract: Lymphatic filariasis (LF) causes disfiguring and disabling lymphoedema, which can lead to mental distress and requires life-long self-care treatment. This study applies syndemic theory to understand the biosocial relationship between LF and mental distress in Malawi. Using in-depth qualitative methods, we critically evaluate experiences of mental distress and LF through 21 life-history interviews, to narrate experiences from the perspective of persons affected by LF, and to understand how enhanced self-care (ESC) for lymphoedema management disrupts the syndemic relationship. Complementary key informant interviews with Ministry of Health LF programme staff were conducted to further understand intervention and health system delivery. All interviews were recorded, transcribed, and translated, and then subject to thematic analysis. Our findings suggest that for persons affected by LF in Malawi, before being trained in ESC, absent referral pathways, inequalities in healthcare provision or available treatment, and limited knowledge of the condition (LF) drove the syndemic of LF and mental distress. Distress was often exacerbated by stigma and social exclusion, and shaped by intersections of gender, generation, poverty, and extreme climate conditions. We argue that addressing the syndemic suffering associated with LF and mental distress through interventions which center the needs of persons affected is critical in effective and equitable LF care delivery.

Keywords: lymphatic filariasis; mental health; mental distress; self-care; lymphoedema management; disease management; disability; inclusion; gender; poverty

1. Introduction

1.1. What Are Syndemics?

Syndemics can be described as the clustering of two (or more) diseases or health conditions in a population, which often emerge in conditions where health, social, and economic inequalities are persistent. Such inequalities increase physical and behavioural vulnerabilities within populations, especially among low-income and marginalised groups, often resulting in adverse disease interactions which can be social, behavioural, or biological [1,2]. Stigma, as a social factor, can drive synergistic interactions between diseases, which further complicate the recognition, treatment, and prevention of disease [3]. In this paper, we consider the clustering of health conditions as a result of social and economic disadvantage, an aspect that is often overlooked within biological and social epidemiology.

The phenomenon of disease clustering is well evidenced, as is the role of social determinants in explaining differences seen in disease within and between populations [4,5]. However, understanding how the biosocial dynamics of disease can cause or exacerbate disease–disease interaction is lacking [2,6].

1.2. Lymphatic Filariasis, Acute Attacks, Disability, and Mental Distress

Lymphatic filariasis (LF) is a neglected tropical disease (NTD) caused by a filarial parasite, transmitted via mosquitoes [7]. An estimated 882 million people in 44 countries remain threatened by LF infection, with 36 million individuals living with LF clinical symptoms. LF leads to disfigurement and disability, which predominantly affect low-income and marginalised populations [7,8]. The second most common clinical symptom of LF is lymphoedema (swelling of the limb or limbs), after hydrocoele (scrotal swelling). Persons affected by lymphoedema are prone to experiencing acute episodes of adenolymphangitis (ADLs), also known as acute attacks, which consist of fever, headaches, and localised inflammation from secondary infection of the already damaged lymphatics [9,10]. Acute attacks have been described as a major contributor to disability and LF severity, as well as causing pain, hindering mobility, and negatively impacting the ability to practice self-care and work, contributing to a loss of earnings [11,12]. Intersections between LF, disability, and mental ill-health are becoming increasingly recognised and evidenced globally [13–16]. Specifically, disability and acute attacks have been found to be associated with higher levels of depression amongst people affected by LF and other skin NTDs [17,18]. However, generally when considering the interaction of mental health conditions and LF, the focus is on epidemiological clustering, with the biosocial context less considered [19–24]. This is despite widespread recognition that understanding the biosocial connections between diseases is crucial in responding to disease interactions [1,13,25,26]. In Malawi, there is evidence highlighting the co-morbidity of LF and mental ill-health based on epidemiological clustering [18]. Current estimates suggest just under 30,000 people are living with symptoms of LF in Malawi that require holistic (physical, mental, and social) care [27].

1.3. WHO 2030 Targets and Disease Management, Disability, and Inclusion (DMDI) Approaches

As outlined in the World Health Organization (WHO) NTD roadmap 2021–2030, a shift from vertical programme delivery to an integrated holistic approach is required to address the physical, mental, and social consequences of disease and maximise resources. The roadmap also highlights the importance of considering the needs of persons affected within elimination and disease control interventions [28]. As Malawi and other LF-endemic countries progress toward the elimination of transmission of LF through the successful delivery of preventative chemotherapy, the focus must shift toward delivering morbidity management and disability prevention (MMDP) services for people with existing disease [29,30]. Currently, the scope of most national MMDP programmes is limited to the provision of hydrocoele surgeries and training for lymphoedema management [31]. Within recent years, a more holistic concept of MMDP has been promoted amongst NTD practitioners, described as disease management, disability, and inclusion (DMDI) [32]. This has an emphasis that' disability' is caused by a condition or impairment within a particular context, and that social manifestations, and other often non-medicalised consequences such as mental health and stigma, are considered as contributors to disability. Additionally, 'inclusion' reflects the need to include persons affected within programme design and implementation. Thus, considering the psychosocial consequences of LF, perspectives of persons affected and the wider biosocial context are essential to achieving person-centred holistic MMDP, henceforth described as DMDI [33].

1.4. The Context of Malawi and the National LF Programme

In Malawi, LF is widespread, with 26/28 endemic districts. The economy is largely reliant on agriculture (over 80%), causing vulnerabilities to extreme climate conditions that may result in damage in agricultural production, e.g., poor crop harvest [34]. The

Malawi National LF Elimination Programme successfully achieved the validation of the elimination of LF as a public health problem from the WHO in 2020 [29]. Elimination was largely achieved through the completion of multiple rounds of preventative chemotherapy through mass drug administration (MDA) in all endemic regions [35]. A key challenge facing the programme moving forward is to deliver the major component of the Global Programme to Eliminate LF (GPELF) strategy, which requires the implementation of MMDP for all those living with the clinical symptoms of LF. Within seven districts in Malawi, a home-based 'enhanced self-care' (ESC) for lymphoedema management has been integrated within the health system through the training of primary health staff [33].

1.5. Enhanced Self-Care Study

In three highly endemic districts for LF in Malawi where the ESC was integrated into the health system, a 6-month prospective study was conducted in 2021, implementing an ESC intervention for lymphoedema management [36]. The study involved training persons affected with LF-related lymphoedema and their primary caregiver in ESC. This included standard WHO-recommended activities including hygiene and skin care practices, daily and overnight elevation of affected limb(s), seated and standing exercises, managing acute attacks with medication, and wearing of appropriate footwear [37]. Enhanced self-care activities included deep-breathing techniques, lymphatic massage, skin mobilisation, walking, drinking water, and eating fresh fruit and vegetables [36]. Activities were designed to impose no financial burden on participants and were easy to practice independently in order to improve physical symptoms of lymphoedema, reduce acute attacks, and improve quality of life.

1.6. Study Contribution and Rationale

This paper presents the use of in-depth qualitative methodology to explore the syndemic relationship between LF and mental distress in Malawi. Drawing on Mendenhall's model of syndemic approaches to health [2], through narratives of persons affected by LF, we consider the following: (1) the lived experiences of the syndemic and current healthcare response; and (2) the impact of an enhanced self-care intervention on the syndemic relationship, with a view to make recommendations to improve the mental and physical wellbeing of people affected by LF in Malawi. This is the first study to consider the syndemic relationship between LF and mental health from the perspective of persons affected in Malawi. Additionally, this research aims to understand how ESC can support health systems to manage LF and mental wellbeing for people affected by LF, focusing specifically on how ESC disrupts this syndemic relationship.

2. Materials and Methods

Life history interviews were conducted with 21 persons affected by LF-related lymphoedema or both hydrocoele and lymphoedema, to explore the syndemic relationship between mental distress and LF, and the impact of the ESC intervention from the perspective of persons affected. In this paper, we refer to mental distress as a continuum of descriptions from stress, anxiety, and depression, to suicidal thoughts within the narratives of persons affected. To complement life history narratives and better understand the context of implementing the ESC within the Malawian health system, key informant interviews were conducted with LF programme staff and LF experts in Malawi.

2.1. Study Setting and Design

This study was conducted in Chikwawa district, Malawi in 2022. This study followed-up a subset of participants who were part of a wider prospective cohort study and trained in ESC conducted in three sites, Karonga (Northern), Nsanje, and Chikwawa (Southern) districts, in Malawi over a 6-month period in 2021. This wider study investigated the physical impact of the ESC intervention for LF-related lymphoedema. Chikwawa was selected as the study site for this qualitative study due to accessibility and finances available and because of the high prevalence of clinical cases of lymphoedema identified in this district. Participants recruitment period was from 2 August 2022 to 11 August 2022.

2.2. Participants, Sampling Procedure, and Data Collection

2.2.1. Life Histories

The use of life history interviews allowed persons affected to narrate their lives and experiences of illness, repositioning them as a storyteller that is best placed to recount their own reality of suffering and resilience. Furthermore, narratives can support individuals to make sense of their illness experience [38,39].

Persons affected by LF-related lymphoedema were purposively selected for life history interviews to ensure maximum variation of characteristics, see sampling matrix in Table 1. Sampling criteria were selected based upon findings from a previous study, identifying associations with higher number of acute attacks and depressive symptoms [18]. This previous study was used to categorise participants into either a "mental distress" group who had recorded a depressive symptoms score (PHQ-9) of above 5, or from descriptions of mental distress collected from an open-ended question: "tell me about your mental health?" where responses were indicative of poor or unchanged mental wellbeing. Depressive symptoms scores were assessed using the Patient Health Questionnaire (PHQ-9) over the study time period of 6 months [18,40]. All other participants fell into the "mental wellbeing improvement" group, indicated from an improvement of depressive symptoms. The change in number of acute attacks was also derived from the same previous study.

Table 1. Sampling matrix for life history interviews.

	Mental Distress		**Mental Wellbeing Improvement**	
	Female	Male	Female	Male
Same or higher acute attacks	2	1	2	2
Reduced acute attacks	3	4	4	2

+1 Male Guardian, trained in the enhanced self-care but was not enrolled onto previous enhanced self-care study.

Sample size was estimated based on the number of life history interviews that was anticipated to reach saturation based on previous research exploring the biographical accounts of persons affected by NTDs. Through our iterative and ongoing approach to analysis, we determined data saturation was reached within our sample and data collection finalised [41]. All persons affected were recruited for this qualitative study due to their previous enrolment in the previous ESC study [18] and were identified through local health facility registers and national programmatic records. One primary caregiver was not enrolled on the ESC study but had received lymphoedema training as part of the ESC study and was therefore included in the life history interviews. Characteristics described in Table 1 were summarised for each participant within Table S1.

Life history interviews took place at the homes of the participants and interview guides were developed prior to interviews aiming to explore the main themes, life histories, experiences of LF (somatic experience), mental wellbeing, stigma, enablers and barriers to the ESC, health-seeking, participation, additional support (i.e., caregivers), and life after the ESC study. A second Malawian researcher (DEM) conducted life history interviews in Chichewa, and translated in real-time to CB to allow follow-up questions. All data collected were audio recorded, transcribed verbatim, and translated into English. To maintain the originality and clarity of information during transcription and translation, 10% of transcripts were randomly selected and cross-checked against audio by DEM for quality assurance purposes.

2.2.2. Key Informant Interviews

Key informant interviews were purposively selected based upon their previous involvement in implementing the ESC study (unpublished data) [18], which included three Ministry of Health (MoH) staff members. The lead author (CB) conducted all key informant interviews in English, which were audio-recorded and then transcribed verbatim.

CB read through all transcripts to ensure completeness for data analysis.

2.3. Data Analysis

All data analysis was guided by framework adapted from Dean et al.'s (2023) describing the syndemic model for NTDs and mental distress, which was informed by Mendenhall's (2017) model of syndemic approaches to health (see Figure 1) [2,15]. This study adapted the framework developed by Dean et al. (2022) that describes the syndemic relationship between NTDs and mental distress in Liberia. Dean et al.'s (2022) original model was informed by Medenhall's (2017) model of syndemic approaches to health. As such, the model of LF and mental distress presented here articulates three main dimensions driving this syndemic within Malawi: (A) the epidemiological co-occurrence and interaction of LF and mental distress; (B) the experiences of persons affected by LF and mental distress grouped into somatic, daily activities, and meaningful experiences; and (C) how the ESC, health, and social systems contribute to responses in LF care. We were specifically exploring how the ESC that was designed to bring lymphoedema care close to the community disrupts this syndemic of LF and mental distress. Thematic analysis was conducted using a deductive coding approach based on topic guides and the adapted framework(s) and additional themes emerging from the data were inductively coded. Analysis was supported by NVivo 12 software.

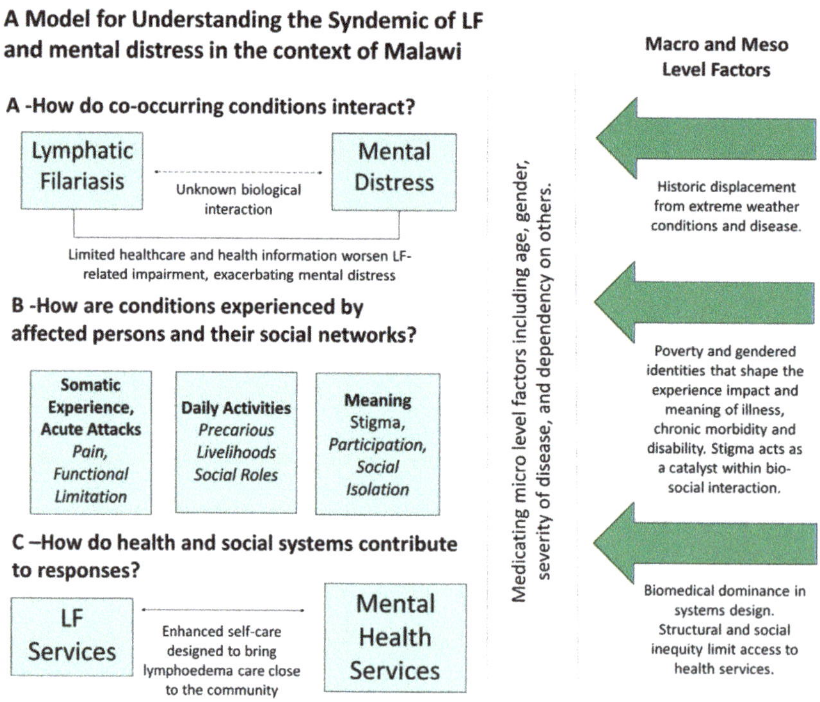

Figure 1. A Model for Understanding the Syndemic of LF and Mental Distress in the Context of Malawi.

2.4. Ethical Statement

Ethical approval was obtained from the Liverpool School of Tropical Medicine, Research Ethics Committee, UK (Research Protocol 22-036) and National Health Sciences Research Committee, Malawi (Number 2615). Written informed consent was obtained from all participants in this study. Consent forms and information sheets, describing the study aims and data collection processes, were translated into Chichewa, the local language, and read out to participants who were less literate. All participants had the opportunity to ask questions and or discuss queries to participation.

3. Results

The pathways reinforcing the syndemic relationship between LF and mental distress in Malawi are shown in Figure 1. We present the study findings aligned to the adapted framework (Figure 1), across three main dimensions: (A) 'How do LF and Mental Distress Interact?'; (B) 'How are Conditions Experienced?'; and (C) 'How do Health and Social Systems Contribute to Responses in LF and Mental Health Services?'. This study found that multiple pathways have played a role in the progression of LF symptoms (especially lymphoedema), disability, chronic illness, and mental distress, largely as a result of underlying health and social inequalities.

Before exploring the syndemic, we first present two narratives from persons affected. Both Chimwemwe's (Figure 2) and Gracious's stories (Figure 3) capture syndemic suffering related to LF and mental distress and highlight how the wider social and environmental context (such as weak health and social systems) intersect with gender, poverty, and disability to exacerbate physical morbidity and mental distress.

Chimwemwe, 43, worked in a factory until he had a stroke at 28 which impacted his speech and functioning on one side of his body. Five years later he noticed his leg starting to swell, an early sign of lymphoedema. Within this same year his wife passed away.

Chimwemwe visited the hospital for his lymphoedema where he was prescribed 36 injections but was not told the cause of his condition. He noticed no improvement in his symptoms and relied on a family member for financial support with the prescribed treatment and associated travel costs. *"When I went to the district hospital they did not give me the results, they gave me 6 injections. Then I told my brother that I was supposed to be given 36 injections of which he accepted and he was giving me transport money to and from the hospital. Then, I finished the dosage and after that dose, nothing changed, there was no improvement."*

Chimwemwe no longer looked after his children as they stayed with their teacher. Following the death of his brother and parents, Chimwemwe needed to be supported so he moved in with his aunt and her second husband where he experienced discrimination, exclusion and abusive behaviour such as denying him of food and chasing him away with a stick. The church he attended began to support him *"they rented a house for me of which they are paying. I sleep over there and they also provide food."*

Chimwemwe experienced pain during his acute attacks, describing that he could not sleep because of the pain, however this changed after he received the enhanced self-care intervention. Chimwemwe described *"I can say I am better right now, but at first I thought of killing myself."* Although, Chimwemwe described improvements in his mental wellbeing following the enhanced self-care, he needed additional support with the enhanced self-care activities *"The exercises, I am able to do [them] ... [my half-brother] assists me with the exercises but when he is away, then I do not do it."* as well as support with supplies *"it is difficult for me to source the soap, sometimes I just wash it with water."*

Following the enhanced self-care Chimwemwe still experienced stigma related to his lymphedema and financial instability which impacted his marital prospects, he said: *"I also fail to marry another woman because of money ...when I was okay, when I was strong enough, ... [I could sell] cattle and after I was diagnosed with this condition, people started stigmatising me."*

Figure 2. Chimwemwe's story.

Gracious, 41, has three children and a grandchild. In 2018, Gracious was diagnosed with lymphoedema which has developed into severe staging. Gracious described experiencing pain in her leg and had tried to seek treatment or a "cure" for her lymphoedema, visiting hospitals, private clinics, traditional and religious healers. None of the treatment she received made her feel better.

Gracious explained that her husband had left her 9 months before and that *"He has gone to find another woman who does not have a disability since I have a disability."*

Gracious was reliant on her children for care and support stating they "*dropped out of school in order to take care of me"* due to her condition. She stated *"My daughter helps me with a lot of chores such as cooking. For example, right now, I would not have been able to run the business since my husband has left me, she is the one [to help]"*

Since the enhanced self-care, Gracious said she was feeling better after being taught how to care for her lymphoedema, she noticed reduce acute attacks (feeling unwell) and improved daily activities like washing her clothes which she was not able to do in the past. Gracious worries a lot about the future and described no longer receiving supplies like soap after the study was a challenge for her *"I am always worried about the healing since the support that we were getting from [the enhanced self-care] was really helping us but now because it is difficult for me to source money even to buy food, then I should also consider buying soap ... I need to use the soap every day from morning, afternoon and evening. So, it is a challenge to me."*

Gracious stated because of her lymphoedema *"I cannot continue with the farming because I struggle to do so since I cannot stand for so long, my leg cannot do that."*

Figure 3. Gracious' story.

3.1. (A) How Do Co-Occurring Conditions Interact?

The first main dimension of the syndemic model of LF and mental distress (Figure 1) explores (A) the co-occurrence and interaction of LF and mental distress. Within this section we describe the interaction between LF and mental distress, the drivers of this related to discovery of lymphoedema, and healthcare availability. Finally, the coping strategies, social systems, and religious support that can disrupt this interaction between LF and mental distress are described.

3.1.1. How Do LF and Mental Distress Interact?

Barrett et al. (2023) explored the co-occurrence of LF and mental health conditions in Malawi. Of 311 people affected by LF-related lymphoedema, 20.3% (95% CI 15.9 to 25.2) reported mild depressive symptoms and 3.2% (95% CI 1.5 to 5.8) reported moderate depressive symptoms assessed using the Patient Health Questionnaire (PHQ-9). For QOL, 28.6% (95% CI 23.7 to 34.0) reported moderately low QOL and 2.9% (95% CI 23.7 to 34.0) reported severely low QOL, using the LF-specific Quality of Life Questionnaire (LFSQQ) [18]. Furthermore, rates of mental distress amongst people affected by LF have been shown to be higher than in the general population in other countries [23,42]. Evidence of the biological interaction between LF and mental distress is lacking, although indication of the bidirectional relationship between depression and inflammation [43] and the social and psychological consequences caused by cancer-related lymphoedema [44] have been made. Within this paper we discuss how the social consequences (particularly around stress-causing stigma and the internalisation of stigma) associated with LF, contribute to the syndemic of concern. Amongst other diseases, stigma and stress can contribute and enhance mental distress, specifically depression and anxiety [3,45]. We suggest that the social consequences of LF, such as stigma (internalised and enacted) and stress related to their condition, are responsible for the interaction of LF and mental distress and exacerbated by progression of disease and degree of disability.

3.1.2. Discovering Lymphoedema and Healthcare Availability

We found that limited knowledge of lymphoedema at the point of diagnosis or symptom onset, alongside the chronic, progressive, and disabling nature of lymphoedema caused mental distress. This was exacerbated by the absence of appropriate healthcare and lack of available treatments or a "cure" for their often-unknown condition. Levels of mental distress varied amongst participants, from feelings of worry, hopelessness, and stress to descriptions of common mental health conditions such as excessive worry (anxiety) and, for some, suicidal ideation.

> *"When I discovered that I have got this problem, my heart sometimes stresses out ... I could think of just dying because I was feeling like I am a failure".* **(Female, 49, Participant 5)**

3.1.3. Coping, Social Systems, and Religious Support

Faith played an important role in coping with LF and mental distress, particularly in times of depression or suicidal ideation. Faith-based organisations offered social support for persons affected; for example, Chimwemwe described the religious group he attended provided him with housing after being 'chased' out of the house he was staying in by a relative, as well as providing him with psychological support from religious group members.

> *"When my husband left me ... I just told God, [and] everything came back to normal. And some people also helped me praying over it, so yes, I am okay".* **(Female, 40, Participant 20)**

Religious teachings promoted acceptance or "being at peace" with their condition or difficult life circumstances, whilst some described increased shame related to suicide ideation as this was a "sin".

> *"... I thought of killing myself. Then I had to comfort myself that I should [not] do that because the bible tells us that committing suicide is a sin and I just accepted to live and struggle like that".* **(Male, 43, Participant 12)**

Outside religious groups, ways of coping with LF, mental distress, and, in some cases, suicidal ideation, were described as self-distraction, community support through talking, and reassurance. Some participants also described alcoholism or a belief 'that others will develop the same condition one day" as coping processes.

3.2. *(B) How Are Conditions Experienced?*

The second main dimension of the syndemic model of LF and mental distress (Figure 1) explores (B): How are Conditions Experienced? Within this section, we discuss how persons affected by LF experience the multi-directional interactions between somatic experience, the ability to complete daily activities, and the social meaning of disease (stigma, participation, and social isolation).

3.2.1. Somatic Experience and Acute Attacks

Somatic experience varied across life-history narratives, depending on pain, functional limitation, and changes in physical appearance, which caused mental distress. For many, prior to the ESC intervention, functional limitations and alterations to physical appearance were more permanent. However, during the first onset of symptoms, this was more transient or temporary. The greatest levels of pain and functional limitation (somatic experience) were experienced during acute attacks. Some described being completely immobile, unable to move from their bed to urinate. These periods were closely associated with experiences of extreme mental distress and many described suicidal ideations during these episodes.

> *"I usually think about ... [suicide] because of the pain ... I feel it is better to die than just to suffer".* **(Female, 36, Participant 9)**

3.2.2. Daily Lives and the Impact of Acute Attacks on Household

Loss of job opportunities, dependency on others, and inability to meet gender roles contributed to mental distress, particularly feelings of failure and worry, due to the somatic experience (physical limitations and pain) associated with LF. Precarious livelihoods centred around day-to-day survival (subsistence farming, foraging, and selling) were a major focus in narratives and a key trigger of distress, particularly where individuals felt unable to achieve essential survival activities.

> *"The depression is there since I have mentioned that I need to search for food so if I do not work, I do not have food. So, food can be unavailable for me to eat and sometimes I am depressed since I do not have any other ways for me to find food".* **(Male, 53, Participant 21)**

Households were impacted during acute attacks, due to participants' dependency on caregivers (often a spouse or family member) and the inability to contribute to household chores or work, such as subsistence farming, which are crucial for day-to-day survival.

> *"After being diagnosed ... I am not able to do most of the chores that I used to do in the past ... I am a failure because for ... [someone] who does not have this condition ... is able to work properly ... while for me I have a limitation".* **(Male, 51, Participant 2)**

> *"... .when I got better [following acute attack], my friends were already at another level with the farming and that meant that I will not have enough food that year. So, because of that, I could think of just dying because I was feeling like I am a failure".* **(Female, 49, Participant 5)**

3.2.3. Social Roles

Here we discuss how social roles, such as the ability to meet gender roles, relationships, and marital prospects, are impacted by LF, which leads to mental distress. Both men and women described their inability to meet expectations of gendered social roles (e.g., as a wife, mother, husband, or father) because of their disability and physical limitation, which led to low self-esteem, feelings of failure, worry, and, in some cases, depression. *"The worrisome moments for me as a man since at times there is no food at home."* (Male, 39, Participant 19). The importance placed on meeting gender roles was greatest amongst younger participants, as described by one participant: *"If the condition develop[s] while you are old, you cannot be that worried."* (Female, 39, Participant 8).

Some women described distress related to their ability to raise and provide for offspring. For example, in Gracious's story, her children acted as the primary caregiver, leading to missed school days or complete suspension of education. For men, this was articulated as a failure to financially provide for their families. Caring responsibilities impacted participation, education, and employment opportunities, highlighting additional gender inequalities associated with lymphoedema where women were largely identified as the primary caregiver [46–48]. For women, and some men, the inability to fulfil gendered ideals often reduced marital prospects. However, one participant experienced stigma from her community when courting her now husband, which didn't impact her marital prospects.

> *"If I am to find a partner, she will mock me saying you have a disability ... Women stigmatise us because of this and they say the way you are looking with your legs; can we be married and move together? So, it is difficult for me to ask a woman out".* **(Male, 53, Participant 21)**

> *"Even when my husband was marrying me, people were telling my husband that if you are getting that girl with big legs, you will have troubles with her but he was telling them that only God knows everything. He was interested in me and not in my legs. He wanted marriage and not the legs".* **(Female, 65, Participant 14)**

Experiences of verbal or physical abuse behaviours from a spouse due to having lymphoedema were generally more normalised amongst females. However, some men decided to separate from their spouse because of intra-marital stigma enacted through verbal or physical abuse; and others reported additional challenges related to hydrocoele symptoms impacting marital and sex life, though improvements were described following surgery.

> *"Ah ... [the condition did not affect my marriage] with the current wife but the first wife whom we separated, we were having quarrels ... she would tell me ... do you think that after leaving me you will get another wife with your condition? ... I decide to just leave her".* **(Male, 39, Participant 19)**

3.2.4. Meaning of Disease

Within this section, we discuss how the social meaning of disease (stigma, participation, and social isolation) can shape individual experiences. Internal stigma ('felt' stigma resulting from either the anticipation of external stigma or internalised stigma/feelings about oneself) or external stigma (actual experiences of stigma described as 'enacted' stigma) [49] were identified amongst people affected by LF and often exacerbated mental distress. Experiences of stigma were shaped by and contributed toward individual physical appearance, inability to meet gender roles, functional limitations, inability to work, and financial instability.

External (Enacted) Stigma

We found that experiences of verbal insults or segregation from the community were common amongst persons affected and a key driver for mental distress.

> *"friends that I used to chat with ... had ... thoughts that I should not ... [go] near them ... they could chase me away [and] say get out, you have got lymphoedema. [That] caused me stress ... people ... [would] say, hey you! Do not chat with this person, he is supposed to be left alone".* **(Male, 39, Participant 19)**

Experiences of stigmatising behaviours, including being laughed at, being singled out, being talked about or being avoided, were often not recognised as 'stigmatising behaviours'. However, some did label extreme levels of discrimination and segregation they experienced from their community as stigmatising. This highlights the differences in definitions of stigma between participants and researchers, or potentially the normalisation of disability-related stigma within participant communities.

Experiences of enacted stigma for those with mild-stage lymphoedema that were less visibly disabled and amongst elderly participants were far less reported. Here, stigma often subsided over time when not particularly problematic at the outset or was only experienced when meeting new community members. Elderly participants reported the fewest experiences of enacted stigma.

> *"[People] were pointing fingers at me to say[ing] ... she has lymphoedema. So, as a woman, I started feeling shy ... of course, there are some people who are just new in the community and they wonder why I have these big legs".* **(Female, 39, Participant 8)**

> *"No, I was living with them freely [following LF diagnosis] and there was no problem. I was able to chat with them as well. I had my peace of mind even up to now".* **(Female, 60, Participant 14)**

Females, those living in poverty, and more visibly disabled individuals recalled the greatest experiences of enacted stigma from the community and in some cases family/relatives. Accounts of challenging enacted stigma were reported by men and not women, potentially attributed to the existing gendered hierarchy. Additionally, such intersections of stigma, gender, poverty, and disability increasingly contributed to mental distress.

> *"They were laughing at me ... They were telling me that it was the beginning of elephantiasis, and I will not get better, that was the beginning of a disability ... [and] the leg will become bigger".* **(Male, 47, Participant 4)**

> *"When I was okay, when I was strong enough, [I] was selling cattle and after I was diagnosed with this condition, people started stigmatising me".* **(Male, 43, Participant 12)**

Some accounts linked stigma with delayed or poor quality of care, as one female described she "was not assisted well" within a healthcare setting. Limited knowledge around causes of lymphoedema contributed to both internal and enacted stigma exacerbating mental distress. Traditional belief systems often exacerbated misinformation around the cause of lymphoedema and associated stigma, rooted within community and personal beliefs which were often reinforced by traditional healers.

> *"Some use the supernatural powers when they want to farm ... people advised me to stop farming on that field ... my penis [started] to swell such that I was struggling with life... [I was advised] to stop using the fields or ... [it] might kill me ... Later on ... my legs started swelling ... it started as if I was bewitched only that the legs were not shrinking even if I went to the hospital".* **(Male, 47, Participant 4)**

Internalised Stigma and Participation

Key drivers of internalised stigma were associated with limited functioning, inability to work, and inability to meet gender social roles (as described above). Greater internalised stigma was associated with repeated experiences of enacted stigma, such as in relationships (abuse or separation) and from community members (social exclusion, verbal insults, or segregation)

> *"... my marriage ended because I am sick...to say the way this person is sick, how useful can he be?"* **(Male, 53, Participant 21)**

Participation, internalised stigma, and mental wellbeing were found to interlink; for example, a lack of participation caused anxiety or worry, described as "stay here and wait" or "thinking a lot". Participants were negatively impacted by their degree of disability, functional limitation, and physical appearance and experienced enacted stigma. Women seemed to experience more shame than men, although females gave fewer accounts of social exclusion, regardless of their lymphoedema. Some adjusted their behaviours, such as by wearing trousers to cover their lymphoedema "So, as a woman, I started feeling shy and I was wearing a wrapper to cover the leg" (Female, 39, Participant 8).

> *"I feel shy sometimes ... I am a chief in this village and I have a name but they nicknamed me chief with a big foot, such that when you are to move around you will hear that name amongst people from this area".* **(Male, 51, Participant 2)**

3.3. Displacement, Poverty, Disease, and Health Inequities

Within our syndemic model of LF and mental distress, we highlight how intersections and influences at the macro and meso level can impact disease interactions and individual experiences. In Malawi, macro and meso factors identified by persons affected were grouped into displacement, poverty, disease, and health inequities. Distressing life events within narratives were described in relation to displacement from annual extreme weather conditions in the Chikwawa. For some, this caused frequent displacement and, when coupled with precarious livelihoods and lymphoedema, caused additional mental distress. As Chimwemwe described, "I was ... [planning] to build a house ... with this condition, I failed to do that..". Financial instability and dependency on others made family illness and death additionally distressing, and often visits to formal health settings were associated with stress.

> *"that missing person is my brother ... he was the one who was taking care of me. ... we found him ... [dead] ... so, from that day, I failed to sleep because ... now, I am the only ... [family member] remaining".* **(Female, 38, Participant 1)**

Additional physical impairments, as well as lymphoedema, resulted in increased dependency on others. This also resulted in extremely poor living conditions and increased vulnerabilities to additional health and social risks.

"I do [think about dying] because living with this condition, even ... [my] guardian gets tired of taking care of me and sometimes if she gets tired, she forgets to provide some other things". **(Female, 62, Participant 16)**

3.4. (C) How Do Health and Social Systems Contribute to Responses in LF and Mental Health Services?

In the following section, we discuss the third main dimension of the syndemic model of LF and mental distress, (Figure 1) (C) How do Health and Social Systems Contribute to Responses in LF and Mental Health Services? Firstly, challenges around accessing available LF and mental health services in Malawi prior to the ESC are discussed. Secondly, how the ESC addresses gaps in LF services, and how the ESC disrupts the syndemic of LF and mental distress, specifically drawing on each person's affected experiences of conditions (somatic, daily activities, and meaning of disease) is discussed. Finally, the sustainability of the ESC is discussed from the perspective of persons affected by LF.

3.4.1. Health Stress, Social, and Structural Barriers

Repeated care-seeking via formal and informal health providers was often a result of weak formal health system capacity to diagnose and treat lymphoedema. This was due to the lack of trained personnel or knowledge of available treatment, unavailable or absent healthcare staff within health facilities, limited supplies, such as painkillers to alleviate acute attacks, and inappropriate and costly treatment which did not improve symptoms. The choice of health-seeking via informal and formal providers was shaped by community or personal beliefs of disease cause and previous care received from providers. Repeated healthcare-seeking visits were often cited as a cause of stress.

"I have been coming [to the hospital] ... several times and the doctor said I can read it from your form". **(Female, 65, Participant 14)**

"After I came back from the hospital and when I noticed that I was not feeling better, I started visiting the traditional healers". **(Female, 40, Participant 20)**

Health-seeking through the formal health system was common, except for one participant who had only accessed traditional care and a pharmacy. Additionally, some elderly participants did not seek any formal or informal care, highlighting potential generational differences in Malawian health-seeking behaviours.

"I just accepted that my leg was swollen because all of my parents also died with this same condition ... they were not seeking medical care from the hospital as we are doing it right now". **(Female, 65, Participant 14)**

All persons affected that were categorised as "mentally distressed" within the sampling matrix (Table 1) reported repeated care-seeking in the first year of symptom onset in an attempt to improve their condition, exhausting all formal and informal options.

"I still visit the hospital [as well as traditional healers] and at times I buy medicine from private clinics ... I have tried going to pastors for prayers and for blessed water ... When I have money, I go and buy the medication and [my leg] ... usually shrinks". **(Female, 40, Participant 20)**

3.4.2. Financial Burden of Healthcare-Seeking, Lymphoedema Management, and Misdiagnosis

Repeated care-seeking brought additional financial stress for individuals, households, and extended families, related to travel and treatment costs and days off work to attend health services. This was exacerbated by a dependency on others for travel to health services and financial support. These barriers and financial stressors were greatest for individuals living in economic instability (poverty), particularly if relatives were in similar financial positions. Consequently, these factors led to delaying seeking healthcare and reducing the ability to access health services.

> *"When I went to the district hospital ... I told my brother that I was supposed to be given 36 injections of which he accepted, and he was giving me transport money to and from the hospital".* **(Male, 43, Participant 12)**

Misdiagnosis and inappropriate prescribed treatment resulted from a lack of trained personnel and knowledge around lymphoedema within formal health settings. However, many were prescribed drugs (painkillers or antibiotics) to manage their acute attacks. Numerous injections were prescribed to some younger participants to treat their lymphoedema, which MoH staff stated were often prescribed to treat cancer-related diagnoses. Chimwemwe and others shared their experiences within a formal healthcare setting where they described a likely misdiagnosis and inappropriate treatment, which imposed a potentially unnecessary financial burden upon a person affected and their family (see Figure 1).

> *"As a young man ... I noticed that my leg has started swelling ... I went to the district hospital, ... [and] I was prescribed 18 injections .... [I was] failing to withstand the budget of staying at the hospital, it was difficult. I needed food and other things ... I continued getting the injection[s] but because I did not have money, I failed to finish all the prescribed injections".* **(Male, 39, Participant 19)**

3.4.3. Resource and Capacity Limitations

Amongst those affected by hydrocoele, cancelled hydrocoelectomy procedures were commonly reported due to prioritisation of emergency surgeries, limited surgical supplies, and unavailability of health staff, resulting in increased morbidity, travel expenses, and missed days off work.

> *"I was feeling tingling, and pain and I went to the hospital because I was failing to sit on the bicycle since my private part was also swollen ... when I went [to the hospital] I was told that I need to be operated. So, they gave me a date and when I went back on that particular date, they told me to go there on another date. I went again, and when I arrived there, after they examined me, they told me that I need to try taking some medication before the operation [and could not have surgery that day]".* **(Male, 70, Participant 6)**

3.5. Mental Health Service Provision in Malawi

Like most LMICs, current resources allocated for mental healthcare in Malawi are limited, reducing treatment and management options [50,51].

> *"There's no ... training for mental health for community health workers and even for the patients I think we overlook this this side of mental health in Malawi ... so for the patients with elephantiasis I think we have been neglected in terms of psychosocial support or mental health because we don't train them or we don't even help them in any way mentally ...... but most of the time when they come with lymphoedema we only look at the clinical part and clinical management".* **(Programme Staff Member)**

3.6. ESC Addressing Gaps in LF Service Provision

The ESC intervention addressed gaps in LF service provision in Malawi. Douglass et al. (2019) designed the ESC intervention with a biological focus to improve the somatic experience of individuals living with lymphoedema, to impose no added financial burden on persons affected, and to be easy to remember for persons affected and their primary caregivers. Participation in the ESC equipped most with knowledge of their condition and diagnosis, alongside skills to manage their symptoms, particularly during acute attacks. This reduced repeated healthcare-seeking, reducing costs associated with travel and inappropriate treatment.

> *"I started practising [the self-care] ... things have improved. Right now, I am able to run which was difficult for me in the past, the skin peeling stopped ... when I started massaging it ... and the exercises ... the pain is gone ... I was unable even to ride a bicycle ... so when [my family] saw me moving about, they were happy".* **(Male 47, Participant 4)**

The management of the physical symptoms of LF was anticipated to indirectly improve daily activities and meaning (i.e., stigma and social isolation) of the persons affected. Supplementary Table S1 summarises each domain (activity) of the ESC and the intended impact of the ESC intervention on the syndemic pathways identified. Evidence of ESC outcomes from the participants' perspective and additional recommendations are also presented.

3.7. The Potential for ESC to Disrupt the Syndemic Relationship between Mental Health and LF

Within this section we discuss how the ESC disrupts the syndemic of LF and mental distress, firstly in relation to the interaction of LF and mental distress and then relating to individual experiences of these conditions (somatic, ability to complete daily activities, and the social meaning of disease). Discovering that treatment, supplies, and financial support for lymphoedema self-management was available through the ESC study led to improved wellbeing, particularly for those who repeatedly sought care. Despite overall improvements in mental wellbeing, for some, the chronic nature of lymphoedema and there being no "cure" still caused distress, particularly for those living with severe staging of lymphoedema, multiple disabilities, and the elderly.

3.7.1. Somatic Experience and Acute Attacks

Improvements in somatic experience, such as less pain, decreased frequency and duration of acute attacks, reduced swelling, and wound healing following the ESC were described, which was attributed to improved mental wellbeing and ESC adherence by participants. All persons affected described a reduction in acute attacks following the ESC, which corroborates Barrett et al.'s (2023) findings that higher depressive symptoms were associated with higher numbers of acute attacks. Reduced acute attacks and participants generally feeling "well" reduced adherence to the ESC, though periods of feeling "unwell" during acute episodes reminded participants to continue to practice ESC.

> *"since from that time, that you taught us the home-based care, I have not been sick [acute attacks] . . . I am able to work as you can see".* ***(Male, 51, Participant 2)***

3.7.2. Daily Activities

Many described a sense of stability in their life following the ESC intervention and that ESC activities were easy to practice within daily life. Livelihood and social activities such as carrying out work (subsistence farming or selling), household activities (chores), and socialising with peers, were barriers to practising the ESC, which was exacerbated by precarious livelihoods and periods of financial instability. This left some participants feeling overwhelmed when balancing lymphoedema care with livelihood activities.

> *"Sometimes because of being so overwhelmed with work, I miss out some days without cleaning it".* ***(Male, 51, Participant 2)***

Improvements in somatic experience, particularly reduced acute attacks and improved functioning, improved participation in daily activities like walking, completing chores, farming, and practising lymphoedema care. These improvements subconsciously improved ESC adherence (i.e., walking and standing exercises). Increased participation enabled the ability to fulfil gender social roles, reduced dependency on others for financial support, and increased days working, thus improving mental wellbeing. However, precarious livelihoods, living with a life-long chronic condition, and the recurrence of dependency on others still caused distress following the ESC.

> *"For me to be able to support my children in terms of education . . . pay[ing] school fees . . . buying them school uniforms and other necessities . . . when I fall sick, I am not able to provide all those things to my children . . . [due to my condition] my life is not the same again".* ***(Female, 53, Participant 3)***

3.7.3. Meaning of Disease-Stigma

Internalised stigma was reported to reduce following the ESC. Information shared about causes of lymphoedema at the start of the ESC intervention challenged self-stigmatising beliefs around causes of lymphoedema such as being "bewitched" or "cursed". However, some mental distress was still ongoing and related to limited knowledge and concerns around lymphoedema.

> *"I was thinking that maybe I inherited [lymphoedema] from my parents . . .. it has been a while since I developed this condition even though I am on treatment but things are not going on okay . . . you might be thinking that you are bewitched and that might just cause enmity between you while the cause is not that".* ***(Male, 70, Participant 6)***

Adherence to the ESC was impacted by the anticipated stigma associated with performing the standing exercises and daytime elevation (see Table S1).

3.8. Sustainability of the ESC

From the perspective of persons affected, challenges related to the sustainability and continued practice of the ESC were attributed to the inability to continue providing medical supplies and halting regular community-based LF-specialist support. This was ultimately limited by internationally funded research coming to an end.

> *"You have found me walking around, and then you have received a report that someone with lymphoedema is sick, how would you help him or her after hearing that she or he is sick? Would you send medicine to his or her house or you say she or he will get the drugs when she gets better and return to the hospital?"* ***(Female, 62, Participant 16)***

Additional care and support with practising the ESC was required for those without a caregiver during acute attacks, the elderly, those with additional disabilities (i.e., physical or learning), and for persons with greater disability. More specialist care for moderate-to-severe staging was needed, which was often not available within the routine health system. Additionally, the financial burden of medical supplies for persons affected was greatest for those affected by severe lymphoedema, who needed medical supplies replaced more regularly. Unsustained support following the ESC left many feeling worried, forgotten, and distressed about the future. Additionally, the anticipation of disease progression causing worsening somatic experience, inability to complete daily activities (including the ability to practice ESC), and experienced stigma contributed to continued mental distress following the ESC study.

> *"I was thinking that maybe they will no longer supply us again since we were told that they were leaving and maybe they have stopped supplying us with the supplies. So, if they have stopped supplying us, how would they know if our conditions are improving or not?"* ***(Female, 49, Participant 5)***

4. Discussion

Syndemics have been rarely discussed in relation to NTDs in comparison to other infectious diseases of poverty such as HIV and TB [1]. The syndemic relationship between NTDs and mental distress has previously been evidenced in Nigeria and Liberia [15,52]. Our study adds to this evidence base, illustrating syndemic interactions between LF and mental distress in Malawi. Within LMICs, the application of syndemic theory should further be explored, as poverty, gender norms, stigma, and weak health systems play an important role within populations' health and in driving syndemic disease interactions [15]. This study considers the wider biosocial context of LF-related lymphoedema management in Malawi from the perspective of persons affected, which has allowed us to highlight the negative psychosocial consequences of LF and the potential impact of enhanced self-care interventions to address these consequences and contribute to holistic person-centred care. This discussion focuses on interventions at the micro (individual) level, whilst acknowledging there are macro and meso level factors, such as social inequalities related to gender, generation, poverty and extreme climate conditions, which act as a catalyst for the syndemic of concern. We recommend that addressing the social mechanisms driving this syndemic, in addition to enhanced self-care to reverse or prevent physical morbidity associated with the disease, will improve social and health outcomes amongst persons affected by LF.

This study places emphasis on the bidirectional relationship between LF and mental distress. Firstly, we describe the social mechanisms, particularly stigma and stress related to LF, that contribute to mental distress in persons affected. Stress related to LF was exacerbated by stigma, financial insecurities and an inability to work, alongside an absence of appropriate healthcare to diagnose and 'cure' their condition. Secondly, we highlight the role of mental distress on the progression of LF symptoms. Depression has been shown to negatively impact health outcomes amongst other chronic diseases, related to health seeking or adherence to treatment [53,54]. Demonstrating this bidirectional relationship between LF and mental distress. Additionally, we found in line with other studies, social determinants such as limited knowledge around the cause of their lymphoedema, and anticipated stigma from healthcare staff were barriers to accessing healthcare [55,56]. Ultimately leading to poor health outcomes for persons affected by lymphedema due to reduced access to diagnosis and treatment [57–60].

To address to the syndemic of LF and mental distress, in Table 2 we give key recommendations for a multi-level system response. Lessons from this work in Malawi can be applied to other endemic countries focusing on holistic care provision for persons affected by LF. In practice, alongside implementing the ESC, we recommend addressing the social mechanisms driving the syndemic. Examples include, establishing peer support groups, stigma reduction interventions and mental health interventions (counselling, peer-counselling, cognitive behavioural therapy, self-help groups and therapeutic workshops) for persons affected and their caregivers, as described in Table 2 [53]. Peer support groups can encourage adherence to self-care, and have been shown to improve wellbeing and self-esteem amongst persons affected by skin-NTDs [61]. Within LF care provision, information and awareness shared with endemic communities and healthcare staff to reduce stigma is crucial in addressing the psychosocial burden of LF.

To address the social forces that contribute to LF and mental distress clustering, looking beyond the health system, to providing social support through already established social structures is critical. As described in Table 2, providing social support for those living with disabilities, through economic support, socio-economic rehabilitation through skills, educational opportunities and enhancing entrepreneurship, particularly for those that are less physically dependent is recommended [62,63]. Caregiver support to help manage lymphoedema self-care and household responsibili-ties for those with disabilities is recommended. The role of religious groups and traditional healers within social structures and mental health support or care provision is critical in the health-seeking journeys of persons affected by LF and should be considered within future research and intervention design in this area [41,64–66].

Table 2. Overview of Multi-level System Response and Recommendations of LF Programmes for Holistic Care Provision for Persons Affected by LF.

	Recommendations
Early Case Detection	• Active case-finding is essential to reduce disease progression, particularly for lymphoedema
Hydrocoele Surgeries	• Increased community sensitisation for men to access clinics for hydrocoele surgeries • Refresher training for health staff conducting hydrocoele surgery • Hydrocoele camps in high endemicity areas
Lymphoedema Management (Self-care)	• Scale-up of enhanced self-care activities in districts without trained health staff • Periodic refresher training for lymphoedema management for staff, persons affected, and their caregivers • Adaption of enhanced self-care activities within the social context of the communities being implemented, i.e., extra provisions for individuals working away on farms to continue practice of self-care • Continued provision of supplies (i.e., soap, antifungal cream, painkillers, antibiotics, or ointment, and less frequently towels) • Provision of footwear (regularly) • Peer-support groups to prioritise and encourage practising of self-care [61] • Patient advocates to promote self-care activities [67]
Psychosocial Support	• Mental health interventions (counselling, peer counselling, cognitive behavioural therapy, self-help groups, and therapeutic workshops) • Stigma reduction interventions, community awareness campaigns [68], stepping stones [69], and community conversations [67] • Training clinicians in MhGAP and strengthening mental health referral pathways • Provision of rehabilitation services including assistive devices
Social Support	• Economic support for persons affected by disabilities • Socio-economic rehabilitation through training in skills, educational opportunities, and enhancing entrepreneurship, for persons affected with disabilities, and to contribute towards stigma reduction • Caregiver support for those with disabilities and without a carer to manage self-care or household responsibilities • Social support given through pre-existing groups or social structures (religious groups, traditional healers, and social groups)
Caregiver Support	• Mental health support for caregivers • Socio-economic rehabilitation though training in skills, educational opportunities, and enhancing entrepreneurship

These study findings have been member-checked to understand the transferability of this work beyond the Malawian context, which align with WHO policy documents [33] and other researchers within the NTD field working in low-resource settings. For example, DMDI interventions that consider the physical health, mental health and psychosocial care for endemic skin conditions collectively, are currently being piloted in Ethiopia, Nigeria, and Liberia [66,70,71]. Addressing the wider biosocial impact of LF beyond healthcare (i.e., lymphoedema management), has been identified as critical across all these studies. to not just improve physical outcomes of lymphoedema whilst raising awareness of cause, treatment and prevention but also to address the psychosocial consequences of LF, such as reducing stigma and improving mental wellbeing [72]. Within Table S1, we summarise each of the ESC domains (i.e., awareness raising and specific ESC activities) and their intended impact to disrupt the syndemic pathway as well as presenting recommendations for practical actions that can support LF programmes to take a more holistic approach to lymphedema care, including the prioritisation of mental wellbeing alongside physical health.

Access to healthcare services for lymphoedema management and mental health services remains a challenge within Malawi [31]. A lack of trained health staff in lymphoedema management available within health facilities was an additional barrier to accessing appropriate healthcare (i.e., diagnosis and treatment), as evidenced in other LMIC (e.g., India and Sri Lanka) settings [19,73–75]. Currently across Malawi, 4000 community health workers and two staff from each health centre (259) have been trained in basic WHO lymphoedema care [29]. Health facility assessments identified that half of the 56 facilities in Malawi had a minimum of one staff member trained in lymphoedema care [29]. More needs to be done in relation to the scale-up of the ESC across all regions as well as regular refresher training of the enhanced self-care. Utilising the community health workforce by upgrading their training to include ESC training should be considered a critical step to improve the availability of accessible, acceptable, and affordable healthcare options for persons affected by lymphedema [75]. Our study has shown that providing ESC support close to communities within highly endemic regions of Malawi [27] can greatly improve mental wellbeing and with appropriate skills building, community health workers may help to address the lack of sustained support in lymphoedema management identified by persons affected in this study. However, such steps should be undertaken with caution so as to adequately support an already highly burdened cadre of the health workforce [76].

This study found that the ESC was able to bring lymphoedema diagnosis and care directly to the community, whilst reducing repeated healthcare-seeking by equipping persons affected with the skills to manage their symptoms [77]. Early case detection for lymphoedema is essential in hindering disease progression to later stages and reducing the severity of disability, functional limitation, and disfigurement [78,79]. Current WHO guidelines are less effective in treating later stages of lymphoedema [36,80,81]. Our findings show that those with more severe staging of lymphoedema experienced increased stigma, mental distress, and disability, as evidenced in previous research [13,14]. Therefore, to meet the needs of persons affected, particularly for those with severe staging of lymphoedema or greater disability, widening the scope of lymphoedema management to include psychosocial support and consider the wider biosocial context within DMDI implementation is critical [82].

The economic context within which DMDI interventions are implemented at the local level is essential [33]. We found key economic barriers to long-term adherence to the ESC, specifically the inability to replace basic supplies for lymphoedema care (e.g., soap, towels, and antifungal cream). Supply replenishment remains a major challenge for many national programmes and is an essential component for providing sustainable DMDI activities [31,77,83,84]. Within settings like Malawi, reducing the economic burden through the provision of medical supplies and suitable footwear to protect feet and prevent infection or wounds is recommended to improve sustained ESC adherence [33]. In addition to this, the promotion of income generation through socio-economic rehabilitation for both persons affected and their caregivers, such as training in skills, educational opportunities, and enhancing entrepreneurship, would also help to address barriers to ESC adherence related to economic instability. Furthermore, lessons from Malawi highlight the importance of supply provision and socio-economic interventions that could be applied to other sub-Saharan endemic countries where persons affected by LF face similar economic climates.

Caregivers should also be recognised as a major contributor to achieving DMDI coverage. Recognising and valuing unpaid care and the domestic work of caregivers and how the absence of this support impacts DMDI coverage is crucial. Significant hardships have been described for the caregivers of persons with lymphedema, most often women [46,85,86]. LF-related lymphoedema has been shown to disproportionately affect women in multiple countries [48,87,88]. For example, in Bangladesh, 3.7 times more women were found to have lymphoedema than men [47]. Such gender inequalities need to be addressed amongst caregivers and persons affected in order to achieve progress towards sustainable development goal 5: "Achieve gender equality and empower all women and girls". These findings highlight the importance of including the caregiver perspectives within intervention design and LF care delivery.

Qualitative research is labour-intensive and requires rapport-building with participants to collect meaningful and honest accounts. The collection of life history narrative data is dependent upon the skill and patience of the research team as well as the willingness of participants when delivering their accounts. CB was present during data collection as an 'outsider' in Malawi; thus, researchers conducted regular debriefs and reflexivity sessions as a team to ensure that honest and transparent interpretations of participant accounts were generated, DEM, as the lead interviewer, established a rapport and trust over time with participants through regular visits during the initial ESC study and in setting up life-history interviews.

5. Conclusions

This work illustrates the syndemic interaction of LF and mental distress in Malawi, demonstrating the importance of addressing both the physical and psychosocial consequences of disease within lymphoedema management. Home-based self-care increases the availability of accessible, acceptable, and affordable healthcare options, offering the huge potential to reduce health inequalities whilst enhancing individual agency. This work supports the design and delivery of holistic person-centred DMDI approaches to improve overall health outcomes for people living with LF and/or mental health conditions. Lessons learned can be applied to other sub-Saharan African endemic countries.

Supplementary Materials: The following supporting information can be downloaded at: https://www.mdpi.com/article/10.3390/tropicalmed9080172/s1, Table S1: Summary of each enhanced self-care (ESC) domain, the intended impact and outcomes of the intervention from the participant perspective.

Author Contributions: Conceptualization, C.B. and L.D.; methodology, C.B., L.D. and L.A.K.-H.; formal analysis, C.B. and L.D.; investigation, D.E.M., J.D. and C.B.; resources, C.B. and L.A.K.-H.; data curation, C.B.; writing—original draft preparation, C.B.; writing—review and editing, All; supervision, J.C., L.D. and L.A.K.-H.; project administration, J.C. and L.A.K.-H.; funding acquisition, C.B. and L.A.K.-H. All authors have read and agreed to the published version of the manuscript.

Funding: This research was funded by a Medical Research Council Doctoral Training Partnership for CB [project number 2267306]. There are no competing financial interests and funders of this study had no role in study design, data collection and analysis, the decision to publish, or in preparation of the manuscript.

Institutional Review Board Statement: The study was conducted in accordance with the Declaration of Helsinki, and approved by the Institutional Review Board (or Ethics Committee) of Liverpool School of Tropical Medicine (protocol code 22-036) and National Health Sciences Research Committee, Malawi (Number 2615).

Informed Consent Statement: Informed consent was obtained from all subjects involved in the study.

Data Availability Statement: All data generated and analyzed during this study are included in this manuscript. Raw qualitative data are not available and will not be publicly shared, as this would compromise the anonymity and protection of our study participants.

Acknowledgments: The authors wish to thank the health surveillance assistants, programme coordinators and managers, district health workers, district and regional officials and participants who made this study possible. We would like to thank the participants who took the time to engage with us as part of this study and for their sharing honest, challenging and personal experiences. The lead author would like to thank Maria Mayisa for her excellent transcription from Chichewa into English.

Conflicts of Interest: The authors declare no conflicts of interest.

References

1. Singer, M.; Bulled, N. Interlocked Infections: The Health Burdens of Syndemics of Neglected Tropical Diseases. *Ann. Anthropol. Pract.* **2012**, *36*, 328–345. [CrossRef]
2. Mendenhall, E.; Kohrt, B.A.; Norris, S.A.; Ndetei, D.; Prabhakaran, D. Non-communicable disease syndemics: Poverty, depression, and diabetes among low-income populations. *Lancet* **2017**, *389*, 951–963. [CrossRef]
3. Ostrach, B.; Lerman Ginzburg, S.; Singer, M. *Stigma Syndemics: New Directions in Biosocial Health*; Lexington Books: Lanham, MD, USA, 2017.
4. Tsai, A.C.; Venkataramani, A.S. Syndemics and health disparities: A methodological note. *AIDS Behav.* **2016**, *20*, 423–430. [CrossRef]
5. Berkman, L.F.; Kawachi, I.; Glymour, M.M. *Social Epidemiology*; Oxford University Press: Oxford, UK, 2014.
6. Tsai, A.C. Syndemics: A theory in search of data or data in search of a theory? *Soc. Sci. Med.* **2018**, *206*, 117–122. [CrossRef]
7. World Health Organization. Lymphatic Filariasis. 2023. Available online: https://www.who.int/news-room/fact-sheets/detail/lymphatic-filariasis (accessed on 1 June 2023).
8. Ramaiah, K.D.; Ottesen, E.A. Progress and Impact of 13 Years of the Global Programme to Eliminate Lymphatic Filariasis on Reducing the Burden of Filarial Disease. *PLoS Negl. Trop. Dis.* **2014**, *8*, e3319. [CrossRef]
9. El-Nahas, H.; El-Shazly, A.; Abulhassan, M.; Nabih, N.; Mousa, N. Impact of basic lymphedema management and antifilarial treatment on acute dermatolymphangioadenitis episodes and filarial antigenaemia. *J. Glob. Glob. Glob. Infect. Dis.* **2011**, *3*, 227–232. [CrossRef] [PubMed]
10. Shenoy, R.K. Clinical and pathological aspects of filarial lymphedema and its management. *Korean J. Parasitol.* **2008**, *46*, 119–125. [CrossRef] [PubMed] [PubMed Central]
11. Kumari, A.; Harichandrakumar, K.; Das, L.; Kaliannagounder, K. Physical and Psychosocial Burden Due to Lymphatic Filariasis as Perceived by Patients and Medical Experts. *Trop. Med. Int. Health* **2005**, *10*, 567–573. [CrossRef]
12. Martindale, S.; Mkwanda, S.Z.; Smith, E.; Molyneux, D.; Stanton, M.C.; Kelly-Hope, L.A. Quantifying the physical and socio-economic burden of filarial lymphoedema in Chikwawa District, Malawi. *Trans. R. Soc. Trop. Med. Hyg.* **2014**, *108*, 759–767. [CrossRef]
13. Bailey, F.; Eaton, J.; Jidda, M.; van Brakel, W.H.; Addiss, D.G.; Molyneux, D.H. Neglected Tropical Diseases and Mental Health: Progress, Partnerships, and Integration. *Trends Parasitol.* **2019**, *35*, 23–31. [CrossRef]
14. Litt, E.; Baker, M.C.; Molyneux, D. Neglected tropical diseases and mental health: A perspective on comorbidity. *Trends Parasitol.* **2012**, *28*, 195–201. [CrossRef] [PubMed]
15. Dean, L.; Theobald, S.; Nallo, G.; Bettee, A.; Kollie, K.; Tolhurst, R. A syndemic born of war: Combining intersectionality and structural violence to explore the biosocial interactions of neglected tropical diseases, disability and mental distress in Liberia. *PLoS Glob. Public Health* **2022**, *2*, e0000551. [CrossRef]
16. Eaton, J. Taking forward a holistic research agenda for mental health of people affected by neglected tropical diseases. *Int. Health* **2023**, *15* (Suppl. S3), iii1–iii2. [CrossRef]
17. Ali, O.; Deribe, K.; Semrau, M.; Mengiste, A.; Kinfe, M.; Tesfaye, A.; Bremner, S.; Davey, G.; Fekadu, A. A cross-sectional study to evaluate depression and quality of life among patients with lymphoedema due to podoconiosis, lymphatic filariasis and leprosy. *Trans. R. Soc. Trop. Med. Hyg.* **2020**, *114*, 983–994. [CrossRef]
18. Barrett, C.; Chiphwanya, J.; Chaponda, L.; Matipula, D.E.; Turner, J.D.; Taylor, M.J.; Read, J.M.; Kelly-Hope, L.A. Mental health conditions in people affected by filarial lymphoedema in Malawi: Prevalence, associated risk factors and the impact of an enhanced self-care intervention. *Int. Health* **2023**, *15* (Suppl. S3), iii14–iii27. [CrossRef] [PubMed] [PubMed Central]
19. Suma, T.K.; Shenoy, R.K.; Kumaraswami, V. A qualitative study of the perceptions, practices and socio-psychological suffering related to chronic brugian filariasis in Kerala, southern India. *Ann. Trop. Med. Parasitol.* **2003**, *97*, 839–845. [CrossRef]
20. Richard, S.A.; Mathieu, E.; Addiss, D.G.; Sodahlon, Y.K. A survey of treatment practices and burden of lymphoedema in Togo. *Trans. R. Soc. Trop. Med. Hyg.* **2007**, *101*, 391–397. [CrossRef] [PubMed]
21. Kanda, K. (Ed.) *The Quality of Life among Lymphedema Patients due to Lymphatic Filariasis in Three Rural Towns in Haiti*; University of South Florida Scholar Common: Tampa, FL, USA, 2004.
22. Wijesinghe, R.S.; Wickremasinghe, A.R.; Ekanayake, S.; Perera, M.S.A. Physical disability and psychosocial impact due to chronic filarial lymphoedema in Sri Lanka. *Filaria J.* **2007**, *6*, 4. [CrossRef] [PubMed]
23. Obindo, J.; Abdulmalik, J.; Nwefoh, E.; Agbir, M.; Nwoga, C.; Armiya'u, A.; Eaton, J. Prevalence of depression and associated clinical and socio-demographic factors in people living with lymphatic filariasis in Plateau State, Nigeria. *PLoS Neglected Trop. Dis.* **2017**, *11*, e0005567. [CrossRef]
24. Molyneux, D.H. Mental health and neglected tropical diseases—The neglected dimension of burden: Identifying the challenges and understanding the burden. *Int. Health* **2023**, *15* (Suppl. S3), iii3–iii6. [CrossRef]
25. Ferlatte, O.; Salway, T.; Trussler, T.; Oliffe, J.; Gilbert, M. Combining intersectionality and syndemic theory to advance understandings of health inequities among Canadian gay, bisexual and other men who have sex with men. *Crit. Public Health* **2018**, *28*, 509–521. [CrossRef]
26. Singer, M.C.; Erickson, P.I.; Badiane, L.; Diaz, R.; Ortiz, D.; Abraham, T.; Nicolaysen, A.M. Syndemics, sex and the city: Understanding sexually transmitted diseases in social and cultural context. *Soc. Sci. Med.* **2006**, *63*, 2010–2021. [CrossRef] [PubMed] [PubMed Central]

27. Barrett, C.; Chiphwanya, J.; Mkwanda, S.; Matipula, D.E.; Ndhlovu, P.; Chaponda, L.; Turner, J.D.; Giorgi, E.; Betts, H.; Martindale, S.; et al. The national distribution of lymphatic filariasis cases in Malawi using case mapping and geostatistical modelling. *PLoS Negl. Trop. Dis.* **2024**, *18*, e0012056. [CrossRef]
28. World Health Organization. *Ending the Neglect to Attain the Sustainable Development Goals: A Road Map for Neglected Tropical Diseases 2021–2030*; World Health Organization: Geneva, Switzerland, 2020.
29. Chiphwanya, J. Elimination of lymphatic filariasis as a public health problem in Malawi. *PLoS Negl. Trop. Dis.* **2023**, *18*, e0011957. [CrossRef]
30. World Health Organization. Global programme to eliminate lymphatic filariasis: Progress report, 2021–Programme mondial pour l'élimination de la filariose lymphatique: Rapport de situation, 2021. *Wkly. Epidemiol. Rec. Relev. Épidémiol. Hebd.* **2022**, *97*, 513–524.
31. Mackenzie, C.D.; Mante, S. Caring for patients in the global programme to eliminate lymphatic filariasis. *Int. Health* **2020**, *13* (Suppl. S1), S48–S54. [CrossRef]
32. Mieras, L.F.; Anand, S.; van Brakel, W.H.; Hamilton, H.C.; Kollmann, K.M.; Mackenzie, C.; Mason, I.; Wickenden, A. Neglected Tropical Diseases, Cross-Cutting Issues Workshop, 4–6 February 2015, Utrecht, the Netherlands: Meeting report. *Int. Health* **2016**, *8* (Suppl. S1), i7–i11. [CrossRef]
33. World Health Organization. *Lymphatic Filariasis: Managing Morbidity and Preventing Disability: An Aide-Mémoire for National Programme Managers*, 2nd ed.; World Health Organization: Geneva, Switzerland, 2021.
34. World Bank. The World Bank in Malawi: The World Bank Group Supports Malawi's Efforts to Reduce Poverty and Promote Economic Growth by Working with the Government, Development Partners, and Civil Society. 2023. Available online: https://www.worldbank.org/en/country/malawi/overview (accessed on 9 November 2023).
35. Neglected Tropical Diseases Support Centre. Malawi Eliminates Lymphatic Filariasis & Other NTD News. 2020. Available online: https://www.ntdsupport.org/news/malawi-eliminates-lymphatic-filariasis-other-ntd-news (accessed on 3 January 2024).
36. Douglass, J.; Mableson, H.E.; Martindale, S.; Kelly-Hope, L.A. An Enhanced Self-Care Protocol for People Affected by Moderate to Severe Lymphedema. *Methods Protoc.* **2019**, *2*, 77. [CrossRef] [PubMed] [PubMed Central]
37. World Health Organization. *Lymphatic Filariasis: Managing Morbidity and Preventing Disability: An Aide-Mémoire for National Programme Managers*; World Health Organization: Geneva, Switzerland, 2013.
38. Mendenhall, E. *Syndemic Suffering: Social Distress, Depression, and Diabetes among Mexican Immigrant Wome*; Routledge: London, UK, 2016.
39. Christensen, A.-D.; Jensen, S.Q. Doing intersectional analysis: Methodological implications for qualitative research. *NORANord. J. Fem. Gend. Res.* **2012**, *20*, 109–125. [CrossRef]
40. Kroenke, K.; Spitzer, R.L.; Williams, J.B. The PHQ-9: Validity of a brief depression severity measure. *J. Gen. Intern. Med.* **2001**, *16*, 606–613. [CrossRef] [PubMed]
41. Dean, L.; Tolhurst, R.; Nallo, G.; Kollie, K.; Bettee, A.; Theobald, S. Neglected tropical disease as a 'biographical disruption': Listening to the narratives of affected persons to develop integrated people centred care in Liberia. *PLoS Negl. Trop. Dis.* **2019**, *13*, e0007710. [CrossRef] [PubMed]
42. Seekles, M.L.; Kadima, J.K.; Ding, Y.; Bulambo, C.B.; Kim, J.J.; Kukola, J.K.; Omumbu, P.O.L.; Mulamba, R.M.; Nganda, M.; Ngenyibungi, S.M.; et al. Mental health, stigma and the quality of life of people affected by neglected tropical diseases of the skin in Kasai Province, Democratic Republic of the Congo: A sex-disaggregated analysis. *Int. Health* **2023**, *15* (Suppl. S3), iii28–iii36. [CrossRef] [PubMed]
43. Beurel, E.; Toups, M.; Nemeroff, C.B. The Bidirectional Relationship of Depression and Inflammation: Double Trouble. *Neuron* **2020**, *107*, 234–256. [CrossRef] [PubMed]
44. McWayne, J.; Heiney, S.P. Psychologic and social sequelae of secondary lymphedema. *Cancer* **2005**, *104*, 457–466. [CrossRef]
45. Lerman, S.; Ostrach, B.; Singer, M. *Foundations of BioSocial Health: Stigma & Illness Interactions*; Lexington Books: Lanham, MD, USA, 2017.
46. Martindale, S.; Mackenzie, C.; Mkwanda, S.; Smith, E.; Stanton, M.; Molyneux, D.; Kelly-Hope, L. "Unseen" Caregivers: The disproportionate gender balance and role of females in the home-based care of lymphatic filariasis patients in Malawi. *Front. Women's Health* **2017**, *2*, 1–3.
47. Karim, M.J.; Haq, R.; Mableson, H.E.; Mahmood, A.S.M.S.; Rahman, M.; Chowdhury, S.M.; Rahman, A.K.M.F.; Hafiz, I.; Betts, H.; Mackenzie, C.; et al. Developing the first national database and map of lymphatic filariasis clinical cases in Bangladesh: Another step closer to the elimination goals. *PLoS Negl. Trop. Dis.* **2019**, *13*, e0007542. [CrossRef] [PubMed]
48. Stanton, M.C.; Mkwanda, S.Z.; Debrah, A.Y.; Batsa, L.; Biritwum, N.-K.; Hoerauf, A.; Cliffe, M.; Best, A.; Molineux, A.; Kelly-Hope, L.A. Developing a community-led SMS reporting tool for the rapid assessment of lymphatic filariasis morbidity burden: Case studies from Malawi and Ghana. *BMC Infect. Dis.* **2015**, *15*, 214. [CrossRef]
49. Weiss, M.G. Stigma and the social burden of neglected tropical diseases. *PLoS Negl. Trop. Dis.* **2008**, *2*, e237. [CrossRef] [PubMed]
50. Udedi, M. Improving access to mental health services in Malawi. *Minist. Health Policy Brief* **2016**, *26*, 505–518.
51. Mafuta, C. *Prevalence of Moderate and High Risk Substance Use and Service Needs among Psychiatric Inpatients at Zomba Mental Hospital in Malawi*; University of Cape Town: Cape Town, South Africa, 2015.
52. Maju, M.; Sharma, A.; Beeram, A.; Ostrach, B. A colonial legacy of HIV/AIDS, NTD, and STI super-syndemics: Eugenicist foreign aid and intertwined health burdens in Nigeria. *Glob. Public Health* **2019**, *14*, 1221–1240. [CrossRef]

53. Koschorke, M.; Hussain Al-Haboubi, Y.; Tseng, P.-C.; Semrau, M.; Eaton, J. Mental health, stigma and neglected tropical diseases: A review and systematic mapping of the evidence. *Front. Trop. Dis.* **2023**, *3*, 808955. Available online: https://sussex.figshare.com/ndownloader/files/41199962 (accessed on 3 January 2024). [CrossRef]
54. Shrestha, M.; Ng, A.; Al-Ghareeb, A.; Alenazi, F.; Gray, R. Association between subthreshold depression and self-care behaviors in people with type 2 diabetes: A systematic review of observational studies. *Syst. Rev.* **2020**, *9*, 45. [CrossRef] [PubMed]
55. Hunter, J.M. Elephantiasis: A disease of development in north east Ghana. *Soc. Sci. Med.* **1992**, *35*, 627–645. [CrossRef] [PubMed]
56. Person, B.; Bartholomew, L.K.; Gyapong, M.; Addiss, D.G.; van den Borne, B. Health-related stigma among women with lymphatic filariasis from the Dominican Republic and Ghana. *Soc. Sci. Med.* **2009**, *68*, 30–38. [CrossRef] [PubMed]
57. Person, B.; Addiss, D.; Bartholomew, L.K.; Meijer, C.; Pou, V.; Gonzálvez, G.; Borne, B.V.D. A qualitative study of the psychosocial and health consequences associated with lymphedema among women in the Dominican Republic. *Acta Trop.* **2007**, *103*, 90–97. [CrossRef] [PubMed]
58. Ahorlu, C.K.; Dunyo, S.K.; Asamoah, G.; Simonsen, P.E. Consequences of hydrocele and the benefits of hydrocelectomy: A qualitative study in lymphatic filariasis endemic communities on the coast of Ghana. *Acta Trop.* **2001**, *80*, 215–221. [CrossRef] [PubMed]
59. Person, B.; Bartholomew, L.K.; Addiss, D.; van den Borne, B. Disrupted social connectedness among Dominican women with chronic filarial lymphedema. *Patient Educ. Couns.* **2007**, *68*, 279–286. [CrossRef] [PubMed]
60. Lu, A.G.; Valencia, L.B.; Llagas, L.D.L.; Aballa, L.; Postrado, L. *Filariasis: A Study of Knowledge, Attitudes and Practices of the People of Sorsogon, Final Report of a Project Supported by the TDR Social and Economic Research Component*; World Health Organization: Geneva, Switzerland, 1988.
61. Chowdhury, S.; Adekeye, O.; McRae, A.; Olorunfemi, T.; Dubukumah, L.; Makinde, O.; Ozokede, E.; Ewemade, J.; Abdulkadir, S.; Ayuba, R.; et al. A holistic approach to well-being and neglected tropical diseases: Evaluating the impact of community-led support groups in Nigeria using community-based participatory research. *Int. Health* **2023**, *15* (Suppl. S1), i87–i99. [CrossRef] [PubMed]
62. Dadun, D.; Van Brakel, W.H.; Peters, R.M.; Lusli, M.; Zweekhorst, M.B.; Bunders, J.G. Irwanto Impact of socio-economic development, contact and peer counselling on stigma against persons affected by leprosy in Cirebon, Indonesia—A randomised controlled trial. *Lepr. Rev.* **2017**, *88*, 2–22. [CrossRef]
63. Ebenso, B.; Fashona, A.; Ayuba, M.; Idah, M.; Adeyemi, G.; S-Fada, S. Impact of socio-economic rehabilitation on leprosy stigma in northern Nigeria: Findings of a retrospective study. *Asia Pac. Disabil. Rehabil. J* **2007**, *18*, 98–119.
64. Alamsyah, T.; Usman, S.; Yusuf, M.; Elvin, S.D. Effectiveness of Traditional Healers in Program to Control Leprosy in Nagan Raya District in Aceh. *Dermatol. Res. Pr.* **2018**, *2018*, 1–6. [CrossRef] [PubMed]
65. REDRESS Liberia. Strengthening People-Centred Health Systems for People Affected by Severe Stigmatising Skin Diseases in Liberia. Available online: https://www.redressliberia.org/ (accessed on 5 January 2024).
66. Semrau, M.; Ali, O.; Deribe, K.; Mengiste, A.; Tesfaye, A.; Kinfe, M.; Bremner, S.A.; Hounsome, N.; Kelly-Hope, L.A.; MacGregor, H.; et al. EnDPoINT: Protocol for an implementation research study to integrate a holistic package of physical health, mental health and psychosocial care for podoconiosis, lymphatic filariasis and leprosy into routine health services in Ethiopia. *BMJ Open* **2020**, *10*, e037675. [CrossRef] [PubMed]
67. Tora, A.; Mengiste, A.; Davey, G.; Semrau, M. Community Involvement in the Care of Persons Affected by Podoconiosis—A Lesson for Other Skin NTDs'. *Trop. Med. Infect. Dis.* **2018**, *3*, 87. [CrossRef] [PubMed]
68. Hofstraat, K.; van Brakel, W.H. Social stigma towards neglected tropical diseases: A systematic review. *Int. Health* **2016**, *8* (Suppl. S1), 53–70. [CrossRef] [PubMed]
69. Jewkes, R.; Nduna, M.; Levin, J.; Jama, N.; Dunkle, K.; Puren, A.; Duvvury, N. Impact of stepping stones on incidence of HIV and HSV-2 and sexual behaviour in rural South Africa cluster randomised controlled trial. *BMJ* **2008**, *337*, 506. [CrossRef]
70. Ministry of Health. Strategic Plan for Integrated Case Management of Neglected Tropical Diseases (NTDs) 2016–2020. 2016. Available online: http://moh.gov.lr/integrated-case-management-ntds-strategic-plan-2016/ (accessed on 3 January 2024).
71. REDRESS. REDRESS Intervention Manual. In *Case Managment of Neglected Tropical Diseases Training Manual: Supporting Health Workers to Identify, Diagnose, Treat and Support Persons Affected by NTDs That Affect the Skin*; National Institute for Health and Care Research: Liverpool, UK, 2023.
72. Ali, O.; Kinfe, M.; Semrau, M.; Tora, A.; Tesfaye, A.; Mengiste, A.; Davey, G.; Fekadu, A. A qualitative study on the implementation of a holistic care package for control and management of lymphoedema: Experience from a pilot intervention in northern Ethiopia. *BMC Health Serv. Res.* **2021**, *21*, 1065. [CrossRef] [PubMed] [PubMed Central]
73. Suma, T.K.; Shenoy, R.K.; Kumaraswami, V. Efficacy and sustainability of a footcare programme in preventing acute attacks of adenolymphangitis in Brugian filariasis. *Trop. Med. Int. Health* **2002**, *7*, 763–766. [CrossRef]
74. Chandrasena, N.; Premaratna, R.; Gunaratna, I.E.; de Silva, N.R. Morbidity management and disability prevention for lymphatic filariasis in Sri Lanka: Current status and future prospects. *PLoS Negl. Trop. Dis.* **2018**, *12*, e0006472. [CrossRef] [PubMed]
75. Torgbenu, E.; Luckett, T.; Buhagiar, M.; Phillips, J.L. Practice points for lymphoedema care in low- and middle- income countries developed by nominal group technique. *BMC Health Serv. Res.* **2023**, *23*, 740. [CrossRef] [PubMed] [PubMed Central]
76. Raven, J.; Akweongo, P.; Baba, A.; Baine, S.O.; Sall, M.G.; Buzuzi, S.; Martineau, T. Using a human resource management approach to support community health workers: Experiences from five African countries. *Hum. Resour. Health* **2015**, *13*, 45. [CrossRef]

77. Ramaiah, K.D.; Guyatt, H.; Ramu, K.; Vanamail, P.; Pani, S.P.; Das, P.K. Treatment costs and loss of work time to individuals with chronic lymphatic filariasis in rural communities in south India. *Trop. Med. Int. Health* **1999**, *4*, 19–25. [CrossRef] [PubMed]
78. BBudge, P.J.; Little, K.M.; Mues, K.E.; Kennedy, E.D.; Prakash, A.; Rout, J.; Fox, L.M. Impact of community-based lymphedema management on perceived disability among patients with lymphatic filariasis in Orissa State, India. *PLoS Negl. Trop. Dis.* **2013**, *7*, e2100. [CrossRef] [PubMed]
79. Douglass, J.; Graves, P.; Gordon, S. Self-care for management of secondary lymphedema: A systematic review. *PLoS Negl. Trop. Dis.* **2016**, *10*, e0004740. [CrossRef] [PubMed]
80. Douglass, J.; Hailekiros, F.; Martindale, S.; Mableson, H.; Seife, F.; Bishaw, T.; Nigussie, M.; Meribo, K.; Tamiru, M.; Agidew, G.; et al. Addition of Lymphatic Stimulating Self-Care Practices Reduces Acute Attacks among People Affected by Moderate and Severe Lower-Limb Lymphedema in Ethiopia, a Cluster Randomized Controlled Trial. *J. Clin. Med.* **2020**, *9*, 4077. [CrossRef] [PubMed] [PubMed Central]
81. Douglass, J.; Mableson, H.; Martindale, S.; Jhara, S.T.; Karim, M.J.; Rahman, M.M.; Al Kawsar, A.; Khair, A.; Mahmood, A.S.; Rahman, A.F.; et al. Effect of an Enhanced Self-Care Protocol on Lymphedema Status among People Affected by Moderate to Severe Lower-Limb Lymphedema in Bangladesh, a Cluster Randomized Controlled Trial. *J. Cin. Med.* **2020**, *9*, 2444. [CrossRef] [PubMed] [PubMed Central]
82. Dixon, R.; Lar, L.; Dean, L. Neglect in the numbers: Leaving no voice behind in disease elimination. *Lancet Glob. Health* **2021**, *9*, e22. [CrossRef] [PubMed]
83. Pryce, J.; Mableson, H.E.; Choudhary, R.; Pandey, B.D.; Aley, D.; Betts, H.; Mackenzie, C.D.; Kelly-Hope, L.A.; Cross, H. Assessing the feasibility of integration of self-care for filarial lymphoedema into existing community leprosy self-help groups in Nepal. *BMC Public Health* **2018**, *18*, 201. [CrossRef] [PubMed]
84. Kollie, K.K.; Jenkins, J.; Theobald, S.; Nallo, G.; Kpadeh, O.; Jones, L.; Borbor, D.; Phillip, M.; Wickenden, A.; Kollie, J.T.; et al. Unpacking the impact of integrating the neglected tropical disease supply chain into the national supply chain system: Illustrative evidence from Liberia. *Parasitology* **2023**, *150*, 1052–1062. [CrossRef] [PubMed] [PubMed Central]
85. Ton, T.G.; Mackenzie, C.; Molyneux, D.H. The burden of mental health in lymphatic filariasis. *Infect. Dis. Poverty* **2015**, *4*, 34. [CrossRef] [PubMed] [PubMed Central]
86. Caprioli, T.; Martindale, S.; Mengiste, A.; Assefa, D.; H/Kiros, F.; Tamiru, M.; Negussu, N.; Taylor, M.; Betts, H.; Kelly-Hope, L.A. Quantifying the socio-economic impact of leg lymphoedema on patient caregivers in a lymphatic filariasis and podoconiosis co-endemic district of Ethiopia. *PLoS Negl. Trop. Dis.* **2020**, *14*, e0008058. [CrossRef] [PubMed]
87. Mwingira, U.; Chikawe, M.; Mandara, W.L.; Mableson, H.E.; Uisso, C.; Mremi, I.; Malishee, A.; Malecela, M.; Mackenzie, C.D.; Kelly-Hope, L.A.; et al. Lymphatic filariasis patient identification in a large urban area of Tanzania: An application of a community-led mHealth system. *PLoS Negl. Trop. Dis.* **2017**, *11*, e0005748. [CrossRef] [PubMed]
88. Kebede, B.; Martindale, S.; Mengistu, B.; Mengiste, A.; H/Kiros, F.; Tamiru, A.; Davey, G.; Kelly-Hope, L.A.; Mackenzie, C.D. Integrated morbidity mapping of lymphatic filariasis and podoconiosis cases in 20 co-endemic districts of Ethiopia. *PLoS Negl. Trop. Dis.* **2018**, *12*, e0006491. [CrossRef]

Tropical Medicine and Infectious Disease

MDPI

Article

Assessing the 1918/19 Pandemic Influenza and Respiratory Tuberculosis Interaction in Malta: Operationalizing a Syndemic During a Crisis Event

Lianne Tripp [1,*], Larry A. Sawchuk [2,†] and Charles J. Farrugia [3]

1 Department of Anthropology, Trent University, Peterborough, ON K9L 1Z8, Canada
2 Department of Anthropology, University of Toronto Scarborough, Toronto, ON M1C 1A4, Canada
3 Department of Library Information and Archive Sciences, University of Malta, MSD 2080 Msida, Malta; charles.j.farrugia@um.edu.mt
* Correspondence: liannetripp@trentu.ca
† Deceased.

Abstract: Studies have indicated that there was a disease interaction of pandemic influenza with respiratory tuberculosis (TB) in Malta, which could explain the heightened mortality recorded in young adults. We revisit the 1918/19 influenza and TB syndemic potential on the island of Malta. Borrowing from crisis studies that explore the harvesting effect, we used the method of assessing changes in pre-pandemic, pandemic, fallow, and post-pandemic mortality/life expectancy to reveal the syndemic experience. Pre-pandemic (1914–1917) life expectancy at birth was significantly higher, at 37.91 years, than during the pandemic (1918), when life expectancy dropped to 33.26 years ($Z = 10.56$, $p < 0.0001$). Post-pandemic (1919) life expectancy rose to 43.49 years, which was an even longer life expectancy than pre-pandemic ($Z = 17.61$, $p < 0.0001$). There were significant changes in TB mortality death rates during the four periods in those of reproductive age. Augmenting our framework for studies of syndemics involving short-term events, we proposed the identification of contributing, driving, and limiting factors. Underlying living conditions contributed to the syndemic. The exacerbation of housing conditions, the economy associated with the First World War, and meteorological measures—temperature, relative humidity, and rainfall—were driving factors. The early implementation of mitigation strategies, such as restrictions on mass gatherings, were limiting factors of the syndemic.

Keywords: syndemic; 1918/19 influenza; respiratory tuberculosis; harvesting effect; life expectancy; crisis events; temperature; relative humidity; rainfall; Malta

1. Introduction

Considerable attention has been directed at the interaction of respiratory tuberculosis with 1918/19 pandemic influenza, which had the potential to result in more than expected deaths from influenza, or from the common secondary infection of pneumonia [1–4]. It is believed that the biological synergism of these diseases resulted from the activation of latent *Mycobacterium tuberculosis* or the acceleration of the progression of illness by the influenza virus [5]. Tuberculosis increased the likelihood of mortality from influenza [2], particularly in people who acquired secondary bacterial pneumonia. Due to the potential synergistic interaction between tuberculosis and the 1918/19 pandemic influenza, which may have manifested more frequently among the impoverished and marginalized, some scholars have characterized this relationship as a syndemic [4,6,7]. In Mamelund's and Dimka's (2019) study [1], they found a significantly higher morbidity rate of influenza-like illness

(20.6%; $p = 0.002$) in females who had respiratory tuberculosis relative to employees in two sanitoria in Norway [1]. Noymer's and Garenne's (2000) study of the USA found that males infection with pandemic influenza had a higher age-standardized death rate from respiratory tuberculosis at 176 per 100,000, and that post-pandemic tuberculosis death rates fell to 107 per 1000, along with there being a temporary increase in life expectancy [2]. In 2009, Noymer found support for passive selection in their study on Union Army veterans; there was a significant effect of TB infection in the company on influenza deaths (hazard ratio= 1.098–1.118, $p = 0.037$–0.018 depending on model), but there was not a significant increase in influenza mortality among those with TB [3]. Tripp, Sawchuk, and Saliba, (2018), in addition to finding excess mortality from TB in Malta during the month of October 1918, also found monthly correlations of tuberculosis cases with influenza morbidity by town in Malta (Rho = 0.58, $p = 0.001$) [4].

The concept of syndemics was proposed by the medical anthropologists Dr. Merrill Singer and Dr. Charlene Snipes in 1992 (Singer had previously presented the term at American conferences in 1991). They recognized that the "synergistic nature of the health and social problems facing the poor and underserved" places those living in inner cities at greater risk of diseases such as AIDs [8] (p. 225). Fundamental to the syndemic concept is the importance of the social environment; in the case of AIDs, this was understood as *S*ubstance *A*buse and *V*iolence and *A*IDs, culminating in the SAVA syndemic [9].

One would expect that our history with diseases and other traumatic events would reveal syndemic occurrences. Singer [7] has proposed numerous examples from famines (such as the Irish famine of 1741) and migrations (such as the Mormons) to wars (such as World War One; see also [10]). For each of these syndemic events to arise, poor economic and social conditions, along with the interaction of malnourishment and infectious disease, drove mortality rates to unprecedented levels. It has also been proposed that potential historical examples of syndemics primarily involving infectious diseases include the following: scarlet fever in 1800s Massachusetts; the 1918/19–20 influenza pandemic around the world (tuberculosis and influenza); and the 1865 cholera epidemic in Gibraltar.

The veracity of these historical events as satisfying the features of a syndemic unfortunately cannot be supported with quantitative evidence, because in many cases it is too onerous or impossible to source reports and data to allow for the exploration of syndemics. Secondly, and more importantly, regardless of the period of the occurrence of the proposed syndemic, there has yet to be a consensus as to a method for "testing" the syndemic criteria or model. Mendenhall and Singer [11] point out an obvious reason for the lack of direction when evaluating a syndemic that is quite often overlooked by health researchers. Syndemic theory originated through ethnography but quickly pivoted to more epidemiological approaches for assessment; over time, numerous approaches have been proposed for the evaluation of syndemics. The diversity in quantitative methods for assessing a syndemic can vary extensively; for syndemic studies on HIV and AIDS alone, various statistical approaches have been utilized: regression analyses, higher-level modeling techniques, frequency and descriptive statistics, longitudinal cohort studies, and social network analyses [11].

At the population level, the comorbidity of two or more diseases or health conditions where the interaction of the diseases "exacerbates the negative health effects of any or all of the diseases involved" [12] (p. 941) is a syndemic, which is a concept that is akin to the ecological concept of synergy. Although the concept has arguably evolved over the last three decades, two constants remain: (1) "noxious social conditions" [9], such as social inequality, be it poverty, overcrowding, stress, or stigma, precipitate increased disease clustering, or physical or behavioral vulnerability [12] and (2), as a result of the synergistical interaction of two or more epidemics [or health problems], there is an "excess burden of disease in a population" [13] (p. 425). Due to the fact that a core element of the syndemic concept is deep-seated inequality, subpopulations that endure a high level of vulnerability are identified.

We borrow the concept of the harvesting effect from studies on crisis events. Otherwise known as forward mortality displacement, harvesting exhibits itself with a temporary increase in the number of deaths of weak, older persons or persons at risk of infection during periods of abnormal stress. Climatic extremes, hunger, bad quality of air, and epidemics can be prime factors in the harvesting effect [14–17]. Harvesting is followed by a period of a decrease in mortality rate, although temporary, in the age group that had been largely removed. The "healthy" or fallow period is another signifier of "excess burden", because without a crisis event, there would not be a subsequent temporary period of enhanced survivorship.

We posit that the identification of a syndemic triggered by a short-term well-defined novel event can be revealed through the presence of the harvesting effect. The application of the harvesting effect for assessing the presence of a syndemic can offer the means for a quantifiable criterion of a syndemic—one that is replicable. Once the occurrence of a syndemic has been established, then the underlying social factors and or health problems contributing to the syndemic can be assessed.

This paper revisits the syndemic potential of 1918/19 influenza and respiratory tuberculosis on the island of Malta, which was reported by two of the authors (see [4]). Because the historical vital statistics for Malta provide death and population counts by age over a long time period, we can utilize a previously proposed methodology to operationalize the syndemic [18]). We use life table analysis to assess whether the *excess burden* of the syndemic was observable from a quantifiable means. This method incorporates the concept of the harvesting effect as a framework to evaluate pre-epidemic/pandemic or baseline mortality, epidemic mortality, and fallow and/or post-epidemic mortality to reveal significant changes in mortality and life expectancy.

We also explore the association of environmental factors such as temperature and relative humidity with the potential syndemic. The underlying social factors that contribute to, drive, and limit the syndemic are discussed. The social risk factors for 1918/19 influenza are debated among scholars. There is, however, an overall consensus that socio-demographic factors such as large population size, high population density, malnutrition, poverty, overcrowded living environments, low education levels, and urbanization, or contradictorily rurality, were contributors (to varying degrees) during epidemics of 1918/19 pandemic influenza, observed in many countries around the world [19–21].

1.1. Core Features of a Syndemic

One can argue that the syndemic approach has a greater potential to better capture and reveal the full range of complex interrelationships that exist in the epidemic experience than what has previously been used by health scholars. At the core of this theoretical construct are four fundamentals: disease clustering, social factors, and their interaction, which yields an excess burden that is greater than the sum of the parts. While numerous scholars have used the syndemic approach to understand health issues, relatively few investigations provide an operational approach to measuring a major element of syndemics: the excess burden of poor health at the population level.

To summarize, Mendenhall and Singer [11] and Gravlee (2020) [22] offer three tenets or core features outlining what constitutes a syndemic, and we have proposed a fourth tenet:

1. Social factors: There are large-scale social forces that precipitate disease clustering, including multigenerational social, economic, and power inequities (e.g., colonialism, enslavement, segregation).

2. Disease clustering (Gravlee [22], refers to this as disease concentration): Two or more diseases cluster together within a population, often described simply as comorbidity or multimorbidity.
3. Interaction: There is interaction either via a biological and/or psychological process between/among the diseases, or interactions across the diseases (biological processes) and the social factors. For example, inflammation is commonly documented in the biological literature, whereas stigma has been reported in anthropology ethnographies. Tsai and co-workers (2017) [23] show that there are different pathways for disease interactions. Sometimes the interactions may not be obvious, and there is not always synergy between/among the diseases.
4. Excess burden: We have added this fourth feature to emphasize that as a result of the three core features above, there is not just simply comorbidity, but the excess burden of poor health and/or diseases is amplified because of the synergy of the diseases, producing "more than the sum of the parts" [22].

In addition to the four requisite core features of a syndemic, we propose that there are three factors or dimensions that modulate the expression of a syndemic. These dimensions—contributing, driving, and limiting—can more readily be assessed for short-term crisis events, such as in the case of an epidemic (see Figure 1).

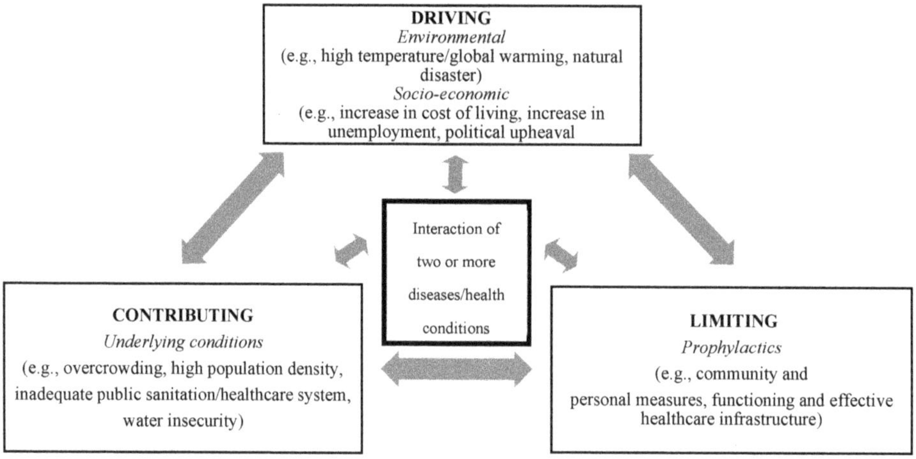

Figure 1. Syndemic paradigm for short-term crisis events, showing the three dimensions.

1.2. Background on Malta in the 20th Century

1.2.1. Overall Health on the Island

During the early 20th century, Malta's standard of living was considered low relative to much of Europe. Throughout the study period, the island's living conditions, sanitation, and health facilities remained persistently inadequate. The working poor constituted the majority of the Maltese population. During the study period, Malta had overcrowding, elevated unemployment rates, large families, and nutritional stress. From 1911 to 1924, the life expectancy at birth for the Maltese was comparatively low at 44 years, in contrast to other European nations [24]). In 1900, the population of Malta had a life expectancy of 40.65 years, while the life expectancy at birth in England and Wales stood at approximately 48.25 years [25]. In 1918, the Maltese exhibited a high infant mortality rate just below 250 per 1000 live births, whereas in another small-scale British colony, Gibraltar, the infant mortality rate was 120 infant deaths per 1000 live births [26]. During this same year, infant mortality rate in England and Wales was much lower at 97.6 per 1000 live births. The diminished survival in Malta during the early 20th century was chiefly attributable to elevated childhood death rates in rural areas [26].

1.2.2. 1918/19 Influenza Pandemic and Early 20th Century Tuberculosis

The influenza epidemic first emerged in Malta at the Cala Frana Seaplane Depot in June 1918, resulting in 31 cases [27]. Between July and August 1918, cases of moderately uncomplicated infection surfaced among the civilian population across six communities on the island: Senglea, Silema, Luca, Tarxien, Paola, Valletta, and Zeitun. According to Dr. Critien, the Principal Medical Officer of Health (PMOH), the herald wave resulted in 34 civilian fatalities [27]. The second wave commenced in mid-August, mostly affecting patients and staff at St. Elmo Hospital, as well as the 1st G.B. Northumberland Fusiliers stationed at Polverista Barracks in Cospicua [27]. The initial documented cases of influenza infection during the second wave occurred within the working classes of Zeitun in September 1918 [27]. The mortality rate for the 1918/19 influenza pandemic in Malta, encompassing both waves, was 3.9 per 1000, comparable to numerous other low mortality rates of influenza deaths recorded in island communities elsewhere during 1918. It was previously observed that on the smaller island of Gozo, children under the age of 5 years transmitted the virus to families, infecting adult females at higher rates relative to adult males [4].

From the early to mid-1900s, tuberculosis mortality rates in the Maltese islands saw a progressive decline. During the First and Second World Wars, the secular trend in tuberculosis mortality was disrupted, resulting in elevated rates of 1.36 deaths per 1000 individuals in 1918, and a decreased rate of 0.84 deaths per 1000 individuals in 1942. Comparable observations of extraordinarily elevated mortality rates during the World Wars have been documented in other studies (see [28–30]). The significantly elevated tuberculosis rates in 1917 and 1918 are attributed by most experts to the intersection of the war and the influenza epidemic. Compared to England, tuberculosis mortality rates in Malta were generally lower but exhibited a similar downward trend, except during the Second World War, when Malta's rates significantly exceeded those of England.

2. Materials and Methods

The main objective of this study was to verify whether there was a period of excess burden of mortality associated with the 1918/19 pandemic, as this is a requisite for a syndemic. We also examined whether there was an association of meteorological measures with the potential 1918 syndemic of influenza and respiratory tuberculosis.

2.1. Data

To assess life expectancy, mortality information from 1914 to 1923 came from two discrete sources. The Annual Health Reports for the Maltese Islands were used to extract information on cause of death by age bands (under 1, 1–4, 5–9, 10–14, 15–19, 20–24, 25–34, 35–44, 45–54, 55–64, 65–74, 75–79, 80–84, 85 plus) for the years 1914 until 1923, with the exception of the year 1918 and part of 1919 [31–38]. Deaths caused by influenza and respective complications (broncho-pneumonia and pneumonia) and respiratory tuberculosis were not recorded in the health reports during the pandemic of 1918/19. Instead, we used the original government nominal death registers to obtain the count of deaths for each of the age bands for this time period and for the aforementioned diseases [39,40]. The death registry provided details on name, age at death, place of birth, place of residence, and name and surname of parents, whether living or dead. The number of annual births for Malta was extracted from the Annual Health Reports for the same years [31–38,41,42] and was used to adjust the population at risk for under 1 year of age.

To estimate the population at risk for the same age bands as the deaths, we undertook a two-stage method. First, we used the raw census numbers for Malta as reported in the 1911 census [43]. From that baseline, we adjusted the number proportionately using the population size cited for Malta in the Annual Health Report for 1918/19 in the Maltese Islands [41]. The census population numbers for the age categories were used to approximate the population size for 1914 to 1917, which was multiplied by 4 to account for the years of the study period.

The second stage was to correct two common problems found in most population census counts; that is, age misreporting and age heaping. Age misreporting is frequently found in populations with low literacy or low educational levels. Another issue that arises during enumeration is when the respondent over- or under-estimates the age. Finally, the census enumerator may simply report the individual's age based on his/her physical appearance. Age heaping is another common problem observed in census counts. The problem arises from the respondent preferring to assign an age with a 0 or ending in 5, rather than a precise age. For example, a 69-year-old or a 71-year-old individual may simply round off the age to 70. To correct for age misreporting and age heaping, we used a smoothing method developed by Arriaga [44]. The "reconstructed and smoothed population structure" for Malta in 1918 was entered into the period life table. The same smoothing method was applied to the year 1919. The 1921 census was used to estimate population size for each of the age categories for the years 1920 to 1923, and the estimate was multiplied by 4 to account for the four years of the study [45].

Because of the relatively small geographical size of the island, Malta had a highly localized micro-climate, meaning that meteorological measures were consistent across the island, and were reliable measures to be examined as potential factors involved in the syndemic.

Three meteorological variables in the assessment of the syndemic period (1918/19) relative to prevailing baseline weather conditions (for the years 1906 until 1917) were extracted from the Annual Health Reports on the Maltese Islands [31–34,41,46–53] The physical properties by month included the following: the absolute minimum and maximum shade temperatures measured in Fahrenheit, the relative humidity given in percent, and the total rainfall amount in inches.

2.2. Analysis

To assess secular trends in respiratory morality over the study period, annual tuberculosis death rates for 1908 until 1938 were generated from the total yearly tuberculosis death counts, divided by the population at risk estimated from the 1911 census [43]. These death rates for the two islands were graphed over time.

A temporally defined period of normal or baseline mortality (BM), the mortality experience as determined by life expectancy at birth, was used to measure changes in survivorship during three periods: P_2, pandemic (1918); P_3, fallow period (1919); P_4, post-pandemic period (1920 to 1923). The war years 1914 to 1917 (P_1) were used to estimate BM.

The Survival Lifetable program (Austin, TX, USA) [54] was utilized to calculate the life table functions (life expectancy at birth ($e_{(0)}$) and probability of dying ($q_{(x)}$)) by employing the period life table methodology, and to evaluate the impact of cause-specific mortality linked to numerous infectious diseases. The period life table provides a cross-sectional view of the mortality and survival experience of a population during a specific year or a group of years. The period life table output was generated using the Survival template by entering the population size counts for each of the age categories and the respective death counts. This was completed for each of the three periods. We also identified and included counts of deaths associated with six distinct cause-specific or disease complexes: (1) influenza pneumonia and bronchopneumonia; (2) respiratory tuberculosis; (3) the diarrhea complex (diarrhea, gastroenteritis, enteritis); (4) the infantile debility complex (marasmus, atrophy, debility); (5) measles; and (6) whooping cough, along with all other causes and residual causes. These disease complexes were chosen because they were known to be common causes of deaths during the study period. The inclusion of the disease complexes allowed for the assessment of the impact of these diseases on life expectancy via the life table function, i.e., the probability of dying ($q_{(x)}$). To quantitatively assess differences in life expectancy across the study periods, two procedures were used. The Z-test, as described by Chiang (1981) [55], was employed to evaluate the importance of life expectancy during the 1918 pandemic, fallow period (1919), and post-pandemic period (1920–23) in comparison to BM (1914–17). The advantages of utilizing the Chiang technique have been detailed in other sources [56,57]. Second, the period life table was complemented by Arriaga's (1984, 1989) decomposition methodology to identify the age band(s) where mortality differentials existed and to elucidate the contributions of variations in age-specific death rates to changes in life expectancy at birth (across two of the study periods) through both direct and indirect effects [58,59]. The Excel template from Auger et al. (2014) [60] was used to construct the decomposition analysis. The direct impact on life expectancy arises from alterations in life years within a specific age range due to the effects of mortality changes in that age range [61]. The indirect impact refers to the increase in life expectancy attributable to the alterations in the number of survivors at the conclusion of an age interval, resulting from changes in mortality within that interval [61]. The Arriaga method also identified the apportion or contribution of cause-specific differences (from the disease complexes) in life expectancy across two of the study periods. p-values indicated whether or not the disease complexes contributed to significant differences in life expectancies. The life table function, showing the probability of dying ($q_{(x)}$) from 1918 influenza and from respiratory tuberculosis during the 1918 influenza pandemic, was graphed to characterize the deaths attributed to each disease by age and sex.

Monthly graphs for the three meteorological measures (temperature, relative humidity, and rainfall) were created for an extended baseline period of 1906 until 1917 to control for the variation that can occur within seasonality. All graphs were created using Statistica (Hamburg, Germany) [62].

3. Results

One of the limitations of this study is that we did not have information to assess the syndemic nature of influenza and respiratory tuberculosis at the individual level. We could only establish an indirect relationship between the two diseases. Our retrospective population-based study does not allow for any detailed account of how rainfall and relative humidity affected influenza transmission, other than a possible relationship of changes in behavioural and inter-personnel responses under cooler temperatures and moisture.

Figure 2 shows Respiratory tuberculosis death rates for the islands of Malta and Gozo from 1908 until 1938. Over the time period, Malta showed higher respiratory tuberculosis rates, in particular during the influenza pandemic. The elevated respiratory tuberculosis mortality rate in 1917 has previously been discussed (see [24]).

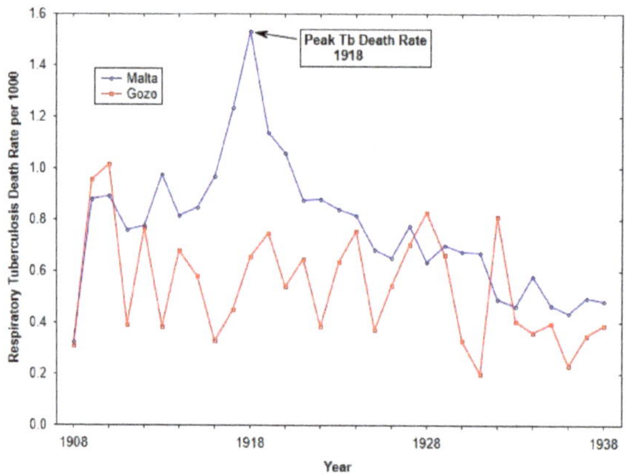

Figure 2. Tuberculosis death rates (per 1000 living) from 1908 to 1938 for Malta and Gozo.

The baseline mortality (BM) period was characterized by a life expectancy at birth of 37.92 ± 0.21 years, with childhood infectious disease epidemics contributing to the low life expectancy (see Table 1). With the appearance of the 1918 pandemic, life expectancy underwent a significant decline to 33.26 ± 0.34 years ($Z = 10.56$, $p < 0.0001$). Even with the continued but muted appearance of influenza in 1919, during this fallow period, there was a dramatic rise in life expectancy to 43.49 years ($Z = 17.61$, $p < 0.0001$). Following the fallow period in 1919, during the post-pandemic period, there was a significant decrease in life expectancy ($Z = 7.08$, $p < 0.0001$), yet life expectancy was higher than that of BM, and as such supports that there was a temporary healthy period following the period of excess burden.

Table 1. Life expectancy at birth during the four periods from 1914 to 1923 in Malta.

Period	Year	Epidemics	LE (ex0)	SE	Z Score	*p*-Value
War (P1)	1914–17	Measles, whooping cough	37.915	0.209		
Pandemic (P2)	1918	Influenza—severe	33.264	0.340	10.56	<0.0001
Fallow period (P3)	1919	Influenza—mild	43.489	0.431	17.61	<0.0001
Post-pandemic (P4)	1920–23	Influenza—slight	40.093	0.212	7.08	<0.0001

Figure 3 shows the impact of influenza and respiratory tuberculosis on the probability of dying in the respective age bands for Malta during the 1918 pandemic. The two diseases have similar patterns for the probability of dying with respect to each of the age categories. And for both diseases, the peak probability of dying occurs in the age band of 25 to 34 years of age.

As with Figure 3, Table 2 shows that there was a significant increase in respiratory tuberculosis mortality among reproductive-age individuals during the 1918 influenza period ($Z = 19.33$, $p < 0.0001$). In contrast, there was not a change in respiratory tuberculosis death among post-reproductive-age individuals ($Z = 1.94$, ns).

The results of the age decomposition in Table 3 show that the largest contribution to the difference between BM and P_2 (pandemic) was due to the indirect effect (90 percent). In contrast, the direct effect was about 10 percent and primarily confined to the 25 to 34 age interval. Approximately two-thirds of the indirect effect fell in the age intervals of 15 to 19 years, 20 to 24 years, and 25 to 34 years. The indirect effect represents the life years added to life expectancy because of the change in the number of survivors at the end of each of the respective age intervals.

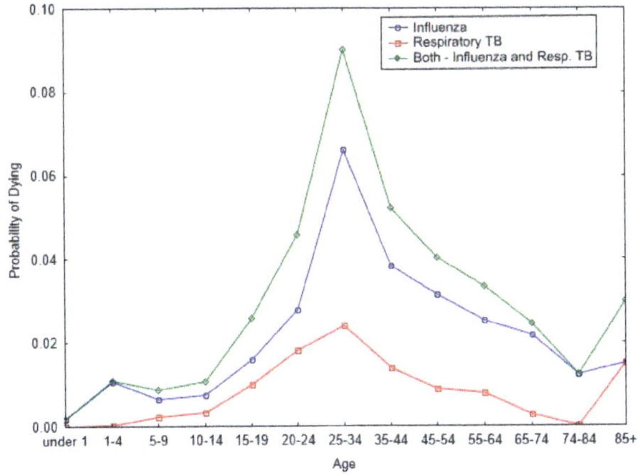

Figure 3. Probability of dying by age categories from 1918/19 influenza and respiratory tuberculosis during the 1918 pandemic.

Table 2. Respiratory tuberculosis death rates (per 1000 living) in Malta for the four time periods.

Age Group	War (P_1)	1918 (P_2)	1919 (P_3)	Post-Pandemic (P_4)
15–44 (reproductive ages)	1.604	2.398	1.736	1.339
45 plus (post-reproductive ages)	0.525	0.823	0.601	0.626

Z-score tests: Reproductive period: P_1 vs. P_2, Z = 19.323, $p < 0.0001$; P_2 vs. P_3, Z = 3.077, $p < 0.003$; P_2 vs. P_4, Z = 6.104. $p < 0.0001$. Post-reproductive period: P_1 vs. P_2, Z = 1.943, ns; P_2 vs. P_3, Z = 1.046, ns; P_2 vs. P_4, Z = 1.239; ns.

Table 3. Age-specific effects on LE differences between war period (1914–1917) and 1918 pandemic period (1918), Malta.

Age	Total Effect	Percent Direct	Percent Indirect
Under 1	−0.17	−0.01	3.65
1 to 4	−0.04	0.04	0.83
5 to 9	−0.13	0.16	2.74
10 to 14	−0.34	0.43	6.91
15 to 19	−1.10	1.47	22.23
20 to 24	−0.75	1.07	15.01
25 to 34	−1.56	4.82	28.75
35 to 44	−0.38	1.48	6.75
45 to 54	−0.30	1.55	4.91
55 to 64	0.17	−1.24	−2.44
65 to 74	−0.09	0.94	1.02
75 to 84	0.05	−0.72	−0.31
85 plus	0.00	−0.06	0.00
Total	−4.65	9.94	90.06

Table 4 shows that the largest significant differences between BM and P_2 (pandemic period) occurred because of the 1918/19 pandemic influenza ($\Delta = 4.052$, $p = 0.001$). There was a significant improvement in the probability of dying during the pandemic due to the diarrhea complex ($\Delta = -0.915$, $p = 0.038$). The lack of significant differences in the contribution of respiratory tuberculosis to the differences in life expectancy between the two periods can be attributed to the fact that tuberculosis affected those primarily in their reproductive prime, and the impact of the disease cannot be observed across the span of 86 years (Figure 3; Table 2).

Table 4. Apportion of cause-specific differences in life expectancy at ages 0 to 85 years between P_1 (war period, 1914–1917) and P_2 (pandemic period, 1918) in Malta.

Cause	LE Difference (Δ)	Probability (*p*-Value)
Influenza	4.052	0. 001
Respiratory tuberculosis	0.592	0.18
Diarrhea, enteritis and gastro-enteritis	−0.915	0.038
Infantile atrophy, debility, and marasmus	0.744	0.092
Measles	−0.461	0.296
Whooping cough	−0.26	0.557
All other causes	0.913	0.039
Residual (distributed among causes)		−0.001
Total	4.664	

Figures 4–6 show the monthly patterns of 1918/19 for the absolute maximum and minimum temperatures, relative humidity, and rainfall against the meteorological baseline of 1906 to 1917. A large deviation in higher relative humidity rates during the 1918/19 pandemic relative to the baseline and post-pandemic periods was observed. The relative humidity remained high in the winter months (third wave of the pandemic) (see Figure 5). While largely subjective, it appears that during the second wave of the influenza pandemic (especially in September and October), maximum temperature, relative humidity, and rainfall total (except for September, where BM rainfall total was higher than pandemic total) were higher than in the BM and post-pandemic periods. Not unexpectedly, the pandemic peaked during the relatively cooler temperatures associated with the fall months (see Figure 4). The post-pandemic period had milder temperatures relative to the pandemic and BM periods, with lower maximum and high minimum shade temperatures.

The epidemic-driven syndemic and its complexities can be dissected further, even beyond the quantitative methodology used. A conceptual framework can be used to assess the syndemic built around three dimensions: driving factors, contributing factors, and limiting factors.

We propose the following as driving factors: environment factors such as relative humidity and rainfall; the First World War and the associated deteriorating economy; and the military presence and interconnectedness with the civilian population. These factors facilitated the elevated rates of both 1918/19 influenza and respiratory tuberculosis. Contributing to the driving factors were the underlying living conditions on the island. Lastly, the magnitude of the syndemic was limited by the numerous mitigation strategies, both at the individual and community level, that were put in place early in the pandemic by government officials. These prevented further transmission of and fatalities from influenza and presumably tuberculosis.

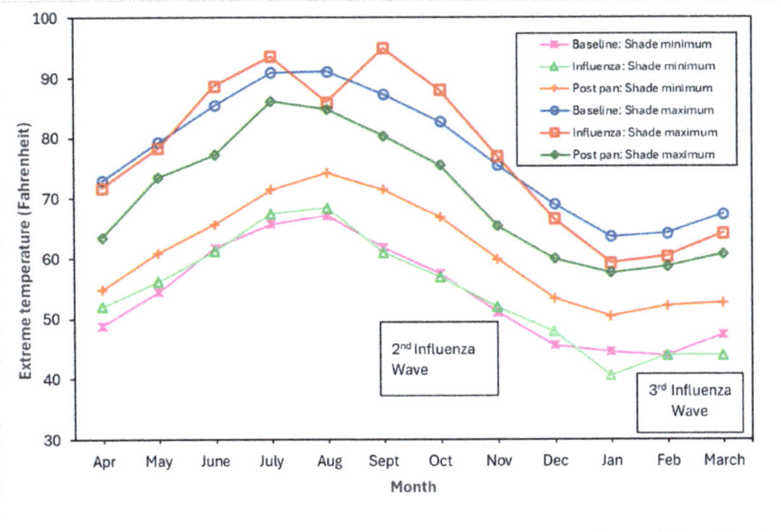

Figure 4. Baseline (1906–1917), pandemic (1918/19), and post-pandemic (1920–1923) minimum shade and maximum shade temperatures.

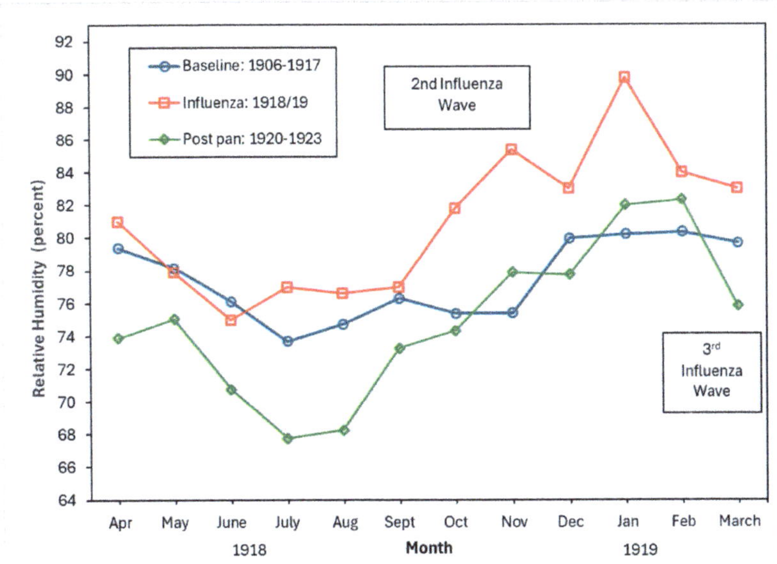

Figure 5. Baseline (1906–1917), pandemic (1918/19), and post-pandemic (1920–1923) relative humidity (percent).

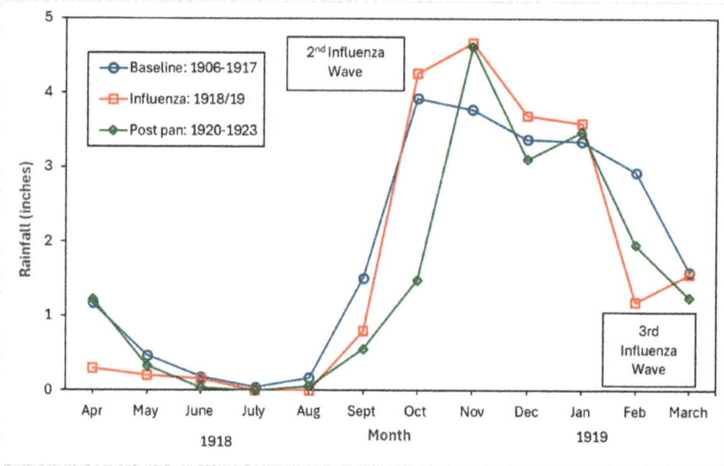

Figure 6. Baseline (1906–1917), pandemic (1918/19), and post-pandemic (1920–1923) rainfall in inches.

4. Discussion

Our study validated the existence of a syndemic during the 1918/19 pandemic. The syndemic of 1918/19 led to a period of unusually low mortality patterns. Beyond the diminished number of deaths due to the influenza complex, we can add that the respiratory tuberculosis death rate among adults (15 to 44 years of age) in 1918 fell from 2.398 per 1000 to 1.736 per 1000 living ($Z = 3.077$, $p < 0.003$). The overall impact was that during the fallow period of 1919, life expectancy at birth increased to 43.49 years from 32.26 years. The life expectancy during the fallow period was also higher than during the war years (37.92 years). In other words, the syndemic period removed the highly vulnerable in the population, corresponding to what scholars who investigate crisis mortality term as short-term mortality replacement followed by a "healthy period".

Unlike its larger sister island of Malta, Gozo did not experience a syndemic of 1918 influenza with tuberculosis, because on the smaller island, tuberculosis deaths rates remained relatively stable over the early part of the 20th century. According to the CMOH at the time, Dr. Critien, the agrarian lifestyle of the Gozitans contributed to the lower rates of respiratory tuberculosis because they were spending more time outside, in addition to the isolative nature of the island [41].

The syndemic nature of tuberculosis and pandemic influenza in Malta was even apparent to the health officials at the time. When summarizing the pattern of 1918 influenza during the pandemic, Doctor Critien (CMOH) acutely observed that influenza was "...in my opinion, connected with diminished physical resistance of the masses brought about by the war. In many cases, also intercurrent influenzal infection must have given a spurt to *tubercular disease* where it was active and contributed to fan it into actively where it was latent" [41].

Based on the proposed conceptual framework, we propose the following as contributing to, driving, or counteracting/limiting the syndemic:

4.1. Contributing Factors: Underlying Living Conditions

Even though there would have been regional variation with regard to the living situations across the island, the general consensus was that the majority of the Maltese were poor. A number of prevailing conditions on the Maltese Islands during our study period created an ideal environment that facilitated the spread of infections, especially frequent childhood epidemics such as measles and whooping cough, as well as endemic diseases such as gastro-enteritis, undulant fever [63], and trachoma [64]. These conditions included the following: first, the standard of housing in most towns and villages was low; second, the houses were small, with overcrowding the norm. For example, in 1911, the average number of persons in a dwelling unit, exclusive of institutions, was 4.84 [43]. Third, family size was large. For women who were married at under 20 years of age, the average number of children was 10, and for women who married between 20 and 25 years of age, the average number of children was 8. Regardless of age at marriage, on average there were 6.51 children per family [65,66]. As such, many children were forced to sleep together in a single room in close contact. Fourth, laid-on water within the household was lacking, and it was often necessary to draw water from public taps and carry it home, thereby limiting personal hygiene and the frequency of laundering. Family members were forced to use the same towels and wash in the same water, such that personal cleanliness was a constant hygiene issue in Maltese households. Fifth, sanitary conditions in and outside the home were abysmal, facilitating the breeding of flies and vermin. Public and household sanitation amenities were poor or virtually absent. In rural settlements, open-air cesspits and latrines were commonplace. Finally, the diet of the lower classes was universally poor: rich in carbohydrates but lacking in fats or meat.

4.2. Driving Factors: Environmental

Despite the vast body of literature on the 1918/19 influenza pandemic and the myriads of factors that played a role in the spread of the pathogen (see, for example, [67]), the importance of meteorological factors such as temperature, rainfall, and relative humidity has received scant attention with regard to pandemic influenza. And although there has been a dearth of studies on the relationship between these meteorological factors and respiratory tuberculosis, the few contemporary studies from China show that there is a correlation between high temperatures, high relative humidity, windspeed, and the incidence of pulmonary tuberculosis [68]. However, some studies found a negative correlation between relative humidity and tuberculosis risk, and that there were lags (in days) in the relationship between meteorological factors and the relative risk of tuberculosis cases [69]. While our research offers only a qualitative perspective, it suggests that unlike the cool and dry conditions proposed as a driver of seasonal influenza [67], higher maximum temperatures, relative humidity, and higher rainfall amounts (compared to the baseline) were clearly associated with the second and third influenza waves (for relative humidity only) of the 1918/19 pandemic. In Malta, during the autumn and winter months with cooler temperatures, the lack of central heating meant that residents of a household would crowd together around a stove fueled by paraffin or propane. Increased familial interpersonal contact under these circumstances would increase the probability of droplet pathogen spread.

4.3. Driving Factors: Declining Economy During the First World War

The national economy of Malta during the war relied heavily on servicing the Royal Navy. As the war progressed, there was a decline in war-related activities, resulting in an increasing number of men and women who were working at lower wages relative to the years before the war, and a significant number of unemployed individuals. The war effort originally generated economic prosperity for the Maltese, but this wealth was short lived. By 1916, the cost of living had doubled, accompanied by increased unemployment rates, employment insecurity, and food shortages. Furthermore, the prices of food items increased; they were of substandard quality and challenging to obtain, even at elevated costs [70]. For instance, between 1914 and 1918, the prices of high-protein food items (fish, meat, cheese, eggs) soared from 200% to 500% [71]. Bread served as a crucial food staple, primarily providing energy for the impoverished. Throughout the First World War, wheat prices surged as flour supplies diminished markedly, resulting in a threefold increase in bread prices by the war's conclusion. The severe bread scarcity incited social discontent and a walkout at the Malta Dockyard in May 1917.

4.4. Driving Factors: Increasingly Poor Housing Conditions, Overcrowding, and Water Insecurity

Additional evidence of the precarious living conditions was the scarcity of available and new dwellings, a deficiency that undoubtedly exacerbated congestion since family sizes in Malta persisted unabated. We contend that household security was undermined not only by increasing unemployment rates, low wages, and precarious employment, but also by the decline in new housing construction throughout the war years, which intensified the prevailing overcrowding issue. The stagnation of housing was apparent in 1915, as the number of houses constructed decreased from 152 in Malta to 17 by 1920–1921. This was exactly the time when respiratory tuberculosis rates increased. Improvements in living conditions occurred only in 1922, with the construction of 5311 dwellings in Malta between 1922 and 1933 [72]. It would appear that there was a decline in population density between 1911 and 1921 (the two census periods). In 1911 (pre-pandemic), population density stood at 1815 persons per square mile, which dipped to 1778 persons per square mile in 1921 (post-pandemic). This small decline, however, was most likely a reflection of the emigration of the population that occurred after the armistice in November 1918, when emigration by the government was encouraged to alleviate overcrowding on the island [73]. By 1931, population density surged to 2016 persons per square mile. Further, overcrowding at the household level (measured by when there are more than two people living in one room in a tenement of fewer than five rooms) was relatively high during the pre-pandemic period in 1911 at 20.9 percent, dropping slightly to 19.07 percent of families being in overcrowded homes in 1921. In keeping with government officials' comments on improvements in living conditions after 1921, household overcrowding dropped to 16.5 percent by 1931 [43,45,74] (Government of Malta: 1912, 1922, 1932). Overcrowding, unemployment, and elevated prices of food and other essentials compromised overall health, while the lack of public welfare for the impoverished further deteriorated the well-being of the Maltese working class.

The Maltese have faced challenges with securing adequate accommodation throughout the centuries, spanning from cave dwellings to present housing. Acquiring accommodation that was spacious, ventilated, well drained, clean, and possessed vital water resources was very important in maintaining the well-being of the Maltese. Access to a plentiful supply of potable water is arguably the most critical component for both cleanliness and for drinking purposes. Due to the size and geography of the islands, water supply was critical for the maintenance of a sanitary home environment, the cleansing of cooking and eating materials, and the washing of clothing. This was particularly important during the long hot summer months, where a shortage of rainwater was a constant source of anxiety and stress. The risk of contracting enteropathogens from their immediate surroundings, given the unhygienic state at the household level, was a constant health risk during the study period.

4.5. Limiting Factors: 1918/19 Influenza Mitigation Strategies

The first mitigation measure was introduced on 9 September 1918, and was printed in the newspaper. The notice included information on droplet transmission and handkerchief use, and emphasized the importance of isolating the sick, as well as fresh air and light for destroying the virus. It instructed readers to avoid gatherings in crowded places. The PMOH, Dr. Critien, recommended that the leaflet be translated into Italian and Maltese [75].

By September 16th, both individual and general prophylaxes had been implemented. At the individual level, there was to be isolation at home or removal to the Manoel Infectious Diseases Hospital for severe cases, and in cases complicated by pneumonia or bronco-pneumonia, in addition to the disinfection of rooms, bedding, and linen.

In cases of influenza that originated in other hospitals, charitable institutions, prisons, ships in harbor, and/or in cases without proper care and accommodation, it was recommended that patients be transported to the Manoel Infectious Diseases Hospital [75].

At the general or community level, the following measures were put in place:

1. Prevention of overcrowding in public places, cinemas, theatres, and other places of amusement; cleanliness, aeration, and disinfection;
2. Disinfection of public places with large amounts of people, such as railway carriages and ferryboats;
3. Reduction in visitations to hospitals and other charitable institutions; discontinuance of pawning off clothes, etc.;
4. Closure of government schools;
5. Increased visiting of dwellings, etc., by sanitary inspectors;
6. Temporary surveillance of all arrivals from abroad and disinfection of personal belongings in certain cases.

For other prophylactic measures that were implemented during the pandemic, please see Supplementary Table S1. Table S1 details the 1918/19 influenza pandemic mitigation strategies in Malta.

5. Conclusions

Following a method to quantitively operationalize short-term syndemics previously proposed by two of the authors [18], we demonstrated that there was a syndemic relationship during the 1918/19 influenza pandemic of the influenza virus with respiratory tuberculosis. Life expectancy during the pandemic significantly dropped (LE = 33.26 $\pm$ 0.340) compared to the pre-pandemic and war years (LE = 37.92 $\pm$ 0.209; Z = 10.56; $p < 0.0001$). Further, in 1919, life expectancy exceeded the pandemic life expectancy (LE = 43.49 $\pm$ 0.431; Z = 17.61; $p < 0.0001$) and surpassed levels observed during the study period, showing evidence of the harvest effect followed by a "healthy period". The fact that the respiratory tuberculosis death rate among those in their reproductive years significantly rose during the pandemic from 1.60 to 2.40 per 1000 living (Z = 19.32; $p < 0.00010$), and significantly declined to 1.74 per 100 living in 1919 (Z = 3.08; $p < 0.003$), is indicative of a crisis event and a syndemic with influenza. We propose that when there is a potential syndemic resulting from a short-term event (such as an epidemic), it would be beneficial to extend our reproducible method to also include an assessment of the dimensions of the syndemic contributing, driving, and limiting factors. In our study of the 1918/19 pandemic in Malta, the contributing factors were the existing inadequate living conditions that were conducive to the spread of infectious diseases, especially childhood infections.

We qualitatively observed environmental factors such as ambient temperature, relative humidity, and rainfall as potentially driving the syndemic. Another driver of the syndemic was the economy associated with the First World War. The exacerbation of living conditions such as overcrowding was an additional driving factor of the syndemic. Finally, the early implementation of effective mitigation measures, despite the lack of knowledge on the transmission of the virus, such as limiting mass gatherings and disinfecting public buildings and institutions, would have worked to limit the extent of the interaction of the two diseases, reducing the transmission of both influenza and tuberculosis.

Our framework to conceptualize the syndemic potential during the 1918 influenza pandemic in Malta contributes to the study of syndemics beyond the small former British colony and beyond studies of past epidemics and pandemics. This framework, which is grounded in crisis mortality and the harvesting effect, can easily be applied to the assessment of other short-term novel events. Further, to capture the factors involved in the syndemic, exploring contributing, driving, and limiting dimensions is useful for deconstructing the components involved in situations where syndemics occur over a limited period of time.

Supplementary Materials: The following supporting information can be downloaded at: https://www.mdpi.com/article/10.3390/tropicalmed10060149/s1, Table S1: Mitigation strategies during 1918/19 influenza pandemic in Malta.

Author Contributions: Conceptualization, L.T. and L.A.S.; methodology, L.T. and L.A.S.; software, L.A.S.; validation, L.T., L.A.S. and C.J.F.; formal analysis, L.T. and L.A.S.; investigation, L.T., L.A.S. and C.J.F.; resources, L.T., L.A.S. and C.J.F.; data curation, L.T., L.A.S. and C.J.F.; writing—original draft preparation, L.T., L.A.S. and C.J.F.; writing—review and editing, L.T. and C.J.F.; visualization, L.T. and L.A.S.; supervision, L.T.; project administration, L.T. and L.A.S.; funding acquisition, L.T. All authors have read and agreed to the published version of the manuscript.

Funding: This research was funded by the Social Sciences and Humanities Research Council (SSRHC) Insight development grant, file number 430-2022-01032.

Institutional Review Board Statement: Not applicable.

Informed Consent Statement: Not applicable.

Data Availability Statement: Data will be made available upon request.

Acknowledgments: We would like dedicate this publication to our dear friend, colleague, and mentor, Larry Sawchuk, without whom this paper would not have been publishable. We miss your guidance and support, collegiality, and above all your friendship for nearly 20 years.

Conflicts of Interest: The authors declare no conflicts of interest. The funders had no role in the design of the study; in the collection, analyses, or interpretation of data; in the writing of the manuscript; or in the decision to publish the results.

Abbreviations

The following abbreviations are used in this manuscript:

TB	Tuberculosis
BM	Baseline mortality

References

1. Mamelund, S.E.; Dimka, J. Tuberculosis as a risk factor for 1918 influenza pandemic outcomes. *Trop. Med. Infect. Dis.* **2019**, *4*, 74. [CrossRef] [PubMed]
2. Noymer, A.; Garenne, M. The 1918 influenza epidemic's effects on sex differentials in mortality in the United States. *Popul. Dev. Rev.* **2000**, *26*, 565–581. [CrossRef] [PubMed]
3. Noymer, A. Testing the influenza–tuberculosis selective mortality hypothesis with Union Army data. *Soc. Sci. Med.* **2009**, *68*, 1599–1608. [CrossRef]
4. Tripp, L.; Sawchuk, L.A.; Saliba, M. Deconstructing the 1918–1919 influenza pandemic in the Maltese Islands: A biosocial perspective. *Curr. Anthropol.* **2018**, *59*, 229–239. [CrossRef]
5. Herring, D.A.; Sattenspiel, L. Social contexts, syndemics, and infectious disease in northern Aboriginal populations. *Am. J. Hum. Biol. Off. J. Hum. Biol. Assoc.* **2007**, *19*, 190–202. [CrossRef]
6. Van Doren, T. Social Inequalities and Mortality During the 1918 Influenza Pandemic on the Island of Newfoundland. Ph.D. Thesis, University of Missouri-Columbia, Columbia, MI, USA, 2022.
7. Singer, M. *Introduction to Syndemics: A Critical Systems Approach to Public and Community Health*; John Wiley & Sons: San Francisco, CA, USA, 2009.

8. Singer, M.; Snipes, C. Generations of suffering: Experiences of a treatment program for substance abuse during pregnancy. *J. Health Care Poor Underserved* **1992**, *3*, 222–234. [CrossRef]
9. Singer, M. A dose of drugs, a touch of violence, a case of AIDS: Conceptualizing the SAVA syndemic. *Free. Inq. Creat. Sociol.* **2000**, *28*, 13–24.
10. Ostrach, B.; Singer, M. Syndemics of war: Malnutrition-infectious disease interactions and the unintended health consequences of intentional war policies. *Ann. Anthropol. Pract.* **2012**, *36*, 257–273. [CrossRef]
11. Mendenhall, E.; Singer, M. What constitutes a syndemic? Methods, contexts, and framing from 2019. *Curr. Opin. HIV AIDS* **2020**, *15*, 213–217. [CrossRef]
12. Singer, M.; Bulled, N.; Ostrach, B.; Mendenhall, E. Syndemics and the biosocial conception of health. *Lancet* **2017**, *389*, 941–950. [CrossRef]
13. Singer, M.; Clair, S. Syndemics and public health: Reconceptualizing disease in bio-social context. *Med. Anthropol. Q.* **2003**, *17*, 423–441. [CrossRef] [PubMed]
14. Revich, B.; Shaposhnikov, D. Excess mortality during heat waves and cold spells in Moscow, Russia. *Occup. Environ. Med.* **2008**, *65*, 691–696. [CrossRef] [PubMed]
15. Smith, R.L. Invited commentary: Timescale-dependent mortality effects of air pollution. *Am. J. Epidemiol.* **2003**, *157*, 1066–1070. [CrossRef] [PubMed]
16. Toulemon, L.; Barbieri, M. The mortality impact of the August 2003 heat wave in France: Investigating the 'harvesting' effect and other long-term consequences. *Popul. Stud.* **2008**, *62*, 39–53. [CrossRef]
17. Zanobetti, A.; Wand, M.P.; Schwartz, J.; Ryan, L.M. Generalized additive distributed lag models: Quantifying mortality displacement. *Biostatistics* **2000**, *1*, 279–292. [CrossRef]
18. Sawchuk, L.A.; Tripp, L.; Samakaroon, M. Assessing a syndemic: Gibraltar in the time of cholera. *Soc. Sci. Med.* **2022**, *295*, 112956. [CrossRef]
19. Chowell, G.; Bettencourt, L.M.; Johnson, N.; Alonso, W.J.; Viboud, C. The 1918–1919 influenza pandemic in England and Wales: Spatial patterns in transmissibility and mortality impact. *Proc. R. Soc. B Biol. Sci.* **2008**, *275*, 501–509. [CrossRef]
20. Chowell, G.; Erkoreka, A.; Viboud, C.; Echeverri-Dávila, B. Spatial-temporal excess mortality patterns of the 1918–1919 influenza pandemic in Spain. *BMC Infect. Dis.* **2014**, *14*, 371. [CrossRef]
21. Grantz, K.H.; Rane, M.S.; Salje, H.; Glass, G.E.; Schachterle, S.E.; Cummings, D.A. Disparities in influenza mortality and transmission related to sociodemographic factors within Chicago in the pandemic of 1918. *Proc. Natl. Acad. Sci. USA* **2016**, *113*, 13839–13844. [CrossRef]
22. Gravlee, C.C. Systemic racism, chronic health inequities, and COVID-19: A syndemic in the making? *Am. J. Hum. Biol.* **2020**, *32*, e23482. [CrossRef]
23. Tsai, A.C.; Mendenhall, E.; Trostle, J.A.; Kawachi, I. Co-occurring epidemics, syndemics, and population health. *Lancet* **2017**, *389*, 978–982. Available online: https://www.ncbi.nlm.nih.gov/pmc/articles/PMC5972361/ (accessed on 27 December 2021). [CrossRef] [PubMed]
24. Tripp, L.; Sawchuk, L.A. Insights into secular trends of respiratory tuberculosis: The 20th century Maltese experience. *PLoS ONE* **2017**, *12*, e0183296. [CrossRef] [PubMed]
25. Kinsella, K.G. Changes in life expectancy 1900–1990. *Am. J. Clin. Nutr.* **1992**, *55*, 1196S–1202S. [CrossRef]
26. Sawchuk, L.A. Deconstructing colonial health differentials: Malta and Gibraltar prior to World War II. *J. Malt. Hist.* **2008**, *1*, 19–32.
27. Bruce, G.R. *Influenza Epidemic Among Officers and Men of H. M.'s Navy and Naval Establishments*; CSG 01.1919 Jan 15; National Archives of Malta: Mdina, Malta, 1919.
28. Cobbett, L. The decline of tuberculosis and the increase in its mortality during the war. *Epidemiol. Infect.* **1930**, *30*, 79–103. [CrossRef]
29. Drolet, G.J. World War I and tuberculosis. A statistical summary and review. *Am. J. Public Health Nations Health* **1945**, *35*, 689–697. [CrossRef]
30. Murray, J.F. Tuberculosis and World War I. *Am. J. Respir. Crit. Care Med.* **2015**, *192*, 411–414. [CrossRef]
31. Government of Malta. *Reports on the Health of the Maltese Islands During 1914–1915*; Government Printing Office: Marsa, Malta, 1915.
32. Government of Malta. *Reports on the Health of the Maltese Islands During 1915–1916*; Government Printing Office: Marsa, Malta, 1916.
33. Government of Malta. *Reports on the Health of the Maltese Islands During 1916–1917*; Government Printing Office: Marsa, Malta, 1917.
34. Government of Malta. *Reports on the Health of the Maltese Islands During 1917–1918*; Government Printing Office: Marsa, Malta, 1918.
35. Government of Malta. *Reports on the Health of the Maltese Islands During 1920–1921*; Government Printing Office: Marsa, Malta, 1921.

36. Government of Malta. *Reports on the Health of the Maltese Islands During 1921–1922*; Government Printing Office: Marsa, Malta, 1922.
37. Government of Malta. *Reports on the Health of the Maltese Islands During 1922–1923*; Government Printing Office: Marsa, Malta, 1923.
38. Government of Malta. *Reports on the Health of the Maltese Islands During 1923–1924*; Government Printing Office: Marsa, Malta, 1924.
39. Government of Malta. *Death Registry of the Maltese Islands for 1918 and 1919*; Government Printing Office: Marsa, Malta, 1919.
40. Government of Malta. *Death Registry of the Maltese Islands for 1919 and 1920*; Government Printing Office: Marsa, Malta, 1920.
41. Government of Malta. *Reports on the Health of the Maltese Islands During 1918–1919*; Government Printing Office: Marsa, Malta, 1919.
42. Government of Malta. *Reports on the Health of the Maltese Islands During 1919–1920*; Government Printing Office: Marsa, Malta, 1920.
43. Government of Malta. *Census of the Islands of Malta, 1911*; Government Printing Office: Marsa, Malta, 1912.
44. Johnson, P.; Spoorenberg, T.; Hertog, S.; Gerland, P. *Method Protocol for the Evaluation of Census Population Data by Age and Sex*; UN DESA/POP/2022/TP/No.5; United Nations Department of Economic and Social Affairs: New York, NY, USA, 2022; pp. 1–47.
45. Government of Malta. *Census of the Islands of Malta, 1921*; Government Printing Office: Marsa, Malta, 1922.
46. Government of Malta. *Reports on the Health of the Maltese Islands During 1906–1907*; Government Printing Office: Marsa, Malta, 1907.
47. Government of Malta. *Reports on the Health of the Maltese Islands During 1907–1908*; Government Printing Office: Marsa, Malta, 1908.
48. Government of Malta. *Reports on the Health of the Maltese Islands During 1908–1909*; Government Printing Office: Marsa, Malta, 1909.
49. Government of Malta. *Reports on the Health of the Maltese Islands During 1909–1910*; Government Printing Office: Marsa, Malta, 1910.
50. Government of Malta. *Reports on the Health of the Maltese Islands During 1910–1911*; Government Printing Office: Marsa, Malta, 1911.
51. Government of Malta. *Reports on the Health of the Maltese Islands During 1911–1912*; Government Printing Office: Marsa, Malta, 1912.
52. Government of Malta. *Reports on the Health of the Maltese Islands During 1912–1913*; Government Printing Office: Marsa, Malta, 1913.
53. Government of Malta. *Reports on the Health of the Maltese Islands During 1913–1914*; Government Printing Office: Marsa, Malta, 1914.
54. Smith, D.P. *Survival 9.2: A Program for Life Tables and Related Measures*; University of Texas Public Health: Austin, TX, USA, 2004.
55. Chiang, C.L. *The Life Table and Its Applications*; Robert E. Krieger Publishing Co.: Malabar, FL, USA,, 1984.
56. Manuel, D.G.; Goel, V.; Williams, J.I. The derivation of life tables for local areas. *Chronic Dis. Inj. Can.* **1998**, *19*, 52–56.
57. Scherbov, S.; Ediev, D. Significance of life table estimates for small populations: Simulation-based study of standard errors. *Demogr. Res.* **2011**, *24*, 527–550. [CrossRef]
58. Arriaga, E.E. Measuring and explaining the change in life expectancies. *Demography* **1984**, *21*, 83–96. [CrossRef]
59. Arriaga, E.E. Changing trends in mortality decline during the last decades. In *Differential Mortality: Methodological Issues and Biosocial Factors*; Ruzicka, L., Wunsch, G., Kane, K., Eds.; Clarendon Press: Oxford, UK, 1989; pp. 105–129.
60. Auger, N.; Feuillet, P.; Martel, S.; Lo, E.; Barry, A.D.; Harper, S. Mortality inequality in populations with equal life expectancy: Arriaga's decomposition method in SAS, Stata, and Excel. *Ann. Epidemiol.* **2014**, *24*, 575–580. [CrossRef] [PubMed]
61. Carolina Population Center (n.d.). Measure Evaluation, Lesson 5: Expectation at Life at Birth. Available online: https://www.measureevaluation.org/resources/training/online-courses-and-resources/non-certificate-courses-and-mini-tutorials/multiple-decrement-life-tables/lesson-5 (accessed on 27 December 2021).
62. StatSoft Inc. *STATISTICA (Data Analysis Software System), Version 10*; StatSoft Inc.: Tulsa, OK, USA, 2011; Available online: http://www.statsoft.com (accessed on 28 December 2024).
63. Tripp, L.; Sawchuk, L.A. Colonialism, Culture, and Compliancy: A case study of Undulant Fever. In *Colonial Encounters: Maltese Experiences of British Rule*; Chircop, J., Ed.; Malta University Press: Msida, Malta, 2015; pp. 211–247.
64. Damato, F.J. The fight against trachoma in the island of Malta. *Br. J. Ophthalmol.* **1961**, *45*, 71. [CrossRef] [PubMed]
65. Ciappara, F. Marriage and the family in a Maltese parish: St. Mary's (Qrendi) in the eighteenth century. *J. Fam. Hist.* **2011**, *36*, 37–51. [CrossRef] [PubMed]
66. Seers, D. A fertility survey in the Maltese islands. *Popul. Stud.* **1957**, *10*, 211–228. [CrossRef]
67. Lowen, A.C.; Steel, J. Roles of humidity and temperature in shaping influenza seasonality. *J. Virol.* **2014**, *88*, 7692–7695. [CrossRef]

68. Nie, Y.; Lu, Y.; Wang, C.; Yang, Z.; Sun, Y.; Zhang, Y.; Tian, M.; Rifhat, R.; Zhang, L. Effects and interaction of meteorological factors on pulmonary tuberculosis in Urumqi, China, 2013–2019. *Front. Public Health* **2022**, *10*, 951578. [CrossRef]
69. Chang, M.; Emam, M.; Chen, X.; Lu, D.; Zhang, L.; Zheng, Y. An investigation of the effects of meteorological factors on the incidence of tuberculosis. *Sci. Rep.* **2024**, *14*, 2088. [CrossRef]
70. Editor of the Daily Malta Chronicle. The Cost of Living in Malta: A comparison. *The Daily Malta Chronicle*, 16 August 1918.
71. Editor of the Daily Malta Chronicle. The Relative Increase in the Cost of Living in England and Malta. *The Daily Malta Chronicle*, 23 December 1918.
72. Government of Malta. *Reports on the Health of the Maltese Islands During 1933–1934*; Government Printing Office: Marsa, Malta, 1934.
73. Bowen-Jones, H.; Dewdney, J.C.; Fisher, W.B. *Malta: Background for Development*; College of the Durham University: Durham, UK, 1961.
74. Critien, A. *Preliminary Report on Influenza*; Influenza, CSG 01 Sept 18; National Archives of Malta: Mdina, Malta, 1918.
75. Government of Malta. *Census of the Islands of Malta, 1931*; Government Printing Office: Marsa, Malta, 1932.

Tropical Medicine and Infectious Disease

MDPI

Article

Serious Bacterial Infections and Hepatitis C Virus Among People Who Inject Drugs: A Syndemic or Intertwined Epidemics?

Thomas J. Stopka [1,*], Robin M. Nance [2], L. Sarah Mixson [2], Hunter Spencer [3], Judith I. Tsui [2], Judith M. Leahy [4], Mai T. Pho [5], Jean DeJace [6], Judith Feinberg [7], April M. Young [8], Wei-Teng Yang [9], Amelia Baltes [10], Eric Romo [11], Randall T. Brown [10], Kerry Nolte [12], William C. Miller [13], William A. Zule [14], Wiley D. Jenkins [15], Joseph A. Delaney [2] and Peter D. Friedmann [16]

1 Department of Public Health and Community Medicine, Tufts University School of Medicine, Boston, MA 02111, USA
2 Department of Medicine, University of Washington School of Medicine, 1959 NE Pacific Street, Seattle, WA 98195, USA; rmnance@uw.edu (R.M.N.); lsmixson@uw.edu (L.S.M.); tsuij@uw.edu (J.I.T.); jadelaney@uw.edu (J.A.D.)
3 Department of Medicine, Oregon Health & Science University, Portland, OR 97239, USA; spencerh@ohsu.edu
4 SOR Harm Reduction and Public Health Strategist, Behavioral Health Division, Oregon Health Authority, Portland, OR 97232, USA; judith.m.leahy@oha.oregon.gov
5 Department of Medicine, Section of Infectious Diseases & Global Health, University of Chicago, Chicago, IL 60637, USA; mpho@bsd.uchicago.edu
6 Division of Infectious Disease, Department of Medicine, University of Vermont, Burlington, VT 05401, USA
7 Departments of Behavioral Medicine and Psychiatry & Medicine/Infectious Diseases, West Virginia University School of Medicine, Morgantown, WV 26505, USA; judith.feinberg@hsc.wvu.edu
8 Department of Epidemiology and Environmental Health, University of Kentucky College of Public Health, Lexington, KY 40536, USA; april.young@uky.edu
9 Division of Infectious Diseases, Perelman School of Medicine, Center for Addiction Medicine and Policy, University of Pennsylvania, Philadelphia, PA 19104, USA; wei-teng.yang@pennmedicine.upenn.edu
10 Department of Family Medicine and Community Health, University of Wisconsin School of Medicine and Public Health, Madison, WI 53705, USA; amelia.baltes@fammed.wisc.edu (A.B.); randall.brown@fammed.wisc.edu (R.T.B.)
11 Department of Family Medicine, Boston Medical Center, Boston, MA 02118, USA; eric.romo@bmc.org
12 Department of Nursing, University of New Hampshire, Durham, NH 03824, USA; kerry.nolte@unh.edu
13 Department of Epidemiology, Gillings School of Global Public Health, Chapel Hill, NC 27514, USA; bill_miller@unc.edu
14 Division of Behavioral Health and Criminal Justice Research, RTI International, Research Triangle Park, NC 27709, USA; bill.zule@yahoo.com
15 Department of Public Health Sciences, Clemson University, Clemson, SC 29634, USA; wileyj@clemson.edu
16 Office of Research and Department of Healthcare Delivery & Population Sciences, University of Massachusetts Chan Medical School—Baystate and Baystate Health, Springfield, MA 01107, USA; peter.friedmann@baystatehealth.org
* Correspondence: thomas.stopka@tufts.edu; Tel.: +1-617-636-2110

Abstract: Limited research has examined the possible synergistic interrelationships between serious bacterial infections (SBIs) of the heart (i.e., endocarditis), bone, spine, brain, or joints (e.g., osteomylelitis) and hepatitis C virus (HCV) infections. We examined whether syndemic interactions existed between SBI, HCV, and substance-use-related factors in rural communities, hypothesizing that injection-mediated risks elevated the likelihood for both SBIs and HCV infections, which could be exacerbated by synergistic biological–biological or biological and social interactions. We calculated the prevalence ratios (PRs) of past-year SBI associated with each risk factor in separate models. Effect modification among significant risk factors was assessed using multiplicative interaction. Among 1936 participants, 57% were male and 85% White, with a mean age of 36 years. Eighty-nine participants (5%) reported hospitalization for an SBI in the year prior to the survey. More than half tested HCV-antibody-positive (58%); 62 (5.6%) of the participants with a positive HCV antibody result reported past-year hospitalization with an SBI. Injection behaviors were correlated with other SBI risk factors, including multiple injections in the same injection event (MIPIE), injection equipment sharing, and fentanyl use. In adjusted models, MIPIE (PR: 1.79; 95% confidence interval [CI]: 1.03, 3.11) and fentanyl use (PR: 1.68; 95% CI: 1.04, 2.73) were significantly associated with past-year SBI. Our analyses pointed to co-occurring epidemics of SBI and HCV, related to the cumulative health effects of fentanyl use contributing to frequent injections and MIPIE. Both the SBI and HCV epidemics present public health challenges and merit tailored interventions.

Keywords: serious bacterial infections; hepatitis C virus; rural; people who inject drugs; syndemic

1. Introduction

The current injection drug use crisis continues to present major challenges to public health in the US. Substance use and other health outcomes are often intertwined, producing synergistic interactions that have been characterized as syndemics [1], helping to reconceptualize how biological and social factors combine to exacerbate health outcomes [2]. Syringe-mediated syndemics, which have been described previously [3], have also begun to take on new meaning, as the ever-changing nonprescribed drug supply impacts injection frequency and practices, which can, in turn, foster new risks and synergies for infectious disease acquisition [4,5]. Moving beyond the early definitions and exploration by Singer and colleagues [1,2,6], the applications of syndemics theory have expanded, with increasing relevance for public health and clinical medicine [7,8] and expanded data and analytical approaches [8–12].

The increased frequency of injection drug use (IDU) has resulted in a range of serious bacterial infections (SBIs). SBIs encompass skin and soft tissue infections (SSTIs), bacteremia, osteomyelitis, septic arthritis, endocarditis, and other deep abscesses [13–16]. The increase in IDU-related infectious complications is multifactorial and may reflect the evolving drug supply, where IDU was previously uncommon [17], as well as changes in the risk environment surrounding IDU (i.e., changes in the drug market, access to harm reduction services) [18,19]. IDU-related SBIs are associated with high morbidity and mortality [20], with a more than fifty-fold increase in death in some studies [21].

Hospitalization rates and hospitalization costs associated with IDU-related SBIs are important measures of the social, economic, and public health burden of IDU [22–24]. They also highlight critical opportunities for substance use disorder (SUD) screening, harm reduction services, and patient engagement—all interventions that can and should happen at both the hospital and community level [25]. Recent reports of increased hospitalizations for SBIs [14,17,24,26] and population-based analyses of hospitalization trends and costs among people who inject drugs (PWID) [17,23,27] indicate an urgent need to optimize resource allocation to the clinical and public health interventions that are best suited to limiting the infectious consequences of IDU. Injection-related infections are especially a concern in rural areas, which may be affected disproportionately [28]. Among rural residents, US hospitalization rates for opioid-use-associated infective endocarditis increased from 0.28 to 3.86 per 100,000 rural residents from 2002 to 2016 [29].

For decades, HCV incidence and prevalence have been exceedingly high among PWID in the US [30,31], with injection-mediated infection occurring relatively early in substance use trajectories [32], leading to high rates of infection in younger populations [33–35]. Historically, HCV treatment among PWID has been poorly addressed. However, evidence that direct-acting antiviral treatment is effective for people who use drugs, as well as ethical and legal arguments, has led to a loosening of restrictions for treatment and successful treatment of active injectors [36–38]. The rural HCV risk environment is compounded by geographic isolation, limited access to transportation, stigma, and less frequent access to harm reduction services; these factors often contribute to high-risk injection events (e.g., syringe sharing, syringe reuse, and multiple injections per injection episode [MIPIE]) [39]. Recent research focused on drug-use-related risks and HCV across eight rural sites in the US found that, compared to people who injected only stimulants, HCV antibody positivity was more prevalent among people who injected opioids alone, injected both opioids and stimulants separately, and injected both drugs with the same syringe [40].

To date, limited prior research has examined SBIs associated with IDU in rural settings or the factors associated with a higher risk of SBIs. The few studies that have assessed SBIs in rural settings have focused on infectious endocarditis [29,41]. Even fewer studies have focused on the possible synergistic interrelationships between SBIs and HCV. Prior research suggests that chronic HCV might be an independent risk factor for bacterial infections, through pathways including reduced bacterial clearance in the setting of cirrhosis or other liver injury [42,43], but the literature is scarce. High levels of streptococcal pneumonia have been documented among people living with HCV [44]. Viral hepatitis is a leading cause of chronic liver disease and cirrhosis, which has been associated with an increased risk of SSTIs [45,46], including those with unusual pathogens [47].

Homelessness, historically considered an urban issue, is a major public health challenge among people who use drugs (PWUD) in rural regions of the US and is associated with a number of drug-related behaviors that increase the risk of acquisition of bloodborne infections [48]. While rural people who inject drugs (PWID) who experience homelessness use syringe services programs (SSPs) at similar rates as those who are housed, housing instability may present barriers to more frequent SSP use [49]. SSPs provide access to alcohol wipes and increasingly to wound care specialists, offering opportunities to improve skin hygiene and reduced risks relating to the progression from SSTIs to SBIs.

Given these initial associations and potential interactions between SBIs and HCV, we sought to (1) examine associations between SBIs and HCV in a large rural sample of PWID, while considering other social factors associated with the two infections and (2) determine whether syndemic interactions (i.e., biological–biological and biological–social) existed between SBI, HCV, and other substance-use-related factors in rural communities. We hypothesized that the four outcomes of interest (drug use, HCV, SBI, and homelessness) were co-occurring and mutually reinforcing, and thus, a syndemic according to the definition given by Singer et al. [1] We operationalized "injection drug use" as the type of substance injected (fentanyl and/or methamphetamine) and IDU-related risk behaviors, including MIPIE and injection equipment sharing. This conceptual hypothesis implies that models predicting any of the four outcomes would find significant interactions between each of the other outcomes (Figure 1).

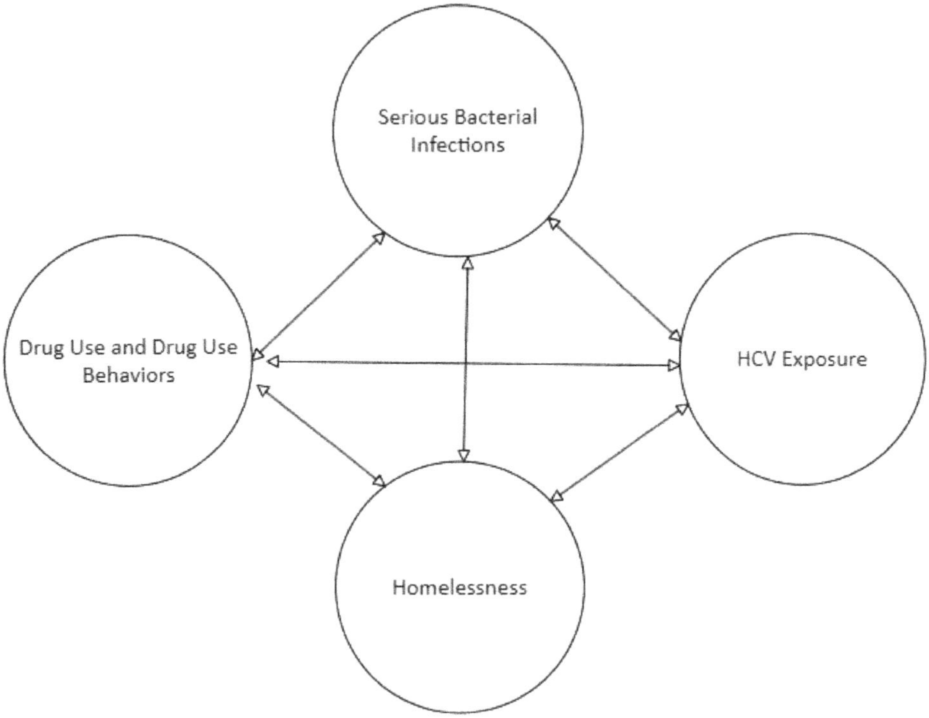

Figure 1. Initial hypothesis. We hypothesized that drug use (including the type of drug injected) and drug use behaviors (practicing multiple injections per injection episode [MIPIE] or injection equipment sharing), serious bacterial infection (SBI), hepatitis C virus infection (HCV), and homelessness existed in a "mutually causal" relationship [9]. Two-sided arrows represent expected relationships and potential interactions between outcomes.

2. Materials and Methods

This study relied on data from seven rural sites that comprised the Rural Opioid Initiative (ROI) consortium across the United States [50]. ROI sites used modified respondent-driven sampling to recruit people reporting their past 30-day use of opioids or injected drugs [51]. Baseline survey and laboratory data were collected between January 2018 and March 2020.

The ROI study locations ranged from Northern New England (Massachusetts, New Hampshire, Vermont) to Appalachia (Kentucky, North Carolina, Ohio, West Virginia), the Midwest (Illinois, Wisconsin), and the Pacific Northwest (Oregon). All study sites were located within counties that were classified as rural as per the US Health Resources and Services Administration definition (https://www.ruralhealthinfo.org/am-i-rural, accessed on 15 August 2024).

We collected survey data from each participant at a baseline visit, which included substance use, IDU-related behaviors, date of last SBI, demographics, and housing. HCV antibody status was also measured via a rapid test or at central lab facilities. Only those participants reporting injection drug use in the past 30 days were included in this analysis.

The primary outcome of this study is a self-report of the past 12-month SBI at baseline: "Have you ever been hospitalized for a serious bacterial infection of the heart, such as endocarditis, or the bone, spine, brain or a joint, such as osteomyelitis?" "When were you last hospitalized for a serious bacterial infection of the heart, such as endocarditis, or the bone, spine, brain, or a joint, such as osteomyelitis? Don't include times when you went to the emergency room and were not admitted to the hospital". The six risk factors of interest were past 30-day fentanyl and/or methamphetamine use, past 30-day sharing of injection equipment, MIPIE, past 6-month homelessness, and current HCV antibody status. We focused on fentanyl and methamphetamine given that these substances were typically injected more frequently due to their short half-life and relatively short euphoric effects. We relied on HCV antibody status as a surrogate for chronic HCV infections, as confirmatory testing was not consistently employed across all sites, and our study population had low HCV treatment rates (12%) [52].

We calculated Pearson correlations between all risk factors, along with *p*-values. We ran relative risk regressions to assess the prevalence ratio (PR) of past-year SBI associated with each risk factor in separate models. We also assessed the effect measure modification between significant risk factors using multiplicative interaction. We ran the same regression models for the secondary outcome, both past-year hospitalization for SBI and HCV-antibody-positive status. We adjusted all models for age, sex, race, and site.

3. Results

The entire ROI cohort included 3048 participants, of whom 1936 reported past 30-day IDU. The participants were 57% male and 85% White, with a mean age of 36 years (Table 1). In the year prior to the baseline survey, 89 participants (5%) reported having been hospitalized for an SBI. All risk factors were commonly reported, ranging from 40% for fentanyl use to 81% for methamphetamine use. More than half tested HCV-antibody-positive (58%); 62 (5.6%) of the participants with a positive HCV antibody test result also reported hospitalization with an SBI in the past year.

Table 1. Characteristics of rural people who injected drugs, Rural Opioid Initiative, United States, 2018–2020.

	No SBI in Past Year	SBI in Past Year	Overall
N	1847	89	1936
Age, mean (SD)	35 (10)	36 (9)	36 (10)
Male	1063 (58%)	44 (49%)	1107 (57%)
White race	1581 (86%)	73 (82%)	1654 (85%)
Site			
IL	100 (5%)	4 (4%)	104 (5%)
KY	212 (11%)	8 (9%)	220 (11%)
NC	163 (9%)	6 (7%)	169 (9%)
NE	341 (18%)	26 (29%)	367 (19%)
OH	165 (9%)	10 (11%)	175 (9%)
OR	127 (7%)	4 (4%)	131 (7%)
WI	739 (40%)	31 (35%)	770 (40%)
HCV-antibody-positive	1055 (57%)	62 (70%)	1117 (58%)
MIPIE	1305 (71%)	73 (82%)	1378 (71%)
Injection equipment sharing	1270 (69%)	69 (78%)	1339 (69%)
Homeless	1052 (57%)	59 (66%)	1111 (57%)
Current fentanyl use	725 (39%)	49 (55%)	774 (40%)
Current methamphetamine use	1503 (81%)	71 (80%)	1574 (81%)

Definitions: Serious bacterial infection (SBI); standard deviation (SD); multiple injections in one injection event (MIPIE); injection equipment sharing: past 30-day distributive and receptive sharing of injection equipment; current fentanyl use: past 30-day fentanyl use; current methamphetamine use: past 30-day methamphetamine use; homeless: past 6-month homelessness; Illinois (IL); Kentucky (KY); North Carolina (NC); New England (NE); Ohio (OH); Oregon (OR); Wisconsin (WI).

The two injection behaviors were correlated with other risk factors (Table 2). MIPIE, injection equipment sharing, and fentanyl use were all correlated, with coefficients > 0.20. Among all participants, 40% reported current fentanyl use, and 71% reported MIPIE (Table 1), and fentanyl was positively and significantly associated with MIPIE (Table 2). Fentanyl use was negatively correlated with methamphetamine use (−0.13), although participants did not always know when they were exposed to fentanyl (Table 2). Fentanyl use, injection equipment sharing, and MIPIE were positively associated with HCV ab+ status, with fentanyl being most strongly associated with HCV (0.24). Methamphetamine use was negatively associated with HCV infection (−0.08). Finally, homelessness was not significantly associated with fentanyl, nor HCV infection (Table 2).

Table 2. Correlation between exposures of interest among rural people who inject drugs, Rural Opioid Initiative, United States, 2018–2020.

	HCV ab+ **	MIPIE	Injection Equipment Sharing	Homeless	Fentanyl
MIPIE	**0.18**				
Injection equipment sharing	**0.17**	**0.32**			
Homeless	−0.02	0.04	**0.07**		
Fentanyl use	**0.24**	**0.24**	**0.21**	0.03	
Methamphetamine use	**−0.08**	−0.02	**0.07**	**0.07**	**−0.13**

Bold entries are significant at $p < 0.05$. ** HCV ab+ infections represent HCV-positive antibody test results at the time of the study survey. Definitions: Multiple injections in one injection event (MIPIE); hepatitis C virus (HCV); antibody (ab); injection equipment sharing: past 30-day distributive and receptive sharing of injection equipment; fentanyl use: past 30-day fentanyl use; methamphetamine use: past 30-day methamphetamine use; homeless: past 6-month homelessness.

In adjusted models, MIPIE (PR: 1.79; 95% confidence interval [CI]: 1.03, 3.11) and fentanyl use (PR: 1.68; 95% CI 1.04, 2.73) were associated with past-year SBI (Table 3). Other risk factors had positive point estimates but did not reach statistical significance (e.g., HCV exposure was not significantly associated with SBI (PR: 1.60; 95% CI: 0.99, 2.59)). There was no significant interaction between MIPIE and fentanyl use. Homelessness was not associated with SBI and HCV. The associations were similar but slightly stronger for the secondary outcome of past-year SBI and positive HCV antibody status, MIPIE (PR: 2.40; 95% CI: 1.13, 5.10), and fentanyl use (PR: 2.35; 95% CI 1.29, 4.29).

Table 3. Multivariable prevalence ratios for serious bacterial infection (SBI) and overlapping SBI and hepatitis C virus (HCV) infections, adjusted for age, sex, race, and study, Rural Opioid Initiative, United States, 2018–2020.

SBI Past-Year Outcome	**PR**	**95% CI**	***p*-Value**
HCV ab+	1.60	0.99, 2.59	0.06
MIPIE	**1.79**	**1.03, 3.11**	**0.04**
Injection equipment sharing	1.48	0.89, 2.46	0.1
Homeless	1.46	0.93, 2.28	0.1
Current fentanyl use	**1.68**	**1.04, 2.73**	**0.04**
Current meth use	1.43	0.78, 2.62	0.3
MIPIE × Current fentanyl	0.75	0.24, 2.29	0.6
SBI and HCV Infections **	PR	95% CI	*p*-value
MIPIE	**2.40**	**1.13, 5.10**	**0.02**
Injection equipment sharing	1.53	0.82, 2.85	0.2
Homeless	1.50	0.88, 2.57	0.1

Table 3. *Cont.*

SBI Past-Year Outcome	PR	95% CI	p-Value
Current fentanyl use	**2.35**	**1.29, 4.29**	**0.005**
Current methamphetamine use	1.10	0.56, 2.16	0.8
MIPIE × Current fentanyl	1.28	0.27, 6.03	0.8

Bold entries are significant at $p < 0.05$. ** SBIs represented the last SBI reported in the past year. HCV infections represented HCV-positive antibody test results at the time of the study survey. Definitions: Multiple injections in one injection event (MIPIE); hepatitis C virus (HCV); serious bacterial infection (SBI); antibody (ab); injection equipment sharing: distributive and receptive sharing of syringes and other injection equipment; prevalence ratio (PR); confidence interval (CI).

4. Discussion

We explored potential syndemic interactions between SBIs, positive HCV antibody status, injection-related behaviors, and rural contextual factors across seven rural sites in the United States. Our modeling results did not support the syndemic hypothesis [1]. Importantly, the lack of significant interaction terms suggested that outcomes were not "mutually causal". Fentanyl use and MIPIE were associated with both SBI and the combined outcome of SBI and HCV, suggesting that fentanyl use and MIPIE were contributing to the co-occurrence of these outcomes. Prior studies point to the short half-life of fentanyl leading to more frequent injection drug use [4], which could inspire MIPIE, a behavior which was documented in an earlier HIV outbreak among people who inject drugs (PWID) [5]. These findings are consistent with co-occurring epidemics in HIV and HCV infections, as well as MIPIE and oxymorphone use in Scott County, Indiana, between 2015 and 2018 [5,18]. Similarly, fentanyl use was associated with increased incidence of HCV exposure among PWID in the San Diego-Tijuana metroplex in 2020–2022 [53], as well as an HIV outbreak among PWID in northeastern Massachusetts between 2015 and 2018 [4].

Further, we did not detect a significant association between HCV exposure and SBI ($p = 0.06$), but the association trended in the direction of a potential mutually reinforcing relationship between these outcomes, meriting further research. While our modeling cannot ascribe causality, we hypothesize that fentanyl use predisposes PWID to MIPIE due to characteristics of the drug (a shorter half-life compared to other opioids) and the practice of injecting a small amount of opioids to determine the potential for fatal overdose risk due to its potency [54,55]. In sum, these findings suggest a new conceptual hypothesis of "parallel epidemics", occurring in a step-wise rather than a mutually reinforcing manner, reflecting the cumulative health effects of one behavior (fentanyl use) contributing to another behavior (more frequent injections and MIPIE) that contributes to health outcomes [9]. Formal mediation and moderation analysis could explore this hypothesis further, given an appropriately large sample [56].

Contrary to our initial hypothesis, we also did not identify significant associations between homelessness and SBIs and HCV infections, despite high levels of homelessness and higher levels of homelessness among participants with past-year SBIs compared to those without SBIs (66% vs. 57%). We anticipated that the risk environment and milieu surrounding drug-related harms [57] among rural study participants with high levels of homelessness would foster less stability and less safe injection behaviors. While we noted modest correlations between homelessness and injection equipment sharing (Table 1), homelessness did not produce meaningful social–behavioral interactions that were associated with SBI and HCV infections in our multivariable models. In comprehensive bivariate analyses of our larger rural sample, Ballard et al. noted marginal associations between homelessness and SBIs, but significant associations between homelessness and overdose risks [48]. This is a reminder that homelessness alone may not produce the social synergistic risks that are needed to drive synergistic infectious interactions among rural PWID but may be associated with other important health outcomes. Bulled and Singer remind us that "in the case of syringe-mediated syndemics, social factors and risky syringe use as well as the nature of interactions among syringe-related infections are two primary areas of concern" [3]. The health care and harm reduction infrastructure in rural communities varies, as does the risk landscape [50]. In New England, we noted significant positive associations between geospatial access to SSPs and HCV infection risks [58], while other sites documented a wide range of social factors, including economic instability and limited economic opportunities, "as well as a lack of physically available HCV prevention and treatment services" [59]. Such varied risk landscapes could impact SBI and HCV co-infection risks and synergies in unique ways, tempering opportunities for syndemic interactions across our entire sample. However, other social factors, including transportation-related access to needed prevention and treatment services, varying health care infrastructures, and poverty levels, among other social factors, may moderate interactions and should be considered in future syndemics research.

Our findings should be considered in light of several limitations. We analyzed the date of last reported SBI hospitalization within one year of the survey date, which implies some level of access to care. We also relied on HCV antibody status via a rapid test or at central lab facilities at the time of the survey. As a result, each infection may not have co-occurred in patients. However, the exposure to both infections likely points to a risk profile that is different from that of PWID patients who did not experience both SBIs and HCV infections. In addition, PWID participants were often recruited through harm reduction programs, which may have contributed to the recruitment of a sample with a different risk profile from the general population of PWID. We did not measure syringe reuse, across all sites, but there is evidence in some rural communities that syringe reuse is common and can be a risk factor for SBIs [60]. Finally, while our focus was on HCV and serious bacterial infections, potential syndemic relationships might exist between other infectious diseases and bacterial infections among rural PWID. HIV prevalence was very low (0.6%) in our sample, and we did not ask participants whether they had ever been infected with tuberculosis or other bacterial infections. Future syndemics-related analyses should consider exploring potential relationships and interactions among other infections.

5. Conclusions

Syndemics theory, since its initial inception 25 years ago [1], has expanded, with increasing relevance for public health and clinical medicine [7,8] and expanded data and analytical approaches [8–12]. We sought to apply syndemics theory to infectious complications related to injection-mediated risks while considering prior described syringe-mediated syndemics [3]. Through surveys and HCV testing completed as part of the Rural Opioid Initiative across several states, we found that HCV infections and SBIs co-existed in some participants. While we hypothesized that HCV and SBIs, together with the local social contextual factor of homelessness, might comprise a syndemic, our analyses instead point to parallel and intertwined epidemics of SBI and HCV, which reflect the cumulative health effects of fentanyl use contributing to frequent injections overall, as well as MIPIE. Both the SBI and HCV epidemics present serious public health and clinical challenges, indicating that prevention and treatment efforts need to be tailored to address both epidemics in concert. Future research in rural communities, informed by syndemics theory, should consider exploring additional associations and interactions among other infections, as well as a wider array of social factors that are unique to the rural risk environment.

Author Contributions: Conceptualization, T.J.S., W.A.Z. and P.D.F.; methodology, T.J.S., P.D.F., R.M.N., L.S.M. and J.A.D.; validation, R.M.N. and L.S.M.; formal analysis, R.M.N. and L.S.M.; data curation, L.S.M., W.-T.Y., W.A.Z., R.T.B. and R.M.N.; writing—original draft preparation, T.J.S.;

writing—review and editing, H.S., J.I.T., J.F., E.R., M.T.P., W.D.J., K.N., A.B., P.D.F., W.-T.Y., W.A.Z., R.T.B., J.D., J.M.L. and L.S.M.; visualization, H.S., R.M.N. and L.S.M.; funding acquisition, T.J.S., P.D.F., J.F., M.T.P., W.D.J., A.M.Y., W.-T.Y., W.A.Z., R.T.B. and W.C.M.; formulation of research goals, W.A.Z.; supervision oversight, W.A.Z. All authors have read and agreed to the published version of the manuscript.

Funding: Primary data collection was supported by grants UG3DA044829/UH3DA044829, G3DA044798/UH3DA044798, UG3DA044830/UH3DA044830, UG3DA044823/UH3DA044823, UH3DA044822/UH3DA044822, UG3DA044831/UH3DA044831, UG3DA044825, UG3DA044826/UH3DA044826, and U24DA044801, co-funded by the National Institute on Drug Abuse (NIDA) with co-funding from the Centers for Disease Control and Prevention (CDC), Substance Abuse and Mental Health Services Administration (SAMHSA), and the Appalachian Regional Commission (ARC). Research presented in this manuscript is the result of secondary data harmonization and analysis and was supported by grant U24DA048538 from NIDA.

Institutional Review Board Statement: All research was conducted in accordance with both the Declarations of Helsinki and Istanbul, and all research were approved by The Baystate Health Institutional Review Board, approval code: #1 BH-17-158.

Informed Consent Statement: Written informed consent was provided by all subjects involved in the study.

Data Availability Statement: We welcome collaboration and encourage mentorship and the use of the ROI data, stripped of all protected health information (PHI), to enable early investigators to address meaningful questions with support to help ensure their success. Additional information can be obtained at the ROI website (ruralopioidinitiative.org) or by contacting the ROI DCC at ruralopioidinitiative@uw.edu. Follow the Rural Opioid Initiative on X @ruralopioids.

Conflicts of Interest: The authors declare no conflicts of interest.

Disclaimer/Publisher's Note: The content is solely the responsibility of the authors and does not necessarily represent the official views of the National Institutes of Health, CDC, SAMHSA, the Department of Health and Human Services, or ARC.

References

1. Singer, M. A dose of drugs, a touch of violence, a case of AIDS: Conceptualizing the SAVA syndemic. *Free. Inq. Creat. Sociol.* **2000**, *28*, 13–24.
2. Singer, M.; Clair, S. Syndemics and public health: Reconceptualizing disease in bio-social context. *Med. Anthropol. Q.* **2003**, *17*, 423–441. [CrossRef]
3. Bulled, N.; Singer, M. Syringe-mediated syndemics. *AIDS Behav.* **2011**, *15*, 1539–1545. [CrossRef] [PubMed]
4. Alpren, C.; Dawson, E.L.; John, B.; Cranston, K.; Panneer, N.; Fukuda, H.D.; Roosevelt, K.; Klevens, R.M.; Bryant, J.; Peters, P.J.; et al. Opioid Use Fueling HIV Transmission in an Urban Setting: An Outbreak of HIV Infection Among People Who Inject Drugs-Massachusetts, 2015–2018. *Am. J. Public Health* **2020**, *110*, 37–44. [CrossRef] [PubMed]
5. Broz, D.; Zibbell, J.; Foote, C.; Roseberry, J.C.; Patel, M.R.; Conrad, C.; Chapman, E.; Peters, P.J.; Needle, R.; McAlister, C.; et al. Multiple injections per injection episode: High-risk injection practice among people who injected pills during the 2015 HIV outbreak in Indiana. *Int. J. Drug Policy* **2018**, *52*, 97–101. [CrossRef]
6. Singer, M.C.; Erickson, P.I.; Badiane, L.; Diaz, R.; Ortiz, D.; Abraham, T.; Nicolaysen, A.M. Syndemics, sex and the city: Understanding sexually transmitted diseases in social and cultural context. *Soc. Sci. Med.* **2006**, *63*, 2010–2021. [CrossRef] [PubMed]
7. Singer, M. Pathogen-pathogen interaction: A syndemic model of complex biosocial processes in disease. *Virulence* **2010**, *1*, 10–18. [CrossRef] [PubMed]
8. Mendenhall, E.; Kohrt, B.A.; Logie, C.H.; Tsai, A.C. Syndemics and clinical science. *Nat. Med.* **2022**, *28*, 1359–1362. [CrossRef] [PubMed]
9. Tsai, A.C. Syndemics: A theory in search of data or data in search of a theory? *Soc. Sci. Med.* **2018**, *206*, 117–122. [CrossRef] [PubMed]
10. Tsai, A.C.; Burns, B.F. Syndemics of psychosocial problems and HIV risk: A systematic review of empirical tests of the disease interaction concept. *Soc. Sci. Med.* **2015**, *139*, 26–35. [CrossRef] [PubMed]

11. Stall, R.; Coulter, R.W.; Friedman, M.R.; Plankey, M.W. Commentary on "Syndemics of psychosocial problems and HIV risk: A systematic review of empirical tests of the disease interaction concept" by A. Tsai and B. Burns. *Soc. Sci. Med.* **2015**, *145*, 129–131. [CrossRef] [PubMed]
12. Shrestha, S.; Bauer, C.X.C.; Hendricks, B.; Stopka, T.J. Spatial epidemiology: An empirical framework for syndemics research. *Soc. Sci. Med.* **2020**, *295*, 113352. [CrossRef] [PubMed]
13. Zibbell, J.E.; Asher, A.K.; Patel, R.C.; Kupronis, B.; Iqbal, K.; Ward, J.W.; Holtzman, D. Increases in Acute Hepatitis C Virus Infection Related to a Growing Opioid Epidemic and Associated Injection Drug Use, United States, 2004 to 2014. *Am. J. Public Health* **2018**, *108*, 175–181. [CrossRef] [PubMed]
14. Ronan, M.V.; Herzig, S.J. Hospitalizations Related To Opioid Abuse/Dependence And Associated Serious Infections Increased Sharply, 2002–2012. *Health Aff.* **2016**, *35*, 832–837. [CrossRef] [PubMed]
15. Conrad, C.; Bradley, H.M.; Broz, D.; Buddha, S.; Chapman, E.L.; Galang, R.R.; Hillman, D.; Hon, J.; Hoover, K.W.; Patel, M.R.; et al. Community Outbreak of HIV Infection Linked to Injection Drug Use of Oxymorphone—Indiana, 2015. *MMWR Morb. Mortal. Wkly. Rep.* **2015**, *64*, 443–444.
16. Springer, S.A.; Korthuis, P.T.; Del Rio, C. Integrating Treatment at the Intersection of Opioid Use Disorder and Infectious Disease Epidemics in Medical Settings: A Call for Action After a National Academies of Sciences, Engineering, and Medicine Workshop. *Ann. Intern. Med.* **2018**, *169*, 335–336. [CrossRef]
17. Schranz, A.J.; Fleischauer, A.; Chu, V.H.; Wu, L.T.; Rosen, D.L. Trends in Drug Use-Associated Infective Endocarditis and Heart Valve Surgery, 2007 to 2017: A Study of Statewide Discharge Data. *Ann. Intern. Med.* **2019**, *170*, 31–40. [CrossRef] [PubMed]
18. Peters, P.J.; Pontones, P.; Hoover, K.W.; Patel, M.R.; Galang, R.R.; Shields, J.; Blosser, S.J.; Spiller, M.W.; Combs, B.; Switzer, W.M.; et al. HIV Infection Linked to Injection Use of Oxymorphone in Indiana, 2014–2015. *N. Engl. J. Med.* **2016**, *375*, 229–239. [CrossRef]
19. Des Jarlais, D.C.; Nugent, A.; Solberg, A.; Feelemyer, J.; Mermin, J.; Holtzman, D. Syringe Service Programs for Persons Who Inject Drugs in Urban, Suburban, and Rural Areas—United States, 2013. *MMWR Morb. Mortal. Wkly. Rep.* **2015**, *64*, 1337–1341. [CrossRef] [PubMed]
20. Horyniak, D.; Stoové, M.; Degenhardt, L.; Aitken, C.; Kerr, T.; Dietze, P. How do drug market changes affect characteristics of injecting initiation and subsequent patterns of drug use? Findings from a cohort of regular heroin and methamphetamine injectors in Melbourne, Australia. *Int. J. Drug Policy* **2015**, *26*, 43–50. [CrossRef] [PubMed]
21. Binswanger, I.A.; Blatchford, P.J.; Mueller, S.R.; Stern, M.F. Mortality after prison release: Opioid overdose and other causes of death, risk factors, and time trends from 1999 to 2009. *Ann. Intern. Med.* **2013**, *159*, 592–600. [CrossRef]
22. Cooper, H.L.; Brady, J.E.; Ciccarone, D.; Tempalski, B.; Gostnell, K.; Friedman, S.R. Nationwide increase in the number of hospitalizations for illicit injection drug use-related infective endocarditis. *Clin. Infect. Dis.* **2007**, *45*, 1200–1203. [CrossRef]
23. Capizzi, J.; Leahy, J.; Wheelock, H.; Garcia, J.; Strnad, L.; Sikka, M.; Englander, H.; Thomas, A.; Korthuis, P.T.; Menza, T.W. Population-based trends in hospitalizations due to injection drug use-related serious bacterial infections, Oregon, 2008 to 2018. *PLoS ONE* **2020**, *15*, e0242165. [CrossRef]
24. Wurcel, A.G.; Anderson, J.E.; Chui, K.K.; Skinner, S.; Knox, T.A.; Snydman, D.R.; Stopka, T.J. Increasing Infectious Endocarditis Admissions Among Young People Who Inject Drugs. *Open Forum Infect. Dis.* **2016**, *3*, ofw157. [CrossRef] [PubMed]
25. Englander, H.; Dobbertin, K.; Lind, B.K.; Nicolaidis, C.; Graven, P.; Dorfman, C.; Korthuis, P.T. Inpatient Addiction Medicine Consultation and Post-Hospital Substance Use Disorder Treatment Engagement: A Propensity-Matched Analysis. *J. Gen. Intern. Med.* **2019**, *34*, 2796–2803. [CrossRef]
26. Keeshin, S.W.; Feinberg, J. Endocarditis as a Marker for New Epidemics of Injection Drug Use. *Am. J. Med. Sci.* **2016**, *352*, 609–614. [CrossRef]
27. McCarthy, N.L.; Baggs, J.; See, I.; Reddy, S.C.; Jernigan, J.A.; Gokhale, R.H.; Fiore, A.E. Bacterial Infections Associated With Substance Use Disorders, Large Cohort of United States Hospitals, 2012–2017. *Clin. Infect. Dis.* **2020**, *71*, e37–e44. [CrossRef] [PubMed]
28. Siddiqi, K.; Freeman, P.R.; Fanucchi, L.C.; Slavova, S. Rural-urban differences in hospitalizations for opioid use-associated infective endocarditis in Kentucky, 2016–2019. *J. Rural Health* **2022**, *38*, 604–611. [CrossRef] [PubMed]
29. Nenninger, E.K.; Carwile, J.L.; Ahrens, K.A.; Armstrong, B.; Thakarar, K. Rural-Urban Differences in Hospitalizations for Opioid Use-Associated Infective Endocarditis in the United States, 2003–2016. *Open Forum Infect. Dis.* **2020**, *7*, ofaa045. [CrossRef] [PubMed]
30. Amon, J.J.; Garfein, R.S.; Ahdieh-Grant, L.; Armstrong, G.L.; Ouellet, L.J.; Latka, M.H.; Vlahov, D.; Strathdee, S.A.; Hudson, S.M.; Kerndt, P.; et al. Prevalence of hepatitis C virus infection among injection drug users in the United States, 1994–2004. *Clin. Infect. Dis.* **2008**, *46*, 1852–1858. [CrossRef] [PubMed]
31. Garfein, R.S.; Doherty, M.C.; Monterroso, E.R.; Thomas, D.L.; Nelson, K.E.; Vlahov, D. Prevalence and incidence of hepatitis C virus infection among young adult injection drug users. *JAIDS J. Acquir. Immune Defic. Syndr.* **1998**, *18* (Suppl. S1), S11–S19. [CrossRef]

32. Hagan, H.; Thiede, H.; Des Jarlais, D. Hepatitis C virus infection among injection drug users: Survival analysis of time to seroconversion. *Epidemiology* **2004**, *15*, 543–549. [CrossRef] [PubMed]
33. Hahn, J.A.; Page-Shafer, K.; Lum, P.J.; Bourgois, P.; Stein, E.; Evans, J.L.; Busch, M.P.; Tobler, L.H.; Phelps, B.; Moss, A.R. Hepatitis C virus seroconversion among young injection drug users: Relationships and risks. *J. Infect. Dis.* **2002**, *186*, 1558–1564. [CrossRef]
34. Onofrey, S.; Church, D.; Kludt, P.; DeMaria, A.; Cranston, K.; Beckett, G.A.; Holmberg, S.D.; Ward, J.W.; Holtzman, D. Hepatitis C virus infection among adolescents and young adults: Massachusetts, 2002–2009. *MMWR Morb. Mortal. Wkly. Rep.* **2011**, *60*, 537–541.
35. Daniel Church, D.; Barton, K.; Elson, F.; DeMaria, A.; Cranston, K.; Harris, N.; Liu, S.; Hu, D.; Holtzman, D.; Holmberg, S. Risk factors for hepatitis C virus infections among young adults—Massachusetts, 2010. *MMWR Morb. Mortal. Wkly. Rep.* **2011**, *60*, 1457–1458.
36. Skeer, M.R.; Ladin, K.; Wilkins, L.E.; Landy, D.M.; Stopka, T.J. 'Hep C's like the common cold': Understanding barriers along the HCV care continuum among young people who inject drugs. *Drug Alcohol Depend.* **2018**, *190*, 246–254. [CrossRef]
37. Greenwald, R.; Waters, P.; Cayer, S. Enforcement of Legal Remedies to Secure Hepatitis C Virus Treatment With Direct-Acting Antiviral Therapies in Correctional Facilities and Medicaid Programs. *Public Health Rep.* **2020**, *135*, 44S–49S. [CrossRef] [PubMed]
38. Litwin, A.H.; Lum, P.J.; Taylor, L.E.; Mehta, S.H.; Tsui, J.I.; Feinberg, J.; Kim, A.Y.; Norton, B.L.; Heo, M.; Arnsten, J.; et al. Patient-centred models of hepatitis C treatment for people who inject drugs: A multicentre, pragmatic randomised trial. *Lancet Gastroenterol. Hepatol.* **2022**, *7*, 1112–1127. [CrossRef] [PubMed]
39. Cloud, D.H.; Ibragimov, U.; Prood, N.; Young, A.M.; Cooper, H.L.F. Rural risk environments for hepatitis c among young adults in appalachian kentucky. *Int. J. Drug Policy* **2019**, *72*, 47–54. [CrossRef]
40. Estadt, A.T.; Miller, W.C.; Kline, D.; Whitney, B.M.; Young, A.M.; Todd Korthuis, P.; Stopka, T.J.; Feinberg, J.; Zule, W.A.; Pho, M.T.; et al. Associations of hepatitis C virus (HCV) antibody positivity with opioid, stimulant, and polysubstance injection among people who inject drugs (PWID) in rural U.S. communities. *Int. J. Drug Policy* **2023**, 104222. [CrossRef]
41. Fatima, S.; Dao, B.; Jameel, A.; Sharma, K.; Strogatz, D.; Scribani, M.; Rammohan, H.R.S. Epidemiology of Infective Endocarditis in Rural Upstate New York, 2011–2016. *J. Clin. Med. Res.* **2017**, *9*, 754–758. [CrossRef] [PubMed]
42. Bruns, T.; Zimmermann, H.W.; Stallmach, A. Risk factors and outcome of bacterial infections in cirrhosis. *World J. Gastroenterol.* **2014**, *20*, 2542–2554. [CrossRef]
43. Chebrolu, P.; Colombo, R.E.; Baer, S.; Gallaher, T.R.; Atwater, S.; Kheda, M.; Nahman, N.S.; Kintziger, K.W. Bacteremia in hemodialysis patients with hepatitis C. *Am. J. Med. Sci.* **2015**, *349*, 217–221. [CrossRef] [PubMed]
44. Marrie, T.J.; Tyrrell, G.J.; Majumdar, S.R.; Eurich, D.T. Concurrent Infection with Hepatitis C Virus and Streptococcus pneumoniae. *Emerg. Infect. Dis.* **2017**, *23*, 1118–1123. [CrossRef] [PubMed]
45. Lin, M.N.; Tsai, C.C.; Hung, T.H. The risk of cellulitis in cirrhotic patients: A nationwide population-based study in taiwan. *Gut Liver* **2012**, *6*, 482–485. [CrossRef]
46. Mohan, P.; Ramu, B.; Bhaskar, E.; Venkataraman, J. Prevalence and risk factors for bacterial skin infection and mortality in cirrhosis. *Ann. Hepatol.* **2011**, *10*, 15–20.
47. Aruch, D.B.; Bhusal, Y.; Hamill, R.J. Unusual cause of cellulitis in a patient with hepatitis C and cirrhosis. *Am. J. Med.* **2011**, *124*, e7–e8. [CrossRef] [PubMed]
48. Ballard, A.M.; Kesich, Z.; Crane, H.M.; Feinberg, J.; Friedmann, P.D.; Go, V.F.; Jenkins, W.D.; Korthuis, P.T.; Miller, W.C.; Pho, M.T.; et al. Rural houselessness among people who use drugs in the United States: Results from the National Rural Opioid Initiative. *Drug Alcohol Depend.* **2024**, *266*, 112498. [CrossRef]
49. Ballard, A.M.; Falk, D.; Greenwood, H.; Gugerty, P.; Feinberg, J.; Friedmann, P.D.; Go, V.F.; Jenkins, W.D.; Korthuis, P.T.; Miller, W.C.; et al. Houselessness and syringe service program utilization among people who inject drugs in eight rural areas across the USA: A cross-sectional analysis. *Harm Reduct. J.* **2023**, *20*, 157. [CrossRef]
50. Jenkins, R.A.; Whitney, B.M.; Nance, R.M.; Allen, T.M.; Cooper, H.L.F.; Feinberg, J.; Fredericksen, R.; Friedmann, P.D.; Go, V.F.; Jenkins, W.D.; et al. The Rural Opioid Initiative Consortium description: Providing evidence to Understand the Fourth Wave of the Opioid Crisis. *Addict. Sci. Clin. Pract.* **2022**, *17*, 38. [CrossRef] [PubMed]
51. Rudolph, A.E.; Nance, R.M.; Bobashev, G.; Brook, D.; Akhtar, W.; Cook, R.; Cooper, H.L.; Friedmann, P.D.; Frost, S.D.W.; Go, V.F.; et al. Evaluation of respondent-driven sampling in seven studies of people who use drugs from rural populations: Findings from the Rural Opioid Initiative. *BMC Med. Res. Methodol.* **2024**, *24*, 94. [CrossRef] [PubMed]
52. Stopka, T.J.; Whitney, B.M.; de Gijsel, D.; Brook, D.L.; Friedmann, P.D.; Taylor, L.E.; Feinberg, J.; Young, A.M.; Evon, D.M.; Herink, M.; et al. Medicaid Policy and Hepatitis C Treatment Among Rural People Who Use Drugs. *Med. Care* **2024**. [CrossRef]
53. Friedman, J.R.; Abramovitz, D.; Skaathun, B.; Rangel, G.; Harvey-Vera, A.; Vera, C.F.; Artamonova, I.; Muñoz, S.; Martin, N.K.; Eger, W.H.; et al. Illicit Fentanyl Use and Hepatitis C Virus Seroconversion Among People Who Inject Drugs in Tijuana and San Diego: Results From a Binational Cohort Study. *Clin. Infect. Dis.* **2024**, *79*, 1109–1116. [CrossRef]
54. Duhart Clarke, S.E.; Kral, A.H.; Zibbell, J.E. Consuming illicit opioids during a drug overdose epidemic: Illicit fentanyls, drug discernment, and the radical transformation of the illicit opioid market. *Int. J. Drug Policy* **2022**, *99*, 103467. [CrossRef]

55. Mixson, L.S.; Whitney, B.M.; Jenkins, W.D.; Stopka, T.J.; Korthuis, P.T.; Drumright, L.N.; Ruderman, S.A.; Friedmann, P.D.; Pho, M.T.; Young, A.M.; et al. Behavioral and Health Outcome Differences by Heroin or Methamphetamine Preference Among People in Rural US Communities Who Use Both Substances. *Subst. Use Res. Treat.* **2024**, *18*, 29768357241272374. [CrossRef] [PubMed]
56. Baron, R.M.; Kenny, D.A. The moderator-mediator variable distinction in social psychological research: Conceptual, strategic, and statistical considerations. *J. Personal. Soc. Psychol.* **1986**, *51*, 1173–1182. [CrossRef]
57. Rhodes, T. Risk environments and drug harms: A social science for harm reduction approach. *Int. J. Drug Policy* **2009**, *20*, 193–201. [CrossRef] [PubMed]
58. Romo, E.; Stopka, T.J.; Jesdale, B.M.; Wang, B.; Mazor, K.M.; Friedmann, P.D. Association of spatial proximity to fixed-site syringe services programs with HCV serostatus and injection equipment sharing practices among people who inject drugs in rural New England, United States. *Harm Reduct. J.* **2024**, *21*, 23. [CrossRef]
59. Walters, S.M.; Frank, D.; Felsher, M.; Jaiswal, J.; Fletcher, S.; Bennett, A.S.; Friedman, S.R.; Ouellet, L.J.; Ompad, D.C.; Jenkins, W.; et al. How the rural risk environment underpins hepatitis C risk: Qualitative findings from rural southern Illinois, United States. *Int. J. Drug Policy* **2023**, *112*, 103930. [CrossRef] [PubMed]
60. Jahangir, T.; Fuller, G.K.; Livingston, M.D.; Freeman, E.; Fanucchi, L.C.; Fallin-Bennett, A.; Cooper, H.L.F.; Young, A.M. Syringe reuse among people who inject drugs in rural Appalachian Kentucky. *Int. J. Drug Policy* **2024**, *128*, 104422. [CrossRef]

Tropical Medicine and Infectious Disease

MDPI

Review

Using a Syndemics Perspective to (Re)Conceptualize Vulnerability during the COVID-19 Pandemic: A Scoping Review

Yisel Hernandez Barrios [1], Dennis Perez Chacon [1], Yosiel Molina Gomez [1], Charlotte Gryseels [2], Kristien Verdonck [2], Koen Peeters Grietens [2,3] and Claudia Nieto-Sanchez [2,*]

[1] Institute of Tropical Medicine Pedro Kourí, Havana 11400, Cuba; yhbarrios@ipk.sld.cu or yhbarrios88@gmail.com (Y.H.B.); dennis@ipk.sld.cu or dennisperezchacon@gmail.com (D.P.C.); yosiel.molina@ipk.sld.cu or yosiel.molina88@gmail.com (Y.M.G.)

[2] Institute of Tropical Medicine—Antwerp, Nationalestraat 155, 2000 Antwerp, Belgium; cgryseels@itg.be (C.G.); tverdonck@itg.be (K.V.); kpeeters@itg.be (K.P.G.)

[3] School of Tropical Medicine and Global Health, Nagasaki University, Nagasaki 852-8501, Japan

* Correspondence: cnieto@itg.be

Abstract: Syndemics theory has been applied to study interactions between biomedical and social factors leading to the clustering of diseases. Because syndemics theory focuses on interactions that enhance risk, the concept of vulnerability is central to this approach. We conducted a scoping review to better understand how this theoretical framework helped to define, operationalize, and tackle issues of vulnerability during the COVID-19 pandemic. Original research, reviews, and opinion pieces elaborating on syndemics, vulnerability, and COVID-19, published between December 2019 and October 2022 and available from PubMed, were eligible. We analyzed 40 records and identified three framings of syndemics operating during this period: (1) interactions between COVID-19, diseases/health conditions, and specific social factors; (2) interactions between COVID-19 and social determinants of health; and (3) impacts of COVID-19 on specific populations. Emerging conceptualizations described vulnerability to COVID-19 as a systemic issue, explained the impact of COVID-19 control measures on increased vulnerability, and presented COVID-19 as a syndemic on its own. However, this theory's potential for deepening our understanding of vulnerability during this pandemic was constrained by superficial explorations of the interactions between biomedical and social spheres, and insufficient theoretical and methodological support from the social sciences.

Keywords: syndemics; vulnerability; COVID-19; syndemic interactions; biosocial interface

1. Introduction

Although interest in the syndemics perspective has grown over the last 25 years [1], this concept gained special traction during the COVID-19 pandemic. At the start of the pandemic, the term "syndemic" was used to describe the unequal distribution of COVID-19 disease outcomes in populations around the world [2–4], and later on, to refer to COVID-19 itself as a syndemic [5,6]. Syndemics theory has been applied since the late 1990s to study linkages between biomedical and social factors leading to disease occurrence in specific populations or geographical regions, so the extended use of the term during the pandemic did not come as a surprise.

Syndemics theory is focused on understanding the synergistic effects of biomedical factors (bio interface) and social conditions (biosocial interface) in the co-occurrence and clustering of diseases [7]. Because of its focus on interactions that enhance risk, the concept of vulnerability has been core to the syndemics approach. The term 'syndemic vulnerability', specifically, defines a predisposition to the development of negative consequences resulting from feedback loops between biomedical and social factors. Therefore, understanding vulnerability under the syndemics perspective implies identifying upstream factors that generate both the environment and the circumstances that fuel synergistic effects, as well as the mechanisms that sustain said predisposition [8].

As social scientists and epidemiologists working in the field of public health, we are interested in understanding how the mechanisms underlying vulnerabilities in health are defined and incorporated into health policies and interventions. Adding a vulnerability angle to health research has proved to be useful to understand the unequal distribution of the risks and consequences of diseases and disasters [9]; more importantly, it has expanded the notion of individual risk factors to include historical contexts, conjunctural circumstances, lifetime trajectories, and differentiated conditions of exposure to specific pathogenic agents to interpret and explain health outcomes [10]. However, using the label 'vulnerable' to define specific groups and vast geographical regions can also lead to stigmatization, obscure institutional arrangements, and contextual elements with a direct impact on vulnerability conditions, and as a result, further increase pre-existing inequities [11,12]. The difficulties in operationalizing this concept have been studied in extensive reviews of recent public health literature [13,14].

Syndemics research is particular in this sense: while solidly established as a theoretical approach suited to study the biosocial nature of health risks, several scholars have criticized the way this theory is applied in research practice [1]. Critics have argued that the interactions between the biomedical and social realms are insufficiently explored, and that syndemics research tends to become 'fuzzy' when trying to explain how simultaneously occurring epidemics work together. Rather than describing causation—as it intends—it has been suggested that syndemics research could be better suited to explain disease distribution [15–17]. The tendency to reduce social realities into mere proxies with limited capacity to explain complex pathways involved in syndemics interactions has also been extensively criticized because of its limited explanatory capacity [18]. In addition, some argue that the critical nature of perspectives such as intersectionality or social justice is often absent from the epidemiological thinking informing syndemics research; as a result, power structures and political arrangements sustaining vulnerability often stay unquestioned [19,20]. Since some of these criticisms contradict core concepts in the original formulation of this approach, the debate about the concrete contributions of syndemics research to address inequities in health remains open [21,22]. Understanding that concrete ideas about how to address vulnerabilities in health emerge from the way they are conceptualized, this review was conceived to address two concerns common to these criticisms: how are syndemic interactions identified and studied? And more specifically, how are the interactions with social dynamics, i.e., the biosocial interface of syndemic relationships approached and explained?

Given the rapid expansion of syndemics research in the medical field during the COVID-19 pandemic and the potential for deepening our understanding of vulnerability in a context of acute risk, we conducted a scoping review to explore how the syndemics perspective contributed to defining, operationalizing, and addressing vulnerabilities in health. Three research questions guided this review: (1) Which social and environmental arrangements (determinants, factors, dynamics, and aspects) were described as part of the biosocial interface of syndemics involving COVID-19? (2) How was that biosocial interface conceptualized and studied (methodological approaches)? (3) What were the main contributions and limitations of the syndemics perspective to the conceptualization of vulnerability in the context of the pandemic?

2. Materials and Methods

We conducted a scoping review, the protocol of which was registered in October 2022 [23]. Where applicable, this review follows the format recommended by PRISMA-ScR (Supplementary File S1) [24]. Using the model of *concept synthesis* [25], we aimed to capture "concepts, viewpoints and ideas" defining vulnerability to COVID-19 under the syndemics perspective.

Consequently, we identified eligible records under three criteria: (1) published as original research, reviews, and opinion pieces; (2) including the words syndemics, vulnerability, and COVID-19 in the title, abstract, or keywords; and (3) published between December 2019 and October 2022.

Our primary data source was PubMed; additional records were identified through manual searches in the lists of references of the included records. No restrictions on language, studied conditions, or geographical locations were applied.

In Boolean terms, the search string for PubMed was ("SARS-CoV-2" [MeSH Terms] OR "COVID-19" [MeSH Terms] OR "COVID" [TextWord]) AND ("vulnerabilities" [All Fields] OR "vulnerability" [All Fields] OR "vulnerable" [All Fields]) AND ("syndemic" [MeSH Terms] OR "syndemic" [All Fields] OR "syndemics" [All Fields]).

All records were managed in Mendeley and imported into Covidence after checking for duplicates (https://www.covidence.org/ accessed on 12 October 2022). Two reviewers (YH and YM) independently screened titles, abstracts, and keywords. They discussed any disagreements and consulted a third reviewer (CN-S) when needed. Articles using the words 'social disadvantage', 'disproportional or unequal impacts', and 'marginalized' were retained considering their close relationship with the term 'vulnerability'. Articles that focused purely on biomedical interactions or did not elaborate on the review topics (syndemics and vulnerability) beyond the initial mention (in titles, abstracts, and keywords), were excluded at the stage of full-text review.

A preliminary data extraction form was tested with 10 randomly selected records. The results of this pilot test were discussed with the review team, and the final version of the data extraction template was completed and applied to all records (Supplementary File S2).

The data extraction was conducted in parallel by four members of the research team (YH, CN-S, DP, and YM) in three moments. First, each researcher extracted data from randomly assigned articles until they were all completed. Second, a different reviewer cross-checked the extracted data for accuracy and completeness. Subsequently, the reviewers collectively discussed and resolved any discrepancies, leading to the consolidation of the final set of extracted data in Covidence. This dataset was then used to address the review questions.

The data were exported to an Excel spreadsheet (Microsoft Office 2010) for qualitative thematic analyses. Records were categorized per type of publication (original research, reviews, and opinion pieces). All data items were thematically coded. Three researchers coded the data (YH, DP, and CN-S) and synthesized them in tables. Additional discussions were held with other members of the research team (KP, KV, and CG) to refine analytical categories.

3. Results

3.1. Search and Selection Process

Figure 1 summarizes the process of the search and selection of sources of evidence in a PRISMA flow chart. Our search strategy yielded a total of 97 articles. Three duplicates were removed in Mendeley before importing the database to Covidence. In the title, keyword, and abstract screening stage, 36 articles were deemed irrelevant. In the full-text review stage, we excluded eighteen additional articles: fifteen lacked sufficient information on syndemics and/or vulnerability, and three were not applied to COVID-19. Hence, this review includes 40 articles.

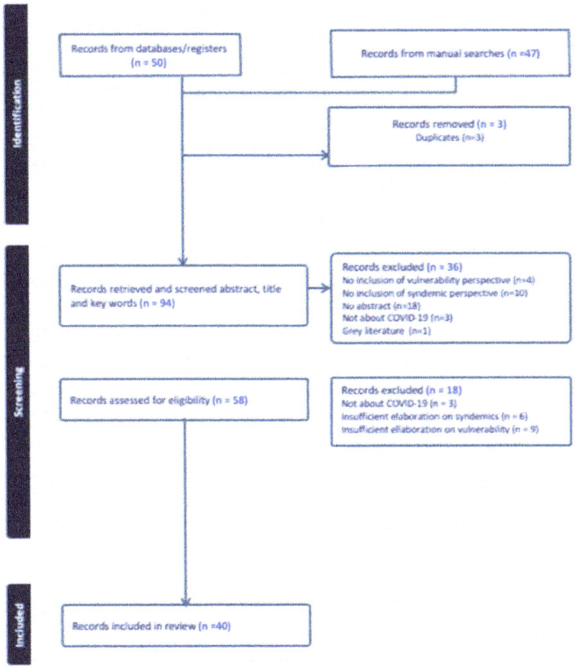

Figure 1. PRISMA flowchart.

Out of 40 articles, 13 were original research studies (conducted in the USA, Canada, England, Brazil, China, South Africa, India, and China), 17 were opinion papers, and 10 were review articles (Table 1). Of the included reviews, three were presented as narrative reviews, and one declared to follow the "guidelines of the Equator Network" [26]. The remaining records included under this category were written as essays based on extended literature reviews.

Table 1. Characteristics of the articles included in the review (n = 40).

Record Characteristics	Records	%
Type of publication		
Opinion pieces	17	42%
Original research	13	32%
Reviews	10	25%
Year of publication		
2020	6	15%
2021	19	47%
2022	15	37%
Setting/Location of study		
Global	13	32%
Specific country	25	62%
Several countries	2	5%

Supplementary File S3 summarizes the applications of the syndemics perspective and associated definitions or operationalizations of vulnerability identified in this review.

3.2. Social Factors Involved in Syndemic Interactions Including COVID-19

We identified three different framings of syndemics in this review: (a) Syndemic interactions between COVID-19 and one or several diseases or medical conditions, and specific social factors; (b) syndemic interactions between COVID-19 and the Social Determinants of Health (SDOH), and (c) syndemic impacts of COVID-19 on specific populations. In this section we summarize factors included as part of the bio–social interface within these framings.

a. Syndemic interactions between COVID-19, one or several diseases or health conditions, and specific social factors

COVID-19 and non-communicable diseases (NCDs): Co-occurrence of NCDs and COVID-19 was the focus of seventeen records (five of them original research studies). In these cases, NCD (e.g., cardiovascular, nervous system, respiratory, kidney, and digestive diseases, as well as cancers and diabetes) were often grouped as comorbidities that, when experienced in contexts characterized by 'socioeconomic inequalities', 'social vulnerability', and 'social disadvantage', enhanced vulnerability to COVID-19. These contexts were generally described in terms of indicators considered to have an impact on patients' capacity to respond to COVID-19 and its control measures. Socioeconomic inequalities, for example, were defined in terms of educational level, employment status, and income at individual, household, and area levels in India and Hong Kong [27,28]. Two publications used pre-existing vulnerability indexes to measure social disadvantage through indicators such as poverty levels, unemployment, population without health insurance, and housing crowding and ownership in specific geographical areas of the USA [29,30]. Susceptibility to COVID-19 in NCD patients was further described in terms of shared risk factors that were exacerbated during the pandemic, including sedentary behaviors and malnutrition [31–35]. Opinion pieces discussed changes in food intake, as well as alcohol and tobacco consumption used as coping mechanisms to deal with control measures, as concrete forms in which COVID-19 affected people living with NCD [35–37].

Pre-existing socio-environmental vulnerabilities were defined in terms of people's exposure to poor sanitation systems and water and air pollutants, as well as consistently deficient access to health services. This included populations considered to be at a higher risk of NCDs, such as undocumented migrants, indigenous communities, and workers linked with unregularized activities such as illegal mining and logging [38]. Urbanization, changing lifestyle habits, climate change, and pollution were also mentioned as factors leading to adverse COVID-19 outcomes in patients with NCDs [31,33,37,39].

COVID-19 and mental health: The impact of COVID-19 on mental health was studied in two original research articles [40,41]. In both cases, syndemics was used as a theoretical framework to explain disproportionate mental impacts in different population groups in Canada. These publications based their results on a cross-sectional monitoring survey administered to 125,000 members of an online panel that included questions on six individual dimensions of mental health. The authors reported on the detrimental impact on mental health of COVID-19 in the general population. However, groups considered to be at higher risk of experiencing structural vulnerability due to their race, ethnicity, socioeconomic status, gender, sexual orientation, mental health, or disability reported an even higher burden of mental health issues and more difficulties coping with pandemic-related challenges. The association between COVID-19's impacts on mental health and the pre-existing forms of social disadvantage concerning income, occupation, social support, living conditions, inequities, and emotional distress was further explored in opinion pieces [42–45]. The confluence of mental illness and substance abuse was suggested to lead to increased susceptibility to adverse consequences of COVID-19 [37,45]. Social exclusion, social isolation, and stigmatization were presented as interfering with access to health services due to the additional mental health burdens generated by the pandemic [43].

COVID-19 and other infectious diseases: Interactions between COVID-19 and other infectious diseases were also described as syndemic in nature. Specifically, interactions between COVID-19 and HIV-related comorbidities, HIV risk factors, and HIV-derived stigmatization, were considered when describing susceptibility to COVID-19 in people living with HIV (PLWH). A scoping review investigated the social and behavioral impacts of COVID-19 on this population during the first year of the pandemic [46]. The syndemics framework was used to explain the mechanisms of interaction between COVID-19 and HIV as interlocking conditions: COVID-19 psychosocial sequelae (i.e., fear and anxiety) exacerbated mental health problems and contributed to structural inequalities affecting people living with unsuppressed HIV. The co-existence of tuberculosis (TB) and COVID-19 among displaced and migrant populations was also presented as a source of dual burden. Authors suggested that pandemic control measures may have increased TB-associated risks by reducing access to health services [47].

b. Syndemic interactions between COVID-19 and social determinants of health (SDOH)

Five records described syndemic interactions involving COVID-19 and socioeconomic indicators grouped under the category of social determinants of health (SDOH). Lee and Ramírez [30] studied the associations between COVID-19 vulnerability and SDOH in Colorado. They used previously existing data on 14 social indicators including socioeconomic status, household composition, housing, and transportation in relation to health-related variables, including mental health, obesity, and substance abuse. Associations were analyzed under a syndemics perspective and the "Hazards of Place Framework" (more details on Section 3.3) to demonstrate that the overlap between mental health and chronic conditions, as well as "inequities in education, income, access to healthcare, and race/ethnicity" at the county level, exacerbated COVID-19 negative outcomes.

Similarly, Siegal et al. [48] sought to describe a syndemic between structural racism and COVID-19 by assessing disparities in selected SDOH in predominantly Black and white neighborhoods in North Carolina (USA). Differences in income levels, employment, job density, and use of public food, nutrition, and health insurance services, as well as the proximity to school-age and early childhood care, low-cost healthcare, grocery stores, and public transit were measured. The authors concluded that racially segregated communities, particularly Black communities in the USA, already experienced detrimental conditions in multiple SDOH before the pandemic and that those inequities were exacerbated by COVID-19.

Some authors proposed using a syndemics approach together with the SDOH framework to describe bidirectional relationships between susceptibility to disease and health inequities experienced by marginalized populations including the elderly, children, people with disabilities, the underinsured, the socioeconomically disadvantaged, the incarcerated, abused individuals, the mentally ill, immigrants, refugees, and racial/ethnic minorities [49–51].

c. Impacts of COVID-19 on specific populations

Thirteen records explored the differentiated impacts of COVID-19 on specific populations. In these cases, the authors emphasized that the conditions of marginalization, disadvantage, or exclusion experienced by some population groups, particularly racial, ethnic, and gender minorities, as well as women and immigrants—not necessarily in relation to specific health conditions—made them increasingly vulnerable to the negative health and social consequences of this pandemic. Intersections between race, gender, and occupation in the generation of marginalization were highlighted. In most cases, syndemics theory was used as a framework to explore the multiple levels of impact of COVID-19 in these populations.

Most of the papers included in this category discussed the role of race and ethnicity in COVID-19 outcomes. Cokley et al. [52] investigated how perceptions of discrimination and police brutality influenced COVID-19 experiences for Black Americans in the USA. Perceptions of police brutality, discrimination, the COVID-19 health threat, COVID-19/race-related stress, and cultural mistrust were assessed among inhabitants of metropolitan and rural areas with high concentration of Black/African population (Black, Black American, African American, African, Afro-Caribbean, and Afro-Latinx). The authors concluded that

COVID-19 concerns were further exacerbated by police violence and poor mental health, which could also have resulted in low vaccination uptake in this population. Concurrently, precarious living conditions experienced by racial and ethnic minorities due to inequities in income, working conditions, access to health care, and housing were considered to be leading to negative COVID-19 outcomes [53,54]. Disparities were described for racial minorities and immigrants employed in crucial sectors such as healthcare [55], hospitality services [45], and transportation [34]. Black women and birthing people (BWBP) and older adults experiencing pre-existing precarities and racial inequities were also presented as populations at risk of severe symptoms and worse COVID-19 outcomes due to their limited access to health care and interruption of services caused by control measures [44,56]. The pervasive effect of racism, race-associated social and health inequities, and racial injustice on health outcomes was extensively described in these publications.

The relationship between occupation, race, gender, and COVID-19 was further explored by Rogers et al. [57], who used syndemics theory as an interpretative lens to study the structural disadvantages putting street-based sex workers in New England at higher risk of COVID-19. Researchers collected data on race, ethnicity, gender, gender identity, sexual orientation, and housing status, and documented changes in sexual and food consumption behaviors during the pandemic. This study concluded that street-based sex workers were at higher risk of COVID-19 and its social impacts due to co-occurring risk factors such as homelessness, food insecurity, mental health problems, substance use disorders, and STIs/HIV. Similarly, Sönmez et al. [58] explained that immigrants represent an important proportion of the workforce of the hospitality services in the USA, and as such were severely impacted by mobility restrictions that put them out of their jobs or reduced their sources of income. The authors argued that immigrant populations linked to these economic activities experienced syndemic risks derived from socioeconomic inequities and excess chronic stress.

Finally, gender-differentiated impacts of COVID-19 were studied by Neto et al. [59] and Duby et al. [60]. The former [59] argued that COVID-19 could have been experienced as a syndemic by gender and sexual minorities in Brazil due to various forms of vulnerability they have historically faced, including racial and gender discrimination, low education levels, precarious working conditions, and reliance on social support systems. The latter [60] took a similar approach to study the impacts of COVID-19 on adolescents, girls, and young women (AGYW) in six districts in South Africa. Thus, syndemics theory was applied to understand how pre-existing situations of poverty, unemployment, food insecurity, and domestic violence in these populations were exacerbated by the pandemic. The authors claimed that their vulnerability was not only derived from gender or age but also from ongoing mental health stressors associated with lack of social support and economic stability; therefore, they proposed to apply an intersectionality lens in combination with syndemics theory to account for the intersecting identities impacting disease outcomes in specific populations.

3.3. Which Methodological Approaches Were Used to Describe These Syndemics?

Out of the thirteen original research studies identified in this review, eight collected primary data [27,40,41,52,57,59–61], four relied exclusively on secondary data [28–30,38], and one combined secondary and primary data [48]. None of the identified publications intended to demonstrate the existence of a particular syndemic; instead, they used syndemic theory as an interpretative lens (an approach, a theory, a concept, or a framework) to conceptualize and analyse emerging data.

Primary data. Five studies reported on data exclusively collected through surveys [40,41,52,57,59], one reported on qualitative data [27], and two more conducted online or telephonic interviews in addition to surveys [60,61]. Participants were drawn from ongoing cohorts organized to follow up on the health needs of the general population [40,41] or specific groups, including Black/African adults in the USA [52] and Brazilian LGBT+ [59]. Respondents were also identified through pre-existing networks and social interventions [57,61]. In all cases, data collection focused on understanding impacts of COVID-19 on specific populations and social groups, as well as their particular needs during the pandemic. Only one group of authors reported on multiple administrations of the same survey [40,41]. Quantitative results were analyzed using binary and multivariate logistic regression models as well as descriptive statistics, while qualitative results relied mainly on thematic coding.

Secondary data. Four studies worked with secondary data. In all cases, researchers used publicly available data collected by health institutions to track COVID-19 incidence, prevalence, and/or mortality rates. Two groups of authors analyzed individual data on NCD pre-existences and mental health indicators to characterize dynamics at the area levels. Using data on cases and deaths from COVID-19 published by the Amazonas State Health Department, Daboin et al. [38] analyzed different municipalities of the Brazilian Amazon region and explored multifactorial correlations between sex, age, indigenous ethnicity, and COVID-19 outcomes. These factors were individually studied and then extrapolated to community (municipality) conditions in relation to poverty, sanitation, and environmental degradation to conclude that "the impact of COVID-19 in the Amazon (...) may present characteristics of a syndemic due to the interaction of COVID-19 with pre-existing illnesses, endemic diseases, and social vulnerabilities". In Hong Kong, Chung and co-authors explored the distribution of severe COVID-19 cases in urban settings in relation to their socioeconomic position and pre-existent multimorbidities [28]. Researchers used the reported address of COVID-19 confirmed cases as published by the Centre for Health Protection (CHP) of Hong Kong to produce "area-level income-poverty rates as the proxy measures of their socioeconomic position".

As mentioned before, social factors were assessed using available census data or previously developed social vulnerability indexes (SVI) [29,30]. An SVI developed by the US Centers for Disease Control and Prevention (CDC) to identify counties particularly vulnerable to environmental disasters in 2018 was used in two publications. In order to characterize health and social vulnerabilities in Colorado, Lee and Ramírez [30] used three different indexes: the CDC's SVI to track specific social determinants (economic stability, education, community, and social context); the health vulnerability index to track underlying health conditions such as diabetes, obesity, and mental health at the county level; and a third index developed during the study to show interactions between these two domains and COVID-19 burden rates. Islam et al. [29] also used the SVI to determine social disadvantage at the county level; these data were included in a model of joint distribution of COVID-19 mortality and five chronic conditions (obesity, diabetes mellitus, chronic obstructive pulmonary disease, heart disease, and chronic kidney disease) in the most vulnerable counties. Neto et al. [59] adapted a vulnerability index previously applied to the LGBT+ population to assess personal and social vulnerability to COVID-19. This index measured what they defined as three vulnerability dimensions: income (defined as living with minimum salary or no income before the pandemic); COVID-19 exposure (described in relation to adherence to preventive measures and contact with people diagnosed with COVID-19), and health (including indicators such as being a user of the public health system and being previously diagnosed with an NCD).

Geo-referenced data were also used to explore clustering of COVID-19. In the USA, Siegal et al. [48] used GIS data (compiled in open mapping and transportation databases) to measure and compare distance to public facilities before COVID-19 in racially segregated communities. The authors proposed a place-based methodological framework to generate "contextually-informed, data-driven and cross-sector responses". Similarly, Lee and Ramírez [30] used data available at the county level in Colorado to explore associations between SDOH and COVID-19 incidence. Due to the absence of data on COVID-19 distribution, the authors used a spatial interpolation model (Empirical Bayesian Kriging) to estimate census tract-level rates of COVID-19. A Hazards of Place Framework was used to identify clusters or "hotspots of persistent risk" in mountainous and urban areas of central and southern counties in the state.

3.4. Conceptualizations of Vulnerability under a Syndemics Perspective

Different definitions of vulnerability around syndemics were identified in the literature reviewed (Supplementary File S3). Most definitions focused on explaining higher risk of infection, illness, or death by COVID-19. In this section, we present three aspects of the vulnerability concept that were particularly salient in the literature about COVID-19 and syndemics: (a) descriptions of vulnerability as a systemic issue, i.e., implying multiple levels and types of interactions; (b) the role of COVID-19 control measures in the generation of new forms of vulnerability; and (c) conceptualizations of COVID-19 as a syndemic in itself. We conclude this section with a summary of theoretical and programmatic discussions proposed around issues of vulnerability in different publications.

(a) Vulnerability as a systemic problem

Multiple authors advocated for the use of the syndemics perspective as an application of systems' thinking when researching vulnerabilities associated with COVID-19. These systemic views were interpreted as wider definitions of health [33] in which disease occurrence cannot be dissociated from the specific context in which it emerges [31]. The syndemics framework was used to describe a relationship in which COVID-19 'increased', 'visualized', 'hindered', 'deepened', 'exacerbated', 'reinforced', or 'perpetuated' pre-existing conditions of social disadvantage, or 'generated' emerging vulnerabilities around the public health measures implemented to control the pandemic. While most articles described bidirectional (mutually reinforcing) relationships between biomedical and social factors leading to syndemic outcomes or occurring in syndemic contexts, two groups of authors engaged in discussions about the causal link between syndemic interactions and COVID-19 outcomes. Daboin et al. [38] referred to a "syndemic context" (described as the product of interactions between pre-existing diseases and social vulnerability) creating difficulties in diagnosing and treating COVID-19 in the Brazilian Amazon, and suggested a direct causal link between this context and high COVID-19 incidence and mortality in the region. Similarly, Mezzina et al. [43] discussed the multifactorial complex nature of causality in health and proposed a descriptive model in which different domains (social determinants, social vulnerability, and social inequalities, among others) act as a "web of determinants" with "non-linear and complex effects" over COVID-19 outcomes.

Individual vulnerability was described in relation to pre-existing health and social conditions enhancing COVID-19 susceptibility. It was often mentioned that these individual vulnerabilities intersect and reinforce each other [40,60,62]. As an example, the vulnerability of girls and women was described as a result of intersecting identities that interact with their socioeconomic status (e.g., living in poverty [44]), living circumstances (in humanitarian settings [42]), income-generation activities (e.g., sex workers [57]), and health-related issues (e.g., HIV-related stigma, birthing conditions [44], mental stressors [60]) to create differentiated layers of risk in this population. While, biologically speaking, COVID-19 did not seem to particularly affect women, records included in this review described "gendered modes of transmission" derived from limited access to health care and social services, the militarization of movement, extended impacts of gender-based violence, and drastic reductions in economic resources.

Subsequently, social vulnerability was characterized as "political decisions and cultural barriers" [59] affecting the course of the pandemic. In this case, the focus of the analysis was not on the individual but on context-specific social circumstances impacting exposure to infections and the development of negative outcomes. Some authors described, for example, how the vulnerability of immigrants, refugees, racial/ethnic minorities, and indigenous communities stemmed from a lack of access to quality healthcare systems. This absence not only predisposed them to particularly negative disease outcomes but also subjected them to substandard services during the pandemic [38,50,55,63]. Thinking of health systems beyond the criteria of clinical cost-efficiency to enable special protection to particularly at-risk populations was recommended as a way to break discriminatory and marginalizing healthcare practices [53,55,56].

The living conditions under which marginalized populations concentrate were also explored in relation to socio-environmental vulnerability [28,29,33,34]. Government-controlled confined spaces such as prisons and detention centers [45,51] were considered particularly conducive to increased SARS-CoV-2 transmission and worsened health outcomes, while humanitarian settings [42,62] were described as contexts where poverty, conflict, displacement, and lack of infrastructure coincided with and co-produced particularly devastating impacts of COVID-19.

At a higher level, structural vulnerability was treated as the "locus of danger, damage, and suffering" [63] experienced by population groups according to their position within specific structures of power. This position was deemed critically relevant to understanding the impacts of COVID-19. Power structures conferring and sustaining privilege during the pandemic based on race [48,52], age [56], socioeconomic position [39], productive sector [36,45,62], and health conditions [40,41,51,63] were extensively described. The structural role of racism, as a socio-political force underlying the conditions of marginalization experienced by racial and ethnic minorities, was mentioned in all publications dealing with this topic [45,55]. In addition, several authors described the important influence of political tensions around pandemic management in countries such as the USA, Mexico, Brazil, India, and Pakistan on negative COVID-19 outcomes and the accentuation of pre-existing structural vulnerabilities [32,38,44,51,55,63,64].

COVID-19 was also analyzed as a global problem that, much like food insecurity, natural and technological disasters, climate change, and population mobility, provided evidence of emerging vulnerabilities. Although these risks were described as latent in the general population, they have also introduced particular forms of vulnerability in groups that have not been traditionally considered at risk. This included people suffering the consequences of the growing incidence of NCDs in high income countries [32,65], those whose income level relies on large-scale food chains [35], and migrants for whom legal irregularity and uncertainties about the future are conducive to increased precariousness in several areas of life, including health care and social support systems [47,51,58].

(b) Emerging vulnerabilities: COVID-19 control measures

The generalized implementation of interventions to control COVID-19 transmission, particularly social (physical) distancing, lockdowns, and mobility restrictions, was described as a COVID-19-specific form of vulnerability [3,5,21,34,40,41,44,49,50]. Among its negative outcomes, researchers mentioned (i) increased poverty and unemployment; (ii) interruption of food supply chains, particularly those involving animal-based products [31,33]; (iii) severe impacts on the population's mental health [40,41]; (iv) increased adoption of unhealthy lifestyles and substance abuse [33,46]; and (v) alterations in the seasonal patterns of respiratory infections [31].

Both stay-home orders and the highly controlled movement of the population were connected to increasing gender-based and other forms of violence [45,52]. Gender-based violence (GBV) was a distinct phenomenon associated with previous outbreaks of infectious diseases such as Zika and Ebola in humanitarian settings [42,62]. It was presented as a pre-existing epidemic that often goes under the radar and worsened with the interruption of attention services due to control measures. Transferring lessons learned from previous epidemics and designing policy responses to tackle the syndemic relationships between infectious diseases and GBV was recommended.

These specific forms of damage derived from government and health systems' responses to the emergency were considered a form of programmatic vulnerability [59]. Importantly, authors who engaged in discussions on this topic mentioned the importance of using a syndemic approach to identify populations and regions that should be prioritized in the response to pandemic threats [29,31,37,40,45,51,56,60,62,63].

(c) "COVID-19 as a syndemic" or "the syndemic nature of the pandemic"

An important feature of the scientific literature produced around the pandemic was the rapid spread of the expression "the COVID-19 syndemic". In our review, five opinion pieces and four reviews (22.5%) adopted this term [32,33,35,37,43,49,53,64,66]. Different from previous uses of the term to describe relationships between specific biomedical and social factors, in this case, the syndemic concept was used to emphasize (a) the large scale and diversity of COVID-19 impacts on vulnerable or marginalized populations; (b) the diverse nature of factors and interactions involved in its occurrence; and (c) the idea that the pandemic was simultaneously cause and consequence of pre-existing vulnerabilities [31–33,35,43,44,50,66]. This framing resembles the use of the expression "the syndemic nature of the pandemic", through which authors emphasized how multiple and extensive interactions between pre-existing social and biomedical conditions resulted in the emergence of COVID-19 [28,31,63,64]. Singer and Rylko-Bauer further explained the use of this expression by describing how COVID-19 made clear the biosocial nature of health by bringing attention to three aspects previously enounced in syndemics theory: (a) interactions between diseases and health conditions that increase overall burden at multiple scales; (b) interspecies interactions; and (c) interactions with social dynamics underlying the clustering of diseases and risks [63].

Concurrently, the COVID-19 pandemic seemed to provide fertile ground to further apply syndemics-related terminology. For example, the term 'syndemics framework' was often employed to explain theoretical, methodological, and analytical decisions supporting the definition of specific interactions. 'Syndemic contexts' were mentioned to describe the resulting composition of social and geographic circumstances in which health conditions overlap [38,59,64]. Some authors described the 'syndemic effects' [31,41,52,61] or the 'syndemic outcomes' of COVID-19 [37,50]. Finally, the term 'syndemic vulnerability' was referred to describe the multiple levels and nature of impacts of the pandemic on vulnerable populations [41,47,51].

(d) Theoretical, methodological, and policy recommendations on syndemics and vulnerability

In terms of theory, four reviews focused specifically on the implications of using syndemics theory in combination with other theoretical frameworks. Singer and Rylko-Bauer [63] used the theoretical lens of syndemics and structural violence to analyze how different socio-environmental configurations engendered different syndemic interactions during the pandemic, exposed the global rise of NCDs and their potential interactions with infectious diseases, and shed light over profound problems in global health systems. According to the authors, while syndemics emphasize the synergistic interactions between biomedical conditions and socio-environmental factors, the concept of structural violence adds a focus on the effects of the 'structures of inequality' that sustain poverty and multidimensional discrimination. In their words, "'structural violence' drives syndemics". These authors proposed that by using these two theoretical frameworks together, both originated in the critical anthropology field, practitioners can bring discipline-specific knowledge to inform contextualized public health responses to this global crisis.

Conceptual arguments around the idea of 'context' in syndemics research were explored by Pirrone et al. [65]. This group of authors conducted a literature review and expert interviews to explore how context has been defined and studied in syndemics research. Focused on syndemics involving NCD and mental health, they concluded that most studies centered on factors that affected populations at micro levels. They argued that, as a consequence, research tends to overlook structural factors shaping said contexts and, in turn, limit the potential contributions of syndemics to COVID-19 management. Since this trend is closely influenced by the methodological designs previously used in the study of syndemics, this review recommended developing longitudinal and population-level analyses that incorporate multiple disciplinary views to study the impacts of context in COVID-19 outcomes. Expanding syndemics-informed research with multi-level and transdisciplinary research designs allowing integration of different datasets was recommended by multiple authors in this review [34,44,48].

Concurrently, Fronteira et al. [31] described COVID-19 as "One Health issue of syndemic nature". These authors referred to the important impacts of COVID-19 control measures on food systems, particularly in areas in which animals play a central role as food sources, income, transportation, fuel, and clothing, among others. Under this rationale, researchers advocated for "syndemic policies" to tackle interconnections between humans, animals, social, and abiotic environments engaged in COVID-19 transmission, which implies (i) learning from documented experiences; (ii) using theoretical frameworks that properly approach the multi-level, interacting, and dynamic nature of the pandemic; and (iii) identifying community responses to COVID-19.

Transfer of knowledge and integration with previous experiences of infectious diseases management was another way of bringing the syndemics angle into programmatic actions. Garcia [50] advocated for using syndemics theory in association with the SDOH framework as an opportunity to generate collaborations between social workers and the public health sector in the development of "biological-social interventions" for vulnerable populations. Additional policy recommendations identified in this review included integrating the management of COVID-19 and other respiratory diseases in migrant populations [46]; informing policies for improving working conditions and workplace regulations considering diseases with syndemic potential [57]; designing pandemic management and preparedness strategies with a focus on vulnerable and at-risk populations [41,53,63]; and formulating public health actions that are grounded in mental health promotion under an equity-oriented lens [58].

4. Discussion

Under the syndemics perspective, vulnerability during the COVID-19 pandemic was extensively described in relation to (a) the risk of being infected, developing illness, or dying from COVID-19, and (b) experiencing negative health, economic, or social outcomes as a result of COVID-19 control measures. Exploring heterogeneous health outcomes, particularly clustering of cases or deaths in specific populations or geographical areas, emerged as the most often claimed argument to apply a syndemics framework during the COVID-19 pandemic.

From these results, two important contributions of syndemic thinking on vulnerability that emerged during the COVID-19 pandemic can be highlighted:

(a) Advances on a biosocial conception of health: All the publications included in this review elaborated on intersections between biomedical and social factors that occurred around COVID-19. A typical application of the syndemics framework during the COVID-19 pandemic would include biomedical factors considered to increase susceptibility to COVID-19, and contextualize, locate, or explain them in the light of socio-environmental factors or dynamics enhancing their negative outcomes. Another common application would describe syndemic interactions or syndemic effects of the pandemic in population groups historically exposed to marginalization based on race, ethnicity, gender, and/or migratory status. The fact that syndemics research has contributed to the definition and understanding of a biosocial conceptualization of health is an important contribution. For too long the public health community has been focusing on downstream "risk factors" and many opportunities for sustainable disease control have been missed. In this review, the syndemics framework helped to illustrate how vulnerabilities to COVID-19 overlapped with vulnerabilities to standardized COVID-19 control measures across contexts, which could provide important arguments to reflect on the profound implications of thinking of these measures simply as 'non-pharmaceutical' interventions. COVID-19 control measures reinforced and engendered new vulnerabilities and provided a clear example of the social ramifications of these measures beyond health-specific spheres.

(b) Syndemics as a language of complexity: The fact that none of the original research studies included in this review focused on demonstrating the existence of a particular syndemic, but rather on applying this concept as a theoretical framework to analyze different datasets, might be an indication of a new phase in syndemics research. Instead of looking into the empirical validity of syndemics's theoretical claims, researchers have appropriated its language to describe complex, i.e., multifactorial, multiscale, intricate, and multidirectional pathways involved in the generation of health and disease, and very

particularly, vulnerability to disease. This coincides with the framing of COVID-19 as a syndemic. Although it has already been argued that extending the use of the term 'syndemic' to all the effects of the pandemic can actually limit the extent to which this perspective can identify interactions that matter amidst a global emergency [21,67], the popularity of Horton's piece [5] (cited over 700 times since its publication) is noteworthy. Uses of this expression in this review referred to COVID-19 as cause and consequence of profound interconnections between different levels of vulnerability and, as a result, facilitated engagement with systemic views in which individual vulnerability was always embedded in larger social, environmental, and political contexts. These discussions linked COVID-19 with new forms of vulnerability at a planetary scale, in which interactions with environmental conditions, non-human species, and economic systems play a fundamental role. Some of the theoretical and policy recommendations already point to the need for interdisciplinary and multisectoral action to tackle the most pressing challenges ahead of us. Syndemics research can definitely contribute to such explorations.

However, we acknowledge that some of the criticism expressed around syndemics remained true for the publications included in this review. We want to focus here on two concrete limitations identified in this study:

(a) Limited exploration of interactions between biomedical and social spheres: Records frequently mentioned that COVID-19 generated multiple forms of interactions with pre-existing medical or social conditions; nevertheless, the most frequently described form of interaction was one in which COVID-19 created additional burdens in patients with comorbidities and populations experiencing different forms of social disadvantage. Although important, it could be argued that this was a somehow expected outcome of the pandemic and that other forms of interactions remained largely unexplored. For example, which interactions moderated the variability of outcomes within these already 'vulnerable' populations? How to account for context-specific circumstances and social responses in populations historically subjected to marginalization or discrimination? In which ways was COVID-19 different from other forms of risk experienced by these populations? Concurrently, social vulnerability or social disadvantages were often described as the main characteristics of syndemic contexts. However, is being part of the context sufficient to establish mutually reinforcing relationships between these forms of marginalization and COVID-19 outcomes? More importantly, what are the implications of considering these distinct phenomena (social vulnerability or social disadvantage) as 'context'?

Limited research on the types of syndemic interactions can be a result of the difficulties in conducting scientific research during the pandemic. However, it could also be argued that there are conceptual limitations in the analytical methods of mainstream epidemiology that limit the possibility of integrating non-epidemiological thinking to explain complex phenomena. As an example, multiple publications emphasized the role of place in the generation of vulnerability. In these cases, most studies focused on understanding COVID-19 clustering around pre-established administrative units (counties, zip code areas, etc.). Using geo-located data, accessed through publicly available datasets, syndemic interactions were often described in relation to the co-existence of specific comorbidities and social conditions within the same geographical space. However, is this co-existence enough to explain the role of 'place' in syndemic interactions? Although somehow mentioned, complex interactions between natural, built, and social environments across geographical scales remained largely unexplored according to this review.

(b) Limited theoretical and methodological developments from the social sciences and other disciplinary fields: In general, socio-environmental factors were treated as 'social' risk factors [1,68], i.e., explored to the extent to which they increased the burden of infection and disease. Issues such as social vulnerability and disadvantage were measured through socioeconomic indicators, inherently limited to portray the material, political, and emotional impacts of complex social phenomena. This was particularly true for studies using the framing of the SDOH. When the SDOH, as a group, were included in syndemic interactions, they acted as a generic framework to account for issues of a very diverse nature, from

precarity in housing to lack of political representation. They were approached by means of indicators from which we can advance, and perhaps confirm, associations between social factors and COVID-19 outcomes; however, they cannot explain the processes of social determination of health that led them to be relevant in specific contexts [69]. Consequently, and contrary to what could be expected, using the SDOH framework, as well as terms such as racism, gender-based violence, and stigmatization, without acknowledging their theoretical foundations, can obscure rather than disentangle the specific mechanisms under which they influence health and disease. While bringing the syndemics perspective is an important step towards more holistic approaches to health, it is not enough to explain the theoretical dimensions of phenomena that are social in essence and for which validated theories, methods, and knowledge exist.

A recent scoping review by Bulled and Singer also focused on applications of syndemics thinking during the COVID-19 pandemic [70], concurring on the conceptual and methodological limitations of current syndemics research. Importantly, the authors made a strong claim to reconsider formulations that conceptualize syndemic interactions as "universal", as the syndemics perspective was conceived precisely to explain the opposite: that health vulnerabilities are highly contextual [67]. Bulled and Singer also identified what they referred to as "misuses" of the term syndemics, when it is applied to research that characterizes independent risk factors without addressing specific interactions. Our review makes an important contribution in this regard: when researchers use the syndemics perspective to explain vulnerability, a more nuanced picture emerges. Although mostly anchored in mainstream statistical methods, all the publications included in our review build on a biosocial conception of health, which could indicate that syndemics is, indeed, a suitable theoretical device to study complex interactions. Although both reviews draw on largely different sets of records (only 14 out of 40 records included here were also included in the review by Bulled and Singer), they arrive at relatively similar conclusions. Nevertheless, we want to highlight two important differences in our findings. First, the fact that spatial analyses were more frequently used in syndemics research during the COVID-19 pandemic is not necessarily an indication of a more rigorous application of the concept. We have already pointed out the lack of engagement with spatial realities identified, which can lead to establishing associations that disregard internal social and geographical heterogeneity in large spatial units of analysis. Second, we agree with the idea that there is a conceptual movement in syndemics research, but for us, this conceptual movement builds on syndemics as a language of complexity. Our review provides a snapshot of how researchers have appropriated the term syndemics—with no evaluative interests involved. The epistemological implications of this movement constitute an interesting area for future research.

5. Conclusions

The syndemic perspective made multiple contributions to understanding vulnerability during the COVID-19 pandemic; nevertheless, current applications of the theory may threaten its empirical foundations and hinder the effective use of this concept in public health policies and practices. During the most recent pandemic, syndemics research advanced a biosocial conception of health that emphasized the role of socio-environmental factors in disease clustering and interaction. Syndemics served as a language of complexity, enabling researchers to describe the multifactorial and multidirectional pathways involved in vulnerability to disease. Despite these contributions, this review identified limitations in its current application. Specifically, there has been limited exploration of the interactions between the biomedical and social spheres. Furthermore, there has been a lack of theoretical and methodological contributions from the social sciences, as we observe socio-environmental phenomena primarily being treated as 'social' risk factors and approached through limited quantitative indicators. Potential ways of overcoming these limitations include enhancing interdisciplinary collaborations to address the complex and multifaceted nature of vulnerability during crises of global scale such as COVID-19; enriching syndemics research with theoretical and methodological developments from the social sciences to deepen the understanding of the social mechanisms through which they shape vulnerability; investigating complex associations between biomedical and social realities; and exploring methodological approaches that facilitate investigation of the intersections between natural, built, and social environments in the generation of disease.

6. Limitations and Strengths of the Review

An important limitation of this study is that we focused our search on publications registered in PubMed. We are aware that other databases—more specialized in multidisciplinary research, for example—could have yielded different results. However, we were interested in understanding the potential contributions of these concepts to the management of the pandemic in the medical field, and for that reason, we considered that PubMed was the best source. As previously mentioned, another review with a similar focus consulted a larger set of sources; our findings provide a focalized analysis zooming into discussions on vulnerability in syndemics research [70]. We also acknowledge that important conceptual discussions around the term 'vulnerability' have occurred in different fields, which, in some cases, have led to a reduced or limited use of the term. That is the case for HIV control and prevention, for example. This conceptual discussion could explain the limited number of HIV-related records identified in this review, despite the extended use of the syndemics perspective in this field. This could also have been the case for other expressions associated with the term vulnerability that could have escaped our search strategy. Another limitation of this study is that it included many opinion pieces, which limits our claims about the theoretical and methodological limitations of syndemics thinking in the pandemic context.

Supplementary Materials: The following supporting information can be downloaded at https://www.mdpi.com/article/10.3390/tropicalmed9080189/s1, Supplementary File S1: PRISMA-ScR checklist; Supplementary File S2: Data extraction form; Supplementary File S3: Table synthesis of results.

Author Contributions: Conceptualization, Y.H.B., C.N.-S., D.P.C. and K.P.G.; methodology, Y.H.B., C.N.-S., D.P.C. and K.V.; validation, C.G., Y.H.B., Y.M.G., C.N.-S., D.P.C. and K.V.; formal analysis, Y.H.B., Y.M.G., C.N.-S. and D.P.C.; investigation, Y.H.B., Y.M.G., C.N.-S. and D.P.C.; resources, Y.H.B., K.P.G. and K.V.; data curation, Y.H.B., Y.M.G., C.N.-S. and D.P.C.; writing—original draft preparation, Y.H.B., Y.M.G., C.N.-S. and D.P.C.; writing—review and editing, CG, Y.H.B., Y.M.G., C.N.-S., D.P.C., K.V. and K.P.G.; supervision, C.N.-S. and K.P.G.; project administration, Y.H.B., D.P.C. and C.N.-S.; funding acquisition, Y.H.B., C.N.-S., D.P.C. and K.P.G. All authors have read and agreed to the published version of the manuscript.

Funding: This research was funded by an ITM-DGD Predoctoral Grant granted to the first author (Dir-AcOff/av/2022/19) financially supported by the Belgian Directorate-General Cooperation and Humanitarian Aid (DGD), the Institute of Tropical Medicine (Antwerp), and the Institute of Tropical Medicine Pedro Kourí (Havana). Additional support was obtained from the Belgian Directorate-general for Development Cooperation and Humanitarian Aid (DGD) via the fifth Framework Agreement (FA5) with the Institute of Tropical Medicine, Antwerp.

Institutional Review Board Statement: Not applicable.

Informed Consent Statement: Not applicable.

Data Availability Statement: The original contributions presented in the study are included in the article; further inquiries can be directed to the corresponding author.

Acknowledgments: We want to thank the Population Data Hub and the Ecohealth Research Group at the Department of Public Health—Institute of Tropical Medicine Antwerp for providing methodological and technical guidance through this process.

Conflicts of Interest: The authors declare no conflicts of interest.

References

1. Singer, M.; Bulled, N.; Ostrach, B. Whither syndemics?: Trends in syndemics research, a review 2015–2019. *Glob. Public Health* **2020**, *15*, 943–955. [CrossRef]
2. Gravlee, C.C. Systemic racism, chronic health inequities, and COVID-19: A syndemic in the making? *Am. J. Hum. Biol.* **2020**, *32*, 23482. [CrossRef]
3. Kantamneni, N. The impact of the COVID-19 pandemic on marginalized populations in the United States: A research agenda. *J. Vocat. Behav.* **2020**, *119*, 103439. [CrossRef]
4. Lund, E.M. Even more to handle: Additional sources of stress and trauma for clients from marginalized racial and ethnic groups in the United States during the COVID-19 pandemic. *Couns. Psychol. Q.* **2020**, *34*, 321–330. [CrossRef]
5. Horton, R. Offline: COVID-19 is not a pandemic. *Lancet* **2020**, *396*, 874. [CrossRef] [PubMed]
6. Irons, R. Pandemic . . . or syndemic? Re-framing COVID-19 disease burden and 'underlying health conditions'. *Soc. Anthropol.* **2020**, *28*, 286–287. [CrossRef] [PubMed]
7. Singer, M.; Bulled, N.; Ostrach, B.; Mendenhall, E. Syndemics and the biosocial conception of health. *Lancet* **2017**, *389*, 941–950. [CrossRef]
8. Willen, S.S.; Knipper, M.; Abadía-Barrero, C.E.; Davidovitch, N. Syndemic vulnerability and the right to health. *Lancet* **2017**, *389*, 964–977. [CrossRef]
9. Faas, A.J. Disaster vulnerability in anthropological perspective. *Ann. Anthropol. Pract.* **2016**, *40*, 14–27. [CrossRef]
10. Marino, E.K.; Faas, A.J. Is Vulnerability an Outdated Concept? After Subjects and Spaces. *Ann. Anthropol. Pract.* **2020**, *44*, 33–46. [CrossRef]
11. Ribera, J.M.; Hausmann-Muela, S. The Straw That Breaks the Camel's Back Redirecting Health-Seeking Behavior Studies on Malaria and Vulnerability. *Med. Anthropol. Q.* **2011**, *25*, 103–121. [CrossRef] [PubMed]
12. Frohlich, K.L.; Potvin, L. Transcending the known in public health practice: The inequality paradox: The population approach and vulnerable populations. *Am. J. Public Health* **2008**, *98*, 216–221. [CrossRef] [PubMed]
13. Jeleff, M.; Lehner, L.; Giles-Vernick, T.; Dückers, M.L.; Napier, A.D.; Jirovsky-Platter, E.; Kutalek, R. Vulnerability and One Health assessment approaches for infectious threats from a social science perspective: A systematic scoping review. *Lancet Planet. Health* **2022**, *6*, e682–e693. [CrossRef] [PubMed]
14. Osborne, J.; Paget, J.; Giles-Vernick, T.; Kutalek, R.; Napier, D.; Baliatsas, C.; Dückers, M. Community engagement and vulnerability in infectious diseases: A systematic review and qualitative analysis of the literature. *Soc. Sci. Med.* **2021**, *284*, 277–9536. [CrossRef]
15. Tsai, A.C. Syndemics: A theory in search of data or data in search of a theory? *Soc. Sci. Med.* **2018**, *206*, 117–122. [CrossRef]
16. Tsai, A.C.; Venkataramani, A.S. Syndemics and Health Disparities: A Methodological Note. *AIDS Behav.* **2016**, *20*, 423–430. [CrossRef]
17. Tsai, A.C.; Burns, B.F.O. Syndemics of psychosocial problems and HIV risk: A systematic review of empirical tests of the disease interaction concept. *Soc. Sci. Med.* **2015**, *139*, 26–35. [CrossRef]
18. Weaver, L.J.; Kaiser, B.N. Syndemics theory must take local context seriously: An example of measures for poverty, mental health, and food insecurity. *Soc. Sci. Med.* **2022**, *295*, 113304. [CrossRef]
19. Sangaramoorthy, T.; Benton, A. Intersectionality and syndemics: A commentary. *Soc. Sci. Med.* **2022**, *295*, 113783. [CrossRef]
20. Weiss, N.M. A Critical Perspective on Syndemic Theory and Social Justice. *Public Anthropol.* **2021**, *3*, 285–317. [CrossRef]
21. Mendenhall, E.; Newfield, T.; Tsai, A.C. Syndemic theory, methods, and data. *Soc. Sci. Med.* **2022**, *295*, 114656. [CrossRef] [PubMed]
22. Bulled, N.; Singer, M.; Ostrach, B. Syndemics and intersectionality: A response commentary. *Soc. Sci. Med.* **2022**, *295*, 114743. [CrossRef]
23. Hernández, Y.; Pérez, D.; Molina, Y.; Peeters Grietens, K.; Nieto-Sánchez, C. (Re)conceptualizing vulnerability in health under the syndemics perspective: Protocol for a scoping review. *F1000Research* **2022**, *11*, 1156. [CrossRef]
24. Tricco, A.C.; Lillie, E.; Zarin, W.; O'Brien, K.K.; Colquhoun, H.; Levac, D.; Moher, D.; Peters, M.D.J.; Horsley, T.; Weeks, L.; et al. PRISMA Extension for Scoping Reviews (PRISMAScR): Checklist and Explanation. *Ann. Intern. Med.* **2018**, *169*, 467–473. [CrossRef]
25. Tricco, A.C.; Antony, J.; Soobiah, C.; Kastner, M.; Cogo, E.; MacDonald, H.; D'Souza, J.; Hui, W.; Straus, S.E. Knowledge synthesis methods for generating or refining theory: A scoping review reveals that little guidance is available. *J. Clin. Epidemiol.* **2016**, *73*, 36–42. [CrossRef]
26. Simera, I.; Moher, D.; Hoey, J.; Schulz, K.F.; Altman, D.G. A catalogue of reporting guidelines for health research. *Eur. J. Clin. Investig.* **2010**, *40*, 35–53. [CrossRef]
27. Singh, K.; Kaushik, A.; Johnson, L.; Jaganathan, S.; Jarhyan, P.; Deepa, M.; Kong, S.; Venkateshmurthy, N.S.; Kondal, D.; Mohan, S.; et al. Patient experiences and perceptions of chronic disease care during the COVID-19 pandemic in India: A qualitative study. *BMJ Open* **2021**, *11*, e048926. [CrossRef]
28. Chung, G.K.K.; Chan, S.M.; Chan, Y.H.; Yip, T.C.F.; Ma, H.M.; Wong, G.L.H.; Chung, R.Y.N.; Wong, H.; Wong, S.Y.S.; Yeoh, E.K.; et al. Differential impacts of multimorbidity on COVID-19 severity across the socioeconomic ladder in Hong Kong: A syndemic perspective. *Int. J. Environ. Res. Public Health* **2021**, *18*, 8168. [CrossRef]

29. Islam, N.; Lacey, B.; Shabnam, S.; Erzurumluoglu, A.M.; Dambha-Miller, H.; Chowell, G.; Kawachi, I.; Marmot, M. Social inequality the syndemic of chronic disease COVID-19: County-level analysis in the USA. *J. Epidemiol. Community Health (1978)* **2021**, *75*, 496–500. [CrossRef]
30. Lee, J.; Ramírez, I.J. Geography of Disparity: Connecting COVID-19 Vulnerability and Social Determinants of Health in Colorado. *Behav. Med.* **2022**, *48*, 72–84. [CrossRef]
31. Fronteira, I.; Sidat, M.; Magalhães, J.P.; de Barros, F.P.C.; Delgado, A.P.; Correia, T.; Daniel-Ribeiro, C.T.; Ferrinho, P. The SARS-CoV-2 pandemic: A syndemic perspective. *One Health* **2021**, *12*, 100228. [CrossRef] [PubMed]
32. Burigo, A.C.; Porto, M.F. 2030 agenda, health and food systems in times of syndemics: From vulnerabilities to necessary changes. *Cienc. Saude Coletiva* **2021**, *26*, 4411–4424. [CrossRef] [PubMed]
33. Di Ciaula, A.; Krawczyk, M.; Filipiak, K.J.; Geier, A.; Bonfrate, L.; Portincasa, P. Noncommunicable diseases, climate change and iniquities: What COVID-19 has taught us about syndemic. *Eur. J. Clin. Investig.* **2021**, *51*, 13682. [CrossRef] [PubMed]
34. Lemke, M.K.; Apostolopoulos, Y.; Sönmez, S. A novel COVID-19 based truck driver syndemic? Implications for public health, safety, and vital supply chains. *Am. J. Ind. Med.* **2020**, *63*, 659–662. [CrossRef] [PubMed]
35. Pryor, S.; Dietz, W. The COVID-19, Obesity, and Food Insecurity Syndemic. *Curr. Obes. Rep.* **2022**, *11*, 70–79. [CrossRef]
36. Melamed, O.C.; Zawertailo, L.; Schwartz, R.; Buckley, L.; Selby, P. Protection des groupes vulnérables contre les méfaits du tabac pendant et après la pandémie de COVID-19. *Health Promot. Chronic Dis. Prev. Can.* **2021**, *41*, 282–287. [CrossRef]
37. Yadav, U.N.; Rayamajhee, B.; Mistry, S.K.; Parsekar, S.S.; Mishra, S.K. A Syndemic Perspective on the Management of Non-communicable Diseases Amid the COVID-19 Pandemic in Low- and Middle-Income Countries. *Front. Public Health* **2020**, *8*, 00508. [CrossRef] [PubMed]
38. Daboin, B.E.G.; Bezerra, I.M.P.; Morais, T.C.; Portugal, I.; Echeimberg, J.D.O.; Cesar, A.E.M.; Cavalcanti, M.P.E.; Jacintho, L.C.; Raimundo, R.D.; Elmusharaf, K.; et al. Deciphering Multifactorial Correlations of COVID-19 Incidence and Mortality in the Brazilian Amazon Basin. *Int. J. Environ. Res. Public Health* **2022**, *19*, 1153. [CrossRef]
39. Ali, I. Syndemics at play: Chronic kidney disease, diabetes and COVID-19 in Pakistan. *Ann. Med.* **2021**, *53*, 581–586. [CrossRef]
40. Jenkins, E.K.; McAuliffe, C.; Hirani, S.; Richardson, C.; Thomson, K.C.; McGuinness, L.; Morris, J.; Kousoulis, A.; Gadermann, A. A portrait of the early and differential mental health impacts of the COVID-19 pandemic in Canada: Findings from the first wave of a nationally representative cross-sectional survey. *Prev. Med.* **2021**, *145*, 106333. [CrossRef]
41. Jenkins, E.K.; Slemon, A.; Richardson, C.; Pumarino, J.; McAuliffe, C.; Thomson, K.C.; Goodyear, T.; Daly, Z.; McGuinness, L.; Gadermann, A. Mental Health Inequities Amid the COVID-19 Pandemic: Findings from Three Rounds of a Cross-Sectional Monitoring Survey of Canadian Adults. *Int. J. Public Health* **2022**, *67*, 1604685. [CrossRef] [PubMed]
42. Meinhart, M.; Vahedi, L.; Carter, S.E.; Poulton, C.; Mwanze Palaku, P.; Stark, L. Gender-based violence and infectious disease in humanitarian settings: Lessons learned from Ebola, Zika, and COVID-19 to inform syndemic policy making. *Confl. Health* **2021**, *15*, 84. [CrossRef] [PubMed]
43. Mezzina, R.; Gopikumar, V.; Jenkins, J.; Saraceno, B.; Sashidharan, S.P. Social Vulnerability and Mental Health Inequalities in the "Syndemic": Call for Action. *Front. Psychiatry* **2022**, *13*, 894370. [CrossRef]
44. Lemke, M.K.; Brown, K.K. Syndemic Perspectives to Guide Black Maternal Health Research and Prevention during the COVID-19 Pandemic. *Matern. Child Health J.* **2020**, *24*, 1093–1098. [CrossRef]
45. Shim, R.S.; Starks, S.M. COVID-19, structural racism, and mental health inequities: Policy implications for an emerging syndemic. *Psychiatr. Serv.* **2021**, *72*, 1193–1198. [CrossRef] [PubMed]
46. Kalichman, S.C.; El-Krab, R. Social and Behavioral Impacts of COVID-19 on People Living with HIV: Review of the First Year of Research. *Curr. HIV/AIDS Rep.* **2022**, *19*, 54–75. [CrossRef]
47. Knipper, M.; Sedas, A.C.; Keshavjee, S.; Abbara, A.; Almhawish, N.; Alashawi, H.; Lecca, L.; Wilson, M.; Zumla, A.; Abubakar, I.; et al. The need for protecting and enhancing TB health policies and services for forcibly displaced and migrant populations during the ongoing COVID-19 pandemic. *Int. J. Infect. Dis.* **2021**, *113*, S22–S27. [CrossRef]
48. Siegal, R.; Cooper, H.; Capers, T.; Kilmer, R.P.; Cook, J.R.; Garo, L. Using geographic information systems to inform the public health response to COVID-19 and structural racism: The role of place-based initiatives. *J. Community Psychol.* **2022**, *50*, 2611–2629. [CrossRef]
49. Caron, R.M.; Aytur, S.A. Assuring Healthy Populations During the COVID-19 Pandemic: Recognizing Women's Contributions in Addressing Syndemic Interactions. *Front. Public Health* **2022**, *10*, 856932. [CrossRef]
50. Caron, R.M.; Adegboye, A.R.A. COVID-19: A Syndemic Requiring an Integrated Approach for Marginalized Populations. *Front. Public Health* **2021**, *9*, 675280. [CrossRef]
51. Garcia, M. This Is America: Systemic Racism and Health Inequities Amidst the COVID-19 Pandemic. *Soc. Work Public Health* **2022**, *37*, 105–121. [CrossRef]
52. Cokley, K.; Krueger, N.; Cunningham, S.R.; Burlew, K.; Hall, S.; Harris, K.; Castelin, S.; Coleman, C. The COVID-19/racial injustice syndemic and mental health among Black Americans: The roles of general and race-related COVID worry, cultural mistrust, and perceived discrimination. *J. Community Psychol.* **2022**, *50*, 2542–2561. [CrossRef] [PubMed]
53. Chaudhuri, E.R. The Syndemic of Inequity and COVID-19 in Virtual Care. *J. Med. Internet Res.* **2022**, *24*, e37717. [CrossRef] [PubMed]
54. Williams, C.; Vermund, S.H. Syndemic Framework Evaluation of Severe COVID-19 Outcomes in the United States: Factors Associated with Race and Ethnicity. *Front. Public Health* **2021**, *9*, 720264. [CrossRef]

55. Poteat, T.; Millett, G.A.; Nelson, L.R.E.; Beyrer, C. Understanding COVID-19 risks and vulnerabilities among black communities in America: The lethal force of syndemics. *Ann. Epidemiol.* **2020**, *47*, 1–3. [CrossRef] [PubMed]
56. Morrissey, M.B.Q.; Rivera, J.L. Protecting the Public's Health in Pandemics: Reflections on Policy Deliberation and the Role of Civil Society in Democracy. *Front. Public Health* **2021**, *9*, 678210. [CrossRef]
57. Rogers, B.G.; Paradis-Burnett, A.; Nagel, K.; Yolken, A.; Strong, S.H.; Arnold, T.; Napoleon, S.C.; Maynard, M.; Sosnowy, C.; Murphy, M.; et al. Sex Workers and Syndemics: A Population Vulnerable to HIV and COVID-19. *Arch. Sex. Behav.* **2021**, *50*, 2007–2016. [CrossRef]
58. Sönmez, S.; Apostolopoulos, Y.; Lemke, M.K.; Hsieh, Y.C.J. Understanding the effects of COVID-19 on the health and safety of immigrant hospitality workers in the United States. *Tour. Manag. Perspect.* **2020**, *35*, 100717. [CrossRef]
59. Neto, A.O.M.E.; Da Silva, S.A.G.; Gonçalves, G.P.; Torres, J.L. COVID-19 vulnerability among Brazilian sexual and gender minorities: A cross-sectional study. *Cad. Saude Publica* **2022**, *38*, e00234421. [CrossRef]
60. Duby, Z.; Bunce, B.; Fowler, C.; Bergh, K.; Jonas, K.; Dietrich, J.J.; Govindasamy, D.; Kuo, C.; Mathews, C. Intersections between COVID-19 and socio-economic mental health stressors in the lives of South African adolescent girls and young women. *Child Adolesc. Psychiatry Ment. Health* **2022**, *16*, 23. [CrossRef]
61. Wildman, J.M.; Morris, S.; Pollard, T.; Gibson, K.; Moffatt, S. "I wouldn't survive it, as simple as that": Syndemic vulnerability among people living with chronic non-communicable disease during the COVID-19 pandemic. *SSM Qual. Res. Health* **2022**, *2*, 100032. [CrossRef] [PubMed]
62. Stark, L.; Meinhart, M.; Vahedi, L.; Carter, S.E.; Roesch, E.; Scott Moncrieff, I.; Palaku, P.M.; Rossi, F.; Poulton, C. The syndemic of COVID-19 and gender-based violence in humanitarian settings: Leveraging lessons from Ebola in the Democratic Republic of Congo. *BMJ Glob. Health* **2020**, *5*, e004194. [CrossRef] [PubMed]
63. Singer, M.; Rylko-Bauer, B. The Syndemics and Structural Violence of the COVID Pandemic: Anthropological Insights on a Crisis. *Open Anthropol. Res.* **2021**, *1*, 7–32. [CrossRef]
64. Borghi-Silva, A.; Back, G.D.; de Araújo, A.S.G.; Oliveira, M.R.; da Luz Goulart, C.; Silva, R.N.; Bassi, D.; Mendes, R.G.; Arena, R. COVID-19 seen from a syndemic perspective: Impact of unhealthy habits and future perspectives to combat these negative interactions in Latin America. *Prog. Cardiovasc. Dis.* **2022**, *71*, 72–78. [CrossRef] [PubMed]
65. Pirrone, I.; Dieleman, M.; Reis, R.; Pell, C. Syndemic contexts: Findings from a review of research on non-communicable diseases and interviews with experts. *Glob. Health Action* **2021**, 14. [CrossRef]
66. Bispo Júnior, J.P.; Dos Santos, D.B. COVID-19 as a syndemic: A theoretical model and foundations for a comprehensive approach in health. *Cad. Saude Publica* **2021**, *37*, e00119021. [CrossRef]
67. Singer, M.; Bulled, N.; Leatherman, T. Are There Global Syndemics? *Med. Anthropol.* **2022**, *41*, 4–18. [CrossRef] [PubMed]
68. Nichter, M. Comorbidity: Reconsidering the Unit of Analysis. *Med. Anthropol. Q.* **2016**, *30*, 536–544. [CrossRef]
69. Breilh, J. The social determination of health and the transformation of rights and ethics1: A meta-critical methodology for responsible and reparative science. *Glob. Public Health* **2023**, 18. [CrossRef]
70. Bulled, N.; Singer, M. Conceptualizing COVID-19 syndemics: A scoping review. *J. Multimorb. Comorbidity* **2024**, *14*, 26335565241249835. [CrossRef]

Tropical Medicine and Infectious Disease

MDPI

Article

Gender and Intersecting Barriers and Facilitators to Access the HIV Cascade of Care in Manitoba, Canada, Before and During the COVID-19 Pandemic: A Qualitative Study

Enrique Villacis-Alvarez [1], Cheryl Sobie [1], Katharina Maier [2], Margaret Lavallee [3], Chantal Daniels [3], Heather Pashe [1], Joel Baliddawa [4], Nikki Daniels [4], Rebecca Murdock [4], Robert Russell [4], Clara Dan [4], Freda Woodhouse [4], Susie Cusson [4], Lisa Patrick [4], Marj Schenkels [4], Michael Payne [5,6], Ken Kasper [6,7], Lauren J. MacKenzie [6,7], Laurie Ireland [5,6,8], Kimberly Templeton [5,6], Kathleen Deering [9,10], Margaret Haworth-Brockman [11,12], Yoav Keynan [1,7,9,11,12] and Zulma Vanessa Rueda [1,13,*]

1 Department of Medical Microbiology and Infectious Diseases, Rady Faculty of Health Sciences, University of Manitoba, Winnipeg, MB R3E 0J9, Canada; villacisenrique@gmail.com (E.V.-A.); yoav.keynan@umanitoba.ca (Y.K.)
2 Criminal Justice, The University of Winnipeg, Winnipeg, MB R3B 2E9, Canada; k.maier@uwinnipeg.ca
3 Ongomiizwin Indigenous Institute of Health & Healing, Rady Faculty of Health Sciences, University of Manitoba, Winnipeg, MB R3E 0W2, Canada
4 Peer Research Team, Alltogether4IDEAS, Winnipeg, MB R3E 0J9, Canada
5 Nine Circles Community Health Centre, Winnipeg, MB R3G 0X2, Canada
6 The Manitoba HIV Program, Winnipeg, MB R3G 0X2, Canada
7 Department of Internal Medicine, Rady Faculty of Health Sciences, University of Manitoba, Winnipeg, MB R3E 0J9, Canada
8 Department of Family Medicine, Rady Faculty of Health Sciences, University of Manitoba, Winnipeg, MB R3E 0J9, Canada
9 Division of Medicine, Department of Medicine, Faculty of Medicine, University of British Columbia, Vancouver, BC V6Z 2K5, Canada; kathleen.deering@cgshe.ubc.ca
10 Centre for Gender and Sexual Health Equity, Faculty of Medicine, University of British Columbia, Vancouver, BC V6Z 2K5, Canada
11 Department of Community Health Sciences, Rady Faculty of Health Sciences, University of Manitoba, Winnipeg, MB R3E 0J9, Canada; margaret.haworth-brockman@umanitoba.ca
12 National Collaborating Centre for Infectious Diseases, Rady Faculty of Health Sciences, University of Manitoba, Winnipeg, MB R3E 0J9, Canada
13 Escuela de Ciencias de la Salud, Universidad Pontificia Bolivariana, Medellin 050021, Colombia
* Correspondence: zulma.rueda@umanitoba.ca

Abstract: Marginalized groups in Manitoba, Canada, especially females and people who inject drugs, are overrepresented in new HIV diagnoses and disproportionately affected by HIV and structural disadvantages. Informed by syndemic theory, our aim was to understand people living with HIV's (PLHIV) gendered and intersecting barriers and facilitators across the cascade of HIV care before and during the COVID-19 pandemic. This study was co-designed and co-led alongside people with lived experience and a research advisory committee. We employed semi-structured interviews with thirty-two participants and three questionnaires. Interviews were audio-recorded, transcribed, and coded, and descriptive statistics were performed on the first two questionnaires. Qualitative data analysis used thematic analysis and focused on identifying categories (individual, healthcare, and social/structural) related to the barriers and facilitators to HIV care. A total of 32 PLHIV completed this study and over 70% of females and 50% of males reported severe and moderate sexual abuse among other traumatic childhood experiences. Barriers to accessing or continuing in the cascade of HIV care included navigating the initial shock of receiving an HIV diagnosis, mental health challenges and inaccessible supports, substance use, violence (including intimate partner), internalized and enacted compounded stigma related to houselessness and substance use, discrimination by primary care service providers and social networks, lack of preventative and social supports, lack of accessible housing, and programmatic issues. COVID-19 increased mental health problems and disrupted relationships with HIV service providers and peers living with HIV. Facilitators to HIV care included stopping substance use, caring service providers particularly during

HIV diagnosis, welcoming healthcare environments, social opportunities and integrated supports, and supportive social networks. Women, men, and non-binary PLHIV experience interconnected factors complicating their experiences with HIV care. Interventions should consider holistic, person-centered, and trauma-informed care options to address the barriers found in this research and appropriately serve PLHIV.

Keywords: HIV; syndemic; barriers to HIV care; person-centered care; qualitative research; community-based research

1. Background

The Joint United Nations Programme on HIV/AIDS estimated that approximately 39 million people worldwide were living with HIV in 2022 [1]. In 2022, the Government of Canada reported a decrease in HIV diagnoses and achievement of the first and third objectives of the 90-90-90 goals [2]. However, the landscape of HIV in Canada is heterogeneous.

The Canadian province of Manitoba reported a 52% increase in new HIV diagnoses between 2018 and 2021, with increased diagnoses among females, those who self-identify as Indigenous, people who engage in heterosexual sex, and those who inject methamphetamines, and an increase in people not returning to HIV care [3–5]. Epidemiological data from new HIV diagnoses reported a disease cluster of increased concurrent sexually transmitted and blood-borne infections (STBBIs) and mental health conditions combined with houselessness (Supplementary File S1) [4,5]. In addition, the COVID-19 pandemic exacerbated health disparities among people living with HIV (PLHIV) [6]. Indigenous people account for 18% of the population of Manitoba [7], yet they are overrepresented in new HIV diagnoses (76% from 2018 to 2021) [4,5], houselessness counts [8], and other health conditions which stem from the past and current harms of colonization and violent structural policies [9].

The biological interactions of the HIV and STBBI disease cluster may lead to worse health outcomes by increasing the transmission of each or exacerbating disease progression. For example, inflammatory immune cell responses induced by STBBIs can increase the risk of HIV transmission [10]. The mutually reinforcing biological implications of HIV and substance use have also been well documented [11–13] and, in particular, methamphetamine use has been associated with a higher rate of HIV viral replication [14]. Preclinical data demonstrate that the use of injection drugs and the presence of STBBIs are powerful independent cofactors that disrupt tissues, favor inflammation, and promote HIV acquisition and poor health outcomes. Specifically, methamphetamine use is associated with changes to mucosal tissues, which are linked to inflammation and immune activation [15–17]. Genital inflammation significantly increases the risk of HIV acquisition due to the recruitment of HIV target cells (activated T cells) to the genital tract. Activated CD4+ T cells are more susceptible to HIV infection than quiescent cells and once infected, produce up to 1000 times more virus [18]. In addition, the recent use of methamphetamine among PLHIV affected T cell function [19,20] and was associated with inflammation and vascular injury [21].

In addition, psychosocial factors such as mental health disorders and trauma, houselessness, marginalization, and stigma and discrimination can negatively impact health outcomes of PLHIV. People experiencing mental health disorders have been overrepresented in HIV diagnoses [22]. The social and structural factors associated with homelessness have been shown to result in altered immune function and high levels of oxidative stress along with impaired NK and interleukin responses [23]. It is plausible that the social, substance use-related, and STBBI-induced immune dysregulation act in concert to increase the risk of HIV acquisition. In addition, researchers have found that people experiencing more severe mental health disorders, homelessness, and blood-borne infections tend to utilize primary and specialized health services at lower rates compared to those with less severe mental health disorders and comorbidities [24]. Qualitative studies have highlighted that substance use and active mental health disorders may increase the risk of apathy about care for PLHIV, resulting in missed appointments and reduced medication adherence [25]. Similarly, stigma and discrimination towards PLHIV are linked to lower retention in HIV care and lower overall healthcare utilization regardless of gender [26,27].

There are numerous facilitators and barriers across the continuum of HIV care. While some affect all sub-groups of PLHIV in Canada [28], others are more specific to contexts and populations. For instance, Gahagan and colleagues documented gender-based testing barriers related to gendered expectations and roles among heterosexual men in Nova Scotia [29]. Barriers for street-involved youth in Canada included intersectional stigma, discrimination, and lack of support for basic needs [30], while affordable and wrap-around services worked as facilitators. In an Ontario-based study, barriers for racial and ethnic minority middle-aged and older men who have sex with men included language, racism, cultural norms, and stigma, while wrap-around community-based services promoting HIV resilience and care engagement enabled their HIV care [31].

Understanding that co-occurring epidemics interact with each other and are shaped by context-specific social factors, our study is informed by syndemic theory originally proposed by Singer [11,32]. The syndemic framework proposes the existence of a cluster of distinct yet interconnected diseases which influence each other at different levels (e.g., biologically, socially, and/or psychologically) within specific social forces that reinforce and maintain these clusters [11,33,34]. Syndemic theory goes further than simply documenting the existence of comorbid diseases as it recognizes that social realities mold the presence of and interactions between diseases which can posit adverse interactions among underserved populations [35]. The present article acknowledges the current cluster of diseases and psychosocial conditions experienced by PLHIV in Manitoba [4,5] and aims to disentangle the gendered and intersecting barriers and facilitators to accessing and remaining in the HIV cascade of care. Our major emphasis is on describing the biological and social interactions that are shaping PLHIV's HIV care utilization to inform public health and clinical interventions across the province.

2. Materials and Methods

2.1. Ethics

The protocol for this research has been published elsewhere [32]. This study was approved by the University of Manitoba Health Ethics Research Board (HS25572; H2022:218), the First Nations Health and Social Secretariat of Manitoba, Nine Circles Community Health Centre, Shared Health Manitoba (SH2022:194), and the 7th Street Health Access Centre.

2.2. Study Setting

This study took place in the province of Manitoba, located in central Canada, which has a population of approximately 1.4 million; the majority of people live in Winnipeg (~900,000) and Brandon (~55,000) [36]. The rest of the population is spread across many smaller towns and communities. Anyone diagnosed with HIV in Manitoba is referred to the centralized Manitoba HIV program. Specialized HIV care is given at three clinics across the province, two located in Winnipeg and one in Brandon. Data were collected at the three Manitoba HIV program sites. At the time of data collection, people with a provincial health card received their specialized HIV care as part of the province's insured services. However, the costs of medications depended on individual situations. For example, people employed with benefits may have had their prescriptions paid for by their employers' health plans. Other employed people may have had their medication costs covered through a provincial insurance plan which requires a deductible each year, depending on annual income.

2.3. Researchers Reflexivity

This study is situated within a larger collaborative multidisciplinary project bringing together academic researchers, people with lived experiences, community-based researchers, and medical and social service providers across Canada. The Alltogether4IDEAS research team came together after initial meetings between the three principal investigators and knowledge users (e.g., HIV physicians and health care personnel, and people living with HIV).

Guidance from the project's research advisory committee, peer research team, cultural advisor, and community members resulted in a recruitment strategy grounded in trauma-informed principles, harm reduction, and cultural safety [32]. Participant engagement reflected a non-judgmental and non-stigmatizing approach, and we offered culturally appropriate supports for Indigenous participants [32] (Figure 1). People with lived experience co-designed and co-authored this research, provided extensive reviews and edits on data collection tools and procedures, participated in the analysis and interpretation of results, and reviewed, edited, and approved this article [32].

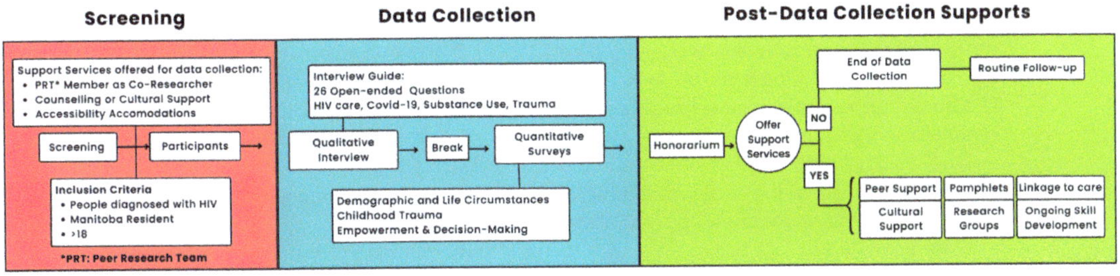

Figure 1. Data collection process. Our approach to inviting people living with HIV to participate in the research project is grounded in cultural safety, trauma-informed care, and harm reduction.

2.4. Participants

The inclusion criteria were PLHIV of 18+ who resided in Manitoba. We used purposive sampling to yield a diverse sample of men, women, and non-binary persons, as well as people from various race/ethnicity backgrounds. Our sampling strategy was carefully designed to hear stories from people diagnosed with HIV. We emphasized including people who have had smooth journeys in connecting and maintaining HIV care, and others who faced more barriers across their HIV care. We wanted to hear stories from people who are representative of the disease clusters recently reported among those with new HIV diagnoses in Manitoba, including experiences of houselessness and substance use [4,5]. The recruitment process included referrals from HIV service providers, posters and flyers in HIV and community organizations, social media, and in-person outreach at Manitoba HIV program sites. We stopped sampling once thematic saturation was reached.

2.5. Data Collection

Data were collected by the research associate (RA), peer co-researchers, and the Indigenous cultural advisor between October 2022, and May 2023. All data collection took place in a private room within at HIV clinics. Participants gave written or verbal informed consent at the start of a session, and then answered questions in an in-depth semi-structured interview inquiring about journey of HIV care, recommendations to HIV care, COVID-19, substance use, harm reduction services, and experiences of trauma. The interview guide was co-developed with people with lived experiences and was published in this study's protocol [32]. After a break, participants responded to the following three survey instruments: a Sociodemographic and Life Circumstances Questionnaire (Supplementary File S2), a Childhood Trauma Questionnaire [37], and an Empower-Making Decisions Survey [38]. The Sociodemographic and Life Circumstances Questionnaire was co-developed through in-depth consultations with people with lived experiences, academic researchers, and HIV knowledge users. Specific questions and goals for understanding key factors related to participants' health and social positions can be found in this study's protocol [32]. All participants had the chance of completing the questionnaires themselves or have the research associate assist with completion orally. All questionnaires were paper-based, and the data were entered in a password-protected database. Data collection sessions took between one and two and a half hours. Interviews were audio recorded, and then transcribed using Otter.ai and reviewed for accuracy by the RA. This qualitative research was part of a broader mixed-methods study; therefore, participant sociodemographic information and responses from the Childhood Trauma Questionnaire are presented below to complement our qualitative findings. The results from the Empower-Making Decisions Survey will be presented in a future paper.

2.6. Data Analysis

Descriptive statistics were calculated for participant demographics. The scoring key for the Childhood Trauma Questionnaire was used to illustrate percentages of severity (e.g., none, low, moderate, severe) across five types of childhood trauma (i.e., emotional abuse, physical abuse, sexual abuse, emotional neglect, physical neglect). Childhood trauma was depicted by sex and gender, and Figure 2 was created using Jamovi® software version 2.5. Along with the syndemic theory described above, we used the World Health Organization's Conceptual Framework for Action on the Social Determinants of Health [32,39] as a theoretical approach to differentiate between the barriers and facilitators at three levels of individual, healthcare, and social and structural. This framework enables researchers to discern the social, economic, and policies that contextualize socioeconomic positions influencing people's opportunities in society [39].

We used NVivo® 12 Pro to thematically analyze the qualitative data. We employed thematic analysis, an approach to analyzing qualitative data originally developed by Braun and Clarke [40]. Since its inception, the methodology has gone through several revisions by its authors, yet this method enables researchers to recognize their own positionality and subjectivity to identify patterns and themes in the qualitative data [41]. The data analysis was led with the open coding of five transcripts by EVA who collected the data and spent extended periods of time in HIV clinics and field sites. CS, ZR, KM, and YK, who are trained researchers with experience in HIV research, reviewed the open coding and collaboratively discussed and compared codes to agree on a framework that would capture barriers and facilitators affecting PLHIV's engagement with HIV care. A framework was developed to code barriers and facilitators at the three levels of individual, healthcare, and social and structural levels. Next, EVA continued coding the remaining transcripts while discussing changes and contradictions between the codes. Once all codes were developed at their responding levels, we created categories and a thematic framework to explain the patterns found. The larger research team, including people with lived experiences in HIV, substance use, houselessness, and violence, reviewed the final themes for consistency and accuracy.

3. Results

3.1. Participant Characteristics

Fifty-four people were screened for participation in this study; 20 did not meet the inclusion criteria at the study start, another 2 were excluded later due to not having an HIV diagnosis, and 1 for feeling too ill to continue data collection. The final sample was 32 participants; 18 participants self-identified as men, 10 as women, 2 participants identified as Two-spirit, and 2 as non-binary or other. Sex at birth was similarly distributed among participants, 46.9% of the group were heterosexual, with 25% saying their orientation was gay, and another 25.1% responding as bi-sexual or other. Table 1 reports the sociodemographic characteristics of the 32 participants.

Table 1. Sociodemographic characteristics of participants in the qualitative interviews.

Variable (N: Participants Who Answered)	Frequency n (%)
Age in years (N = 32)	
Mean (Range)	44.03 years (24–63)
Gender Identity (N = 32)	
Woman	10 (31.3)
Man	18 (56.3)
Trans Woman	0
Trans Man	0
Non-Binary	1 (3.1)
Two-Spirit	2 (6.3)
Other	1 (3.1)
Prefer not to say	0
Sex (N = 32)	
Male	21 (65.6)
Female	10 (31.3)
Intersex	0
Prefer not to say	1 (3.1)
Sexual Orientation (N = 32)	
Lesbian	0
Gay	8 (25)
Bisexual	6 (18.8)
Asexual	0
Heterosexual	15 (46.9)
Pansexual	0
Other	2 (6.3)
Prefer not to say	1 (3.1)
Cultural Background (N = 32)	
Indigenous–First Nations	15 (46.9)
Indigenous–Métis	4 (12.5)
White/European	4 (12.5)
Southeast Asian	4 (12.5)
Other	5 (15.6)
Marital Status (N = 27)	
Single	18 (56.3)
Married	0
Divorced	2 (6.3)
Common Law	7 (21.9)
Widowed	0
Other	0
Highest Level of Education (N = 30)	
K-12	21 (65.6)
Certificate, Diploma, vocational course from an educational institution	6 (18.8)
Bachelor's Degree	3 (9.4)
Master's Degree	0
Doctorate	0
Other	0
Income (N = 31)	
<10,000 CAD/Year	12 (37.5)
10,000–19,999 CAD/Year	8 (25)
20,000–29,999 CAD/Year	2 (6.3)
30,000–39,999 CAD/Year	3 (9.4)
40,000–49,999 CAD/Year	3 (9.4)
>50,000 CAD/Year	1 (3.1)
Prefer not to say	2 (6.3)

Table 1. *Cont.*

Variable (N: Participants Who Answered)	Frequency n (%)
Housing Situation *	
Living Alone (N = 32)	10 (31.25)
Living with Partner (N = 32)	6 (18.75)
Living with Children (N = 32)	3 (9.38)
Living with Roommates (N = 32)	5 (15.63)
Living with Extended Family (N = 31)	8 (25)
Experiencing Housing Instability (insecure housing, shelter, transitional housing, houseless) (N = 32)	14 (43.75)

* Non-mutually exclusive categories.

3.2. Childhood Trauma Questionnaire

Figure 2 presents the results from the Childhood Trauma Questionnaire by sex (Figure 2A) and by gender (Figure 2B). Only five persons did not experience any type of abuse. People experienced multiple types of abuse, and 70% of females and 50% of males reported severe and moderate sexual abuse. Females also experienced significant emotional abuse (60%) compared to males (38.5%).

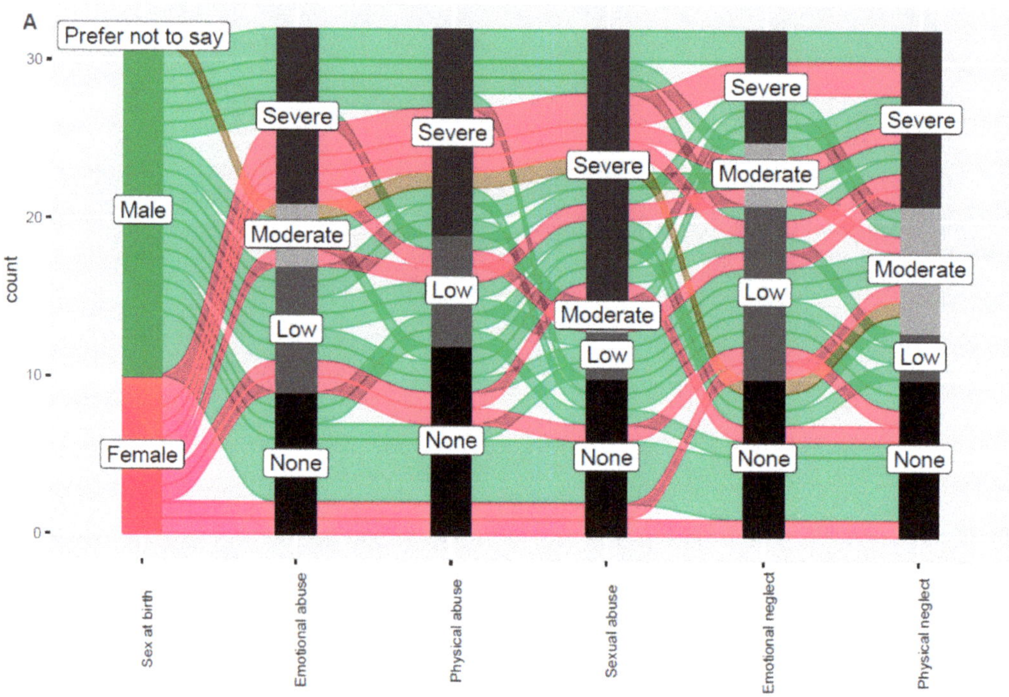

Figure 2. *Cont.*

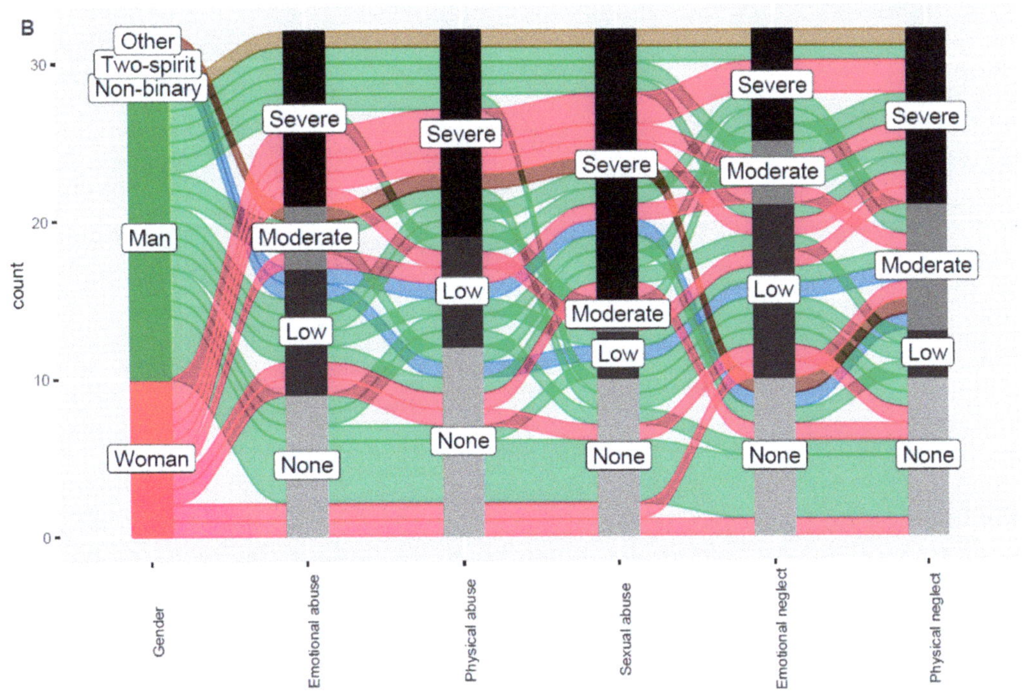

Figure 2. Severity of trauma for each of type of childhood trauma experienced by people living with HIV in Manitoba by sex (**A**) and gender (**B**). Severity score of trauma: none, low, moderate, and severe. Type of childhood trauma: emotional, physical and sexual abuse, and emotional and physical neglect.

3.3. Barriers

Participants reported numerous barriers to HIV care at the individual, healthcare, and social and structural levels, as seen in the statements shown in Table 2.

Table 2. Representative quotes on the barriers experienced by men, women, and non-binary people living with HIV in Manitoba by individual, healthcare, and social and structural factors.

Category	Quote #	Quote	Participant Age and Gender
		Individual Factors	
HIV Diagnosis	1	I was so in the clouds about it. I don't even remember them talking to me about any support or anything . . . I do remember . . . I felt like garbage and like, as if nobody wanted to be around me, or I felt gross and felt really suicidal. It really embarrassed me to even talk about it.	Participant 39 Woman
Mental Health Challenges	2	I have flashbacks, and like, it interferes with my work in school, because then I'm spacing out, and it has to do with me not talking about it [sexual abuse] either because I think that if I just keep myself busy, that'll distract whatever is going on in my head.	Participant 39 Woman
	3	I don't know what to do with myself, and I just feel if I do anything . . . (soft cry), I'm just scared to do anything. I'm scared to reach out and start doing things with my life because I always end up backwards headwind, and it just goes away. So, I just think what's the point? What's the point in trying to do the same thing? . . . It's just recently I've been wanting to [get back on HIV treatment] because I just felt like there was no point in trying to fight this disease because there wasn't much to live for.	Participant 46 Woman

Table 2. *Cont.*

Category	Quote #	Quote	Participant Age and Gender
Mental Health Challenges	4	It was really hard to lose your best friend [mother] and someone who was, your rock, you know. I just turned into an adult [and] I was grieving. I didn't understand grief and loss. I didn't realize that there's a cycle and you can actually deal with it without turning to drugs and alcohol because . . . I missed my mom, I needed my mother.	Participant 40 Woman
Substance Use Deterring HIV Care	5	When they say it's [having substance use disorder] like, a flu, or whatever. It's kind of like a flu and it's not because it is definitely worse. Like you can't even move. You can't get up to feed yourself or you can't get up to even bathe yourself or anything.	Participant 43 Woman
	6	I wasn't consistent [with HIV medications], you know, like you gotta take it every day. And I wasn't, you know, it'd be going off and be like, I didn't go a week without it, but maybe three days. Sometimes it was like, 'Oh, my God, what am I doing?' but I was using [methamphetamine] a lot. So, when you using too and you don't care, your health, like your health doesn't really matter.	Participant 64 Man
	7	I just have addictions, like, you know, a lot of my days are based around what I do get like [high].	Participant 55 Woman
	8	Like, going to get into an [medical] appointment? Feeling the social anxiety oh no, no. Oh, they think I'm high or they know I'm high or whatever.	Participant 39 Woman
COVID-19	9	Healthcare settings, there was a fear of going to . . . because I didn't want to go in because even though my CD4, is okay, I still have this fear of getting in, getting sick.	Participant 33 Man
Experiences of violence	10	I feel pretty drained I guess tired. I really wanted to get on my [HIV] medication, but it's just like, with my boyfriend around, I could never get to go do what I need to do . . . I connected with them [HIV care] once my boyfriend went into jail . . . but before that I didn't see them for like two years.	Participant 46 Woman
Internalized Stigma	11	I am ashamed of myself. I could say that. I would say to myself I am no longer clean I am dirty and contaminated with the virus.	Participant 35 Man
		Healthcare Factors	
Programmatic/ Administrative	12	The only thing is sometimes the waiting . . . It could take a week, two weeks, or three months to get an appointment for something that you might want to be able to see someone like that day.	Participant 57 Two-Spirit
	13	Have an HIV clinic on the reserve, or more services for HIV in the reserve . . . I was flying in and out to get here for appointments. . . It would be expensive because we would be using money everyday here, and we had to bring the kids over here.	Participant 49 Man
Lack of follow-up care and supports during HIV diagnosis	14	Because I was homeless at the time, so I had a lot that I was missing to actually be focusing on one thing [HIV diagnosis] so that's why my head was like everywhere . . . I think I was looking for someone to tell me that everything was going to be okay and that what I needed to do was do these steps to-to get where I'm trying to go and not give up. I honestly can't remember when they told me I had HIV. I'm pretty sure they just gave me a phone number and where to call and if I needed support and someone to talk to and that was it.	Participant 39 Woman
Stigma, Discrimination, and Insecurity in Health Settings	15	They [prison staff] come in and they're like 'hey Mr. you know you [got] AIDS right? Do you know you have AIDS right?' I thought he was joking or whatever but then he is not. . . A little bit of support a little bit of sympathy like, buddy, you just told me I have fucking AIDS and you just come here like nothing like 'Hey you know you got AIDS right'. How much of a slap in the face do you think that is? I was a kid man, 23 years old.	Participant 52 Man
	16	The hospitals are fucking ridiculous. I can't go to emergency rooms, and some of those nurses are vicious because they're judgmental. You hear them talking because I got HIV, they treat us different because we're addicted. They treat us differently just because we have addictions . . . Those chicks [nurses] are mean I hate going to emergency rooms now because a lot of my other friends said the same thing before, they won't go to hospitals and like the emergency rooms because they treat us so shitty there.	Participant 55 Woman
Lack of Social Supports	17	The environment here [hospital] is very sterile sometimes . . . Well, we started it [food bank] and we had coffee out, and people would sit down, and they were talking, and you would network. I had more confidence in not thinking that I was going to die anytime I had the flu, or anytime I had a spot. Because I met people at the food banks, while I was volunteering, that were there for like 10 years, 20 years, 30 years, you know, I met people there and we all sat around and we talked and we got to know each other. And if somebody passed away, we knew they were dead. Now. You [don't] hear about it? Maybe on Facebook.	Participant 54 Woman

Table 2. *Cont.*

Category	Quote #	Quote	Participant Age and Gender
Lack of Social Supports	18	Definitely someone who's got it [HIV], someone's got already. A nurse and doctor no-no, someone who's got already . . . More believable, yes. I mean I believe doctors, but you know they still got their own jargon . . . I want to hear it from someone who's gone through it.	Participant 58 Man
COVID-19	19	Because there was places that weren't even open. And you had to have a phone, you had to have internet.	Participant 39 Woman
Lack of Prevention Strategies	20	I rarely ever see, tables for resources [in shelters] . . . Like, this [educational materials] wasn't there when I was on the streets and stuff. They [shelters] kind of just had a place for people to come in eat, you know, sit around and chat. There was no resources being handed out. There was posters hung up. But, I like I would change the fact that people get greeted at the door with people with a whole table of pamphlets like this. 'Are you struggling with addiction? This is what you can do to help. And this is what you can do to get there'.	Participant 40 Woman
	21	You got to have more outreach going to these people [experiencing houselessness] and saying, 'Hey how are you guys doing?' I've never seen that here in Winnipeg. Out of all the people in like back lanes and stuff I've never seen anybody talk to him like a human being. 'How are you doing? Are you okay? Is everything okay with you? Sure. Do you need anything? No. Just checking in to make sure because you're a human being'. . . . They don't outreach you gotta reach out to them.	Participant 52 Man
Inaccessible Mental Health Services	22	I used to have a hard time getting into detox, I would spend nights at hospitals in the waiting room trying to get into [a] detox place. 'What am I doing wrong?' I'm saying that I'm trying to get out of this, and they seem to not be taking me serious or something, or seem to think I could do it by myself . . . It was discouraging for me to speak up for myself. Yeah, like different hospitals. Sometimes, I'll just give up and just go back to drugs.	Participant 39 Woman
	23	If I want to talk to a psychologist and fuck it's two years . . . And then suddenly you get a psychologist. He's like, yeah, you don't need me because you're gay or because you're this.	Participant 51 Man
		Social and Structural Factors	
Housing	24	Because I was homeless at the time so that's why my head was like everywhere . . . Well I don't have a phone, I don't know where to go, you know, I'm homeless, struggling with an addiction and you're just gonna set me off on the street expect me to figure out things by myself.	Participant 39 Woman
	25	I had a rooming house experience, but I left it. Fucking awful, overrun with mice. Addictions and homelessness, just like confusion . . . I've been trying to get a place which is a lot. Yeah, I just was trying to survive out there.	Participant 55 Woman
	26	Having a place to go at night. It's called mine. Not stay out [at] somebody else's place. . . . Like people who are homeless and HIV and all like it's really important for them to be in stabilized situation to where they don't get sick and their immune system is like not sick.	Participant 41 Woman
	27	They [HIV doctors] only give me a week's worth [of medication] at a time because I live on the streets, and bags get stolen a lot so, they don't want me to have all my meds on me and when I fall asleep and my bag goes missing . . . Having the stability of my own place having a steady routine that's how you get into not forgetting and take your pill every day. Because you have a home you go home that you can fell sleep.	Participant 42 Non-Binary
	28	When my pills got stolen, they were in my room. I was in this rooming house, they were in a bag, my bag that I take with me everywhere. And they got stolen. And I wasn't able to go on my meds for two weeks, because they were only given to you once a month. Tried coming here [HIV health centre]. Come here, I couldn't see the doctor, of course.	Participant 59 Man
Stigma and Discrimination	29	After that [HIV diagnosis], everyone started treating me different. You know, everyone wanted to stay away, like, didn't want to shake my hand and didn't want to be around me. It was just really hard.	Participant 46 Woman
Lack of Structural Supports	30	Zero [money] it's hard for fucking four months already and got no support, no money, no fucking nothing . . . I try to fucking walk around and I get paid just fucking beating somebody in streets	Participant 32 Other

3.3.1. Individual Factors

HIV Diagnosis

Most participants described their HIV diagnosis as a "death sentence". They expressed feeling overwhelmed with shock, disbelief, confusion, and denial. Women experiencing houselessness and substance use dependence shared that their diagnosis was profoundly confusing and overwhelming. For example, participant 39 recalled feeling "confused" and "spaced out" (Table 2; Quote 1). Others felt embarrassment and internalized stigma. Men were more likely to recall feeling angry leading some to suicidal ideation and attempts. Participants explained that the combination of these emotions made it difficult to focus on the supports offered and prepare for next steps.

Mental Health Challenges

Many participants reported experiencing unresolved traumatic experiences beyond their HIV diagnosis. They shared the profound impact of these experiences on their mental health, which, in turn, hindered their ability to cope with and navigate their day-to-day functioning (Table 2; Quote 2). Women, men, and non-binary persons shared ongoing feelings of loneliness and hopelessness. For example, participant 46 shared how feeling hopeless led her to think "what's the point?" in even starting HIV treatment (Table 2; Quote 3), while participant 58 experienced a loss of hope as "[losing] my mojo. I've lost my umph, my energies" which made him miss half of his HIV appointments. Women reported experiencing trauma related to separation from family members such as mothers and children and for some, substance use became a coping strategy to process traumatic experiences such as losing a mother (Table 2; Quote 4).

Substance Use Deterring HIV Care

Participants who used substances reported that their substance dependence directly interfered with their day-to-day functioning and, for some, their HIV care (Table 2; Quotes 5–7). Health was not a priority for many people who actively used substances. HIV care was affected as many reported being unable to focus on anything beyond acquiring and using their substance, leading them to forget appointments, or feeling increasingly anxious when attending medical appointments (Table 2; Quote 8).

COVID-19

Men and women reported the COVID-19 pandemic affected their health and mental well-being. They recounted increased feelings of isolation, depression, worry, and anxiety due to fear of acquiring COVID-19 or other illnesses with a compromised immune system (Table 2; Quote 9), and loss of income.

Experiences of Violence

Several participants commented on violence across their lives (e.g., intimate partner violence, sexualized). Participant 39, who was houseless and struggling with substance use at the time of diagnosis, shared a particularly harrowing story of constant sexual assaults where she was "praying that I would catch it [HIV], … I thought, if I have HIV, then there's automatic consequences for the guys that want to do whatever to my body that I don't agree to". Women and non-binary participants discussed how experiences of intimate partner violence and abusive relationships impacted their HIV care. For participant 42, testing for and preventing HIV acquisition became hard as their partner would refuse to be tested for STBBIs, leaving them frustrated and alone because of the "lies and the cheating and the manipulation towards me". Participant 46 noted that her engagement with HIV care broke down because her boyfriend was "abusive, so he keeps me tied in a lot" (Table 2; Quote 11).

3.3.2. Healthcare Factors

Programmatic/Administrative

Participants shared some inconveniences with the delivery of primary and HIV services. Men, women, and non-binary persons discussed problems with appointment waiting times which sometimes deterred them from attending primary care clinics: "just because of the waiting period, I just decided I'm not even gonna bother getting checked out" (Table 2; Quote 12). Men and women shared they were hampered by a lack of service options for their HIV care outside "9–5 business hours". Men remarked that the ability to obtain HIV drugs "should not be based on someone's salary" and commented on the need for HIV services outside metropolitan areas (e.g., rural communities; Table 2; Quote 13).

Lack of Follow-Up Care and Support During HIV Diagnosis

As reported above, some participants felt lost and unsure of what to do after diagnosis. These feelings were exacerbated by the lack of follow-up care, education, and treatment relating to HIV from primary care providers. Participants desired more information and guidance after being diagnosed as "that was the moment when I really needed someone" and many were "expecting to feel a little empathy" as they went through emerging emotions. Women discussed the intersecting experiences of being houseless and using substances at the time of diagnosis more, leaving them even more confused during the process and overwhelmed as to where to ask for help (Table 2; Quote 14).

Compounded Stigma, Discrimination, and Insecurity in Health Settings

Participants reported routinely feeling stigmatized and discriminated against by healthcare providers outside of the HIV care teams, such as nurses, pharmacists, staff in hospitals, emergency rooms, and prisons. Across genders, participants described coldness, prejudice, lack of empathy or support from service providers in primary care settings, hindering their engagement in care (Table 2; Quote 15). Disappointment, frustration, and distrust were shared mainly among women who used substances because of the negative experiences they reported while seeking healthcare. These women recounted experiencing compounded stigma about their intersectional identities of HIV status, substance use, and houselessness as primary service providers would not prioritize their needs, they mocked them, or discussed their stories out loud (Table 2; Quote 16). Participant 55 remarks that she received vicious treatment not only because she had HIV but also because she was "addicted". She explained that it is those who experience HIV and substance use dependence who are subjected to the worst treatment in emergency rooms as "they make US sit there forever. Like, just US, I've seen them put up through other people". Men recounted discriminatory experiences within the criminal justice system as prison staff would disclose their HIV status without consent, leaving them angry and resentful, and discouraging them from future HIV care. Women recounted unsafe experiences in emergency and primary healthcare environments, while one man described being harassed by a security guard while trying to attend his HIV appointment.

Lack of Social Supports

Participants identified the reduction in HIV social support groups as another barrier to care. Participants of all genders described a time when several social groups were supporting PLHIV beyond biomedical care. While participants noted that these groups slowly disappeared before the COVID-19 pandemic, they mentioned there were even fewer after the onset of the pandemic. They described these "social gatherings" as an invaluable aspect of their maintenance in care because they offered informal mental health support for people during their journey with HIV (Table 2; Quote 17). Participants also shared disappointment about the lack of peer support for their HIV medical care, particularly during diagnosis. Having someone "that has the same thing I do" was understood as providing closer and more intimate understanding and community than medical professionals (Table 2; Quote 18).

COVID-19

Participants described reduced service availability (Table 2; Quote 19) during the COVID-19 pandemic, and people without a phone or internet access were particularly affected by this change. Disrupted care meant people could no longer interact in a space they relied on for social connection and support. Men and non-binary persons reported no disruptions to their biomedical care (i.e., could continue medication), yet they expressed a sense of grief in "losing this [social space] . . . it was our meeting place in a sense" leaving many feeling even more "segregated" during the pandemic as "this [HIV care site] is the only place that you can go to connect". Likewise, men and women felt a loss of personal connection with their HIV service providers, as many organizations shifted their services to virtual appointments or hybrid care. While this change did not impede participants from remaining linked to medical care, it did create a loss of connection with HIV service providers.

Lack of Prevention Strategies

Participants shared concerns over the lack of STBBI education and prevention strategies for people who are most at risk (Table 2; Quote 20). Participants also emphasized a concern over the lack of outreach, street-based nursing, and providing care that meets people where they are at, given the number of people experiencing houselessness in Manitoba who are unable to attend traditional HIV care (Table 2; Quote 21).

Inaccessible Mental Health Services

Women shared stories of facing many bureaucratic hurdles to getting into substance dependence programs and a number had unsuccessful and frustrating experiences, deterring them from trying again (Table 2; Quote 24). Participant 39 described her journey of sleeping in hospital emergency rooms for six months while waiting to enter detox as "discouraging", at times pushing her to "go back to drugs". Women emphasized that emergency departments should aim to "[not] turn them [people with substance dependence] away. They could actually be in danger of harming themselves or others". Men in our study were more likely to note long wait times and a limited number of mental health professionals, which frustrated participants seeking mental health supports (Table 2; Quote 25).

3.3.3. Social and Structural Factors

Housing

Many participants did not have stable and long-term housing. In particular, for women struggling with substance use dependence, the instability associated with houselessness made it hard to focus on their HIV care, as their priorities were on "surviving out there" (Table 2; Quotes 24–26). Additionally, participants of all genders reported increased victimization, such as constant thefts of their belongings, including their HIV medications, while experiencing houselessness (Table 2; Quotes 27–28). They explained that if their medication is stolen, it can take a long time to replace it because of the steps involved in calling care providers, dealing with pharmacies, and applying for medication funding. Participants mentioned increased anxiety due to the possibility of an increased viral load, heightened infection progression, or a greater ability to transmit HIV.

Stigma and Discrimination

Many participants experienced enacted stigma and discrimination in their social circles because of their HIV status leaving them without adequate social circles to support their HIV care. Women and non-binary persons described feeling frustrated when people shared their HIV status without their consent and a number of participants said they felt alone, insecure, and unsure about who they can share their HIV status with those social circles without potential repercussions (Table 2; Quote 29).

Lack of Social and Structural Supports

Men and women shared that a lack of comprehensive social and structural supports such as financial assistance hinders their HIV care. For some participants, being unable to acquire financial assistance and an increased cost of living has forced them to find other ways to "survive" such as boosting (stealing) or fighting people (Table 2; Quote 30). Men and women also expressed a lack of affordable transportation options to attend their HIV appointments as the reason "why I miss them [appointments]".

Figure 3 provides a holistic conceptualization of the interconnected barriers experienced by PLHIV in this study.

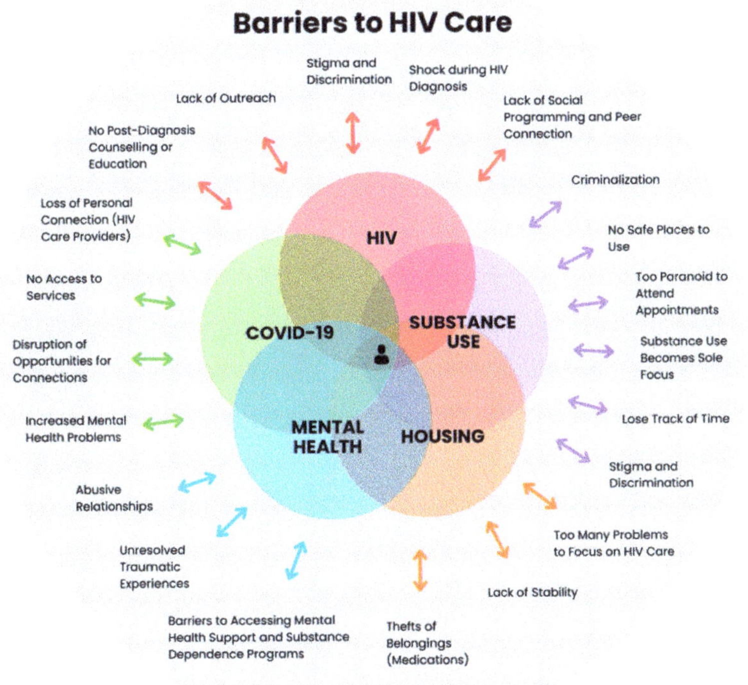

Figure 3. Barriers to HIV care in Manitoba. Model of understanding the interconnected barriers in HIV care experienced by people living with HIV in Manitoba.

3.4. Facilitators

Table 3 summarizes the most representative quotes by each level of facilitators reported by participants.

Table 3. Participants' quotes regarding facilitators to HIV care, by individual, healthcare, and social and structural factors.

Category	Quote #	Quote	Participant Age and Gender
		Individual Factors	
Stopping Substance Use	31	Things are starting to get a lot better because I have stopped doing drugs like I used to inject. So, I quit like eight weeks ago now. So, things are getting a lot better for me.	Participant 46 Woman

Table 3. *Cont.*

Category	Quote #	Quote	Participant Age and Gender
Will to Survive	32	You have to learn how to have a thick skin. Take things with salt. You sort of have to look at it. If I was in that situation, what would I do? To help people and stuff like that.	Participant 48 Man
		Healthcare Factors	
HIV Service Providers	33	I'm very close with my nurse, my doctor. So, I'm close with a lot of the receptionist. A lot of them know me by name. And we laugh and we joke and it's just-it's just like I said, just having an extended support circle of family, like I wouldn't even call them friends, they're more like family because they know my story because they've known me for so long.	Participant 40 Woman
HIV Healthcare Environments	34	Only here [HIV care site] is where I got help. If I wasn't for this place, I would probably be dead right now. I really don't know where I would be because I have nobody for talking.	Participant 58 Man
	35	It's just an accepting, loving environment . . . like it's-it's very friendly and welcoming, there's no judgment here. They understand everything, you know, it's a lot more [welcoming] than others [healthcare settings].	Participant 40 Woman
	36	I think it's great because they're more concerned about me as a whole, not just one little piece of me, and that one little piece of me [HIV] is really almost, I know this might not sound right., but it's okay. It's almost like that's been put on the backburner, you know, they look at the results. You don't see anything that scares them . . . It's like, you know, 'how you're feeling otherwise, how's your aches and pains falls?'	Participant 44 Man
Social Supports	37	How they had their little workshops and programs. I really liked one of their programs that I did . . . I came to all 10-10 classes . . . It told me a lot about my disease, and plus I got to meet people that had it too. And I really liked that too, because I felt so alone. When I first got it, I just thought I'm the only one out there [with HIV].	Participant 46 Woman
	38	And the only reason I came here was because I'd run out of food at home, and I was hungry. And I had this piece of paper from the hospital saying, I was entitled to a food bank here. I was like what the hell, I'll go down and see if I can find out.	Participant 44 Man
Post-HIV Diagnosis Emotional Support and Education	39	They made me feel really [safe] . . . I was broke down crying. They were talking to me and telling me 'it's okay, this isn't, you know, the end of it' . . . she's like, 'it's okay, there's treatment and stuff'. Because when you hear HIV, people are like, 'Oh, my God, I'm dying', right? So, it's like, that's initially what I thought . . . then they-they pretty much calmed me down, made me feel safe, and eventually they were able to tell me that this is, you know, I have an appointment and stuff so and they were willing to pick me up and take me to my appointment.	Participant 40 Woman
		Social and Structural Factors	
Support Networks	40	I told my cousin's wife first. Of course, and I broke down, and she came over to hug me. 'You are just sick, that's all. Don't worry there are lots of treatments out there available, you're still young'. And then I told my sister there, and she's like-she's like, 'I don't care, you're still my brother. Just take your meds.'	Participant 49 Man
	41	For myself, I didn't like being looked at weird, you know, I know my mom never looks at me any different like she's always there for me. You know so I wish more people were like my mom and just loved us unconditionally.	Participant 62 Woman
Structural Supports	42	So, I got in contact with people there [housing services] because I was homeless, I was struggling to stay sober. . . But when I got my own place [without wrap-around supports], I just went off the handle . . .My first month's rent money went to alcohol, drugs, more alcohol, it was-it was crazy . . . So, and then I got addicted to meth like right before I was kicked out . . . I've been there since the program opened [new recovery home with wrap around services]. . . I really have, where I live is a support. Like I have an unending circle of support . . . So, when I get the [HIV care] appointments, I-I write them down, and then make sure to put it in my calendar. And I made sure to tell them so that they know ahead of time. They're like, 'does she need a ride?'	Participant 40 Woman

3.4.1. Individual Factors

Stopping Substance Use

Some participants mentioned that ending substance use helped them focus on their HIV care. They described stopping substance use as a welcome change because they were better able to focus on other priorities and plan their lives, which they described as an "impossible task" when using substances (Table 3; Quote 31).

Will to Survive

Some participants of all genders described how having an innate will to survive is what has kept them motivated to engage with HIV care. This intrinsic motivation to stay alive was necessary for them to maintain their HIV care despite many challenges in their lives such as the trauma associated with the death of friends and family members (Table 3; Quote 32).

3.4.2. Healthcare Factors

HIV Service Providers

At the healthcare level, the primary facilitator for all participants was the non-judgmental and above-and-beyond care they received from HIV service providers. Many participants were moved to tears when describing the importance of providers to their care and their lives. Being close with their service providers allowed participants to be "honest about what's going on in [their] life", without feeling judged (Table 3; Quote 33). Participants who used substances felt these relationships as "somebody cares about me", because at times they feel that "nobody gives a shit about me, they don't. Nobody cares, because I'm a drug user". Participants were clear in differentiating that the care from their HIV service providers is unique and unlike the care from other medical services. Men were more appreciative of HIV service providers who involved them in designing treatment plans as they would empower them to participate in their HIV care.

HIV Healthcare Environments

Participants also noted the importance of welcoming HIV healthcare settings (Table 3; Quotes 34–36). Many participants shared that they felt safe at these sites because their interactions with providers were accepting and non-judgmental. Participants said staff welcomed anyone who needed help, regardless of how they presented to care, were friendly from the moment people walked through the door, remembered people's names, and offered snacks or basic supplies. Similarly, participants felt more connected with their care when they received services for other health needs beyond their HIV care (Table 3; Quote 36).

Social Supports

Participants reported that incorporating social support as part of their services was beneficial for their wellbeing. Men, women, and non-binary persons emphasized social programs and opportunities for connections with peers allowed them to understand their disease better and remain hopeful about their care. They described educational workshops as empowering, especially among people newly diagnosed, as this engagement fostered a sense of community and enabled knowledge sharing among peers (Table 3; Quote 37). For many, these programs are "like the best medicine, the social part". Similarly, other resources outside of HIV biomedical care such as help with transportation costs and using a food bank at an HIV care site motivated people to return (Table 3; Quote 38).

Post-HIV Diagnosis Emotional Support and Education

Participants who received emotional and educational support post-diagnosis described feeling more informed and able to connect and maintain engagement in HIV care. For women, this support created emotional safety and instilled hope to continue their lives. Men appreciated genuine service providers who did not rush to get them out of the door, thus ensuring that they "understood what was going to happen". Men and non-binary persons found it easier to make the first connection with their HIV care when service providers were clear and organized in guiding them through the process (Table 3; Quote 39).

3.4.3. Social and Structural Factors

Support Networks

Participants greatly emphasized the role their support networks (e.g., family, friends, partners) play in initiating and maintaining their HIV care. Support networks that are open, understanding, and non-judgmental about participants' HIV diagnosis and care needs (e.g., reminding of medications) were described as the most important in sustaining motivation (Table 3; Quotes 40–41).

Structural Supports

Women who received housing and financial support were better able to focus on their HIV care. For example, participants described housing options that supported their HIV care through wrap-around services including culturally safe care, sharing appointment reminders, and arranging transportation for their medical needs. One participant's story highlights the importance of the holistic care she received in a recovery home with wrap-around services supporting her substance use dependence, Child and Family Services journey, and HIV diagnosis (Table 3; 42).

Figure 4 summarizes the barriers and facilitators in each step of an extended HIV care cascade. Participants remarked on the importance of expanding the traditional HIV cascade of care to include prevention strategies and long-term social support for a more person-centered HIV care in Manitoba.

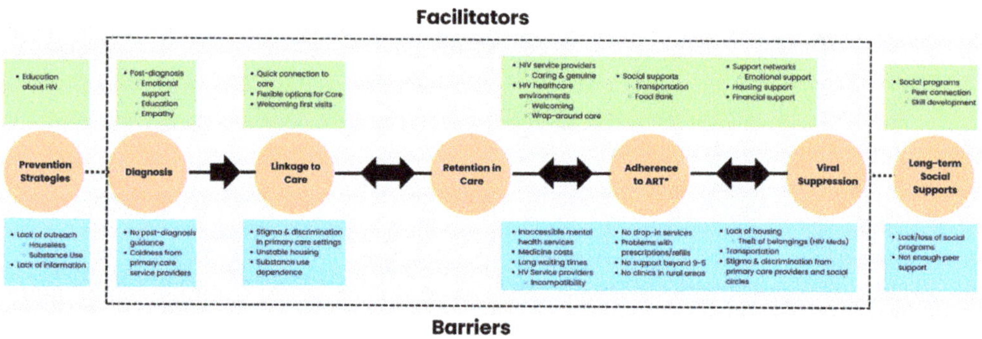

Figure 4. Barriers and facilitators to HIV care in Manitoba. Facilitators and barriers across an extended cascade of HIV care.

4. Discussion

The experiences of women, men, and non-binary PLHIV interviewed in this study point to a complex syndemic of health and social conditions that cluster with HIV to facilitate or impede access to and maintenance of HIV care in Manitoba.

Mental health challenges including traumatic experiences (e.g., sexualized violence), problematic substance use, houselessness, stigma and discrimination, and inaccessible healthcare and social services interacted and exacerbated negative health outcomes. The findings from our study highlight how trauma and mental health challenges can affect people's day-to-day functioning and, therefore, their HIV care. The literature suggests the negative biological interactions of these intersecting conditions. Mental health diagnoses commonly associated with experiences of trauma, such as depression and post-traumatic stress disorder, have been found to enhance inflammation and suppress antiviral immune responses potentially increasing the risk of acquiring other diseases [42,43]. Participants described receiving their HIV diagnosis as traumatic, with some men reporting suicidal ideation and attempts. Similarly, traumatic experiences, particularly those experienced during childhood, have been linked with accelerated HIV disease progression and overall negative quality of life [44]. Mental health challenges and traumatic experiences have also been found to diminish HIV treatment outcomes (e.g., viral suppression, mortality) for women [45], men and trans women [22,46], and those experiencing houselessness [24,25]. The harrowing and common experiences of interpersonal and sexualized violence among women in this study along with the increased childhood experiences of sexual and emotional abuse among females should be regarded as a concerning public health issue. Past research on the syndemic of gender-based violence, HIV, and substance use suggests that these forms of violence might increase the risk of HIV and STBBI transmission [47].

Many participants in this study resorted to substances to cope with their stressors, trauma, and lack of mental health services. Increased substance use closely interacts with trauma, mental health disorders, and HIV [34,48]. Our findings have highlighted the challenges that substance use can create for people to engage with HIV care such as being too physically unwell to attend an HIV clinic. However, it is crucial to note the biological impacts that increased substance use could have on PLHIV's health. Approximately 71.8% of females and 43.4% of males among those with new HIV diagnoses in Manitoba reported injection substance use with methamphetamine as the substance of preference (62.4%) [4]. Substance use, including methamphetamines, can increase HIV transmission, lead to more rapid HIV progression and overall worse health outcomes for PLHIV [13,14,49].

Beyond the biological implications of the cluster of diseases described above, our findings portray how these experiences are shaped by social processes that hinder participants' engagement with HIV care. Despite having histories of childhood trauma and mental health challenges, many participants mentioned several barriers to mental health services they needed, particularly those with substance dependence. Participants spoke positively about past peer support groups, many of which no longer exist, and reported limited peer social spaces where they could support each other's mental health and HIV journey, interventions which have been described as cost-effective ways to improve HIV indicators [50]. These findings show a need for increased investment in psychosocial interventions to support PLHIV who have experienced trauma which can improve psychological wellbeing and health outcomes [44,51].

The COVID-19 pandemic amplified the interconnected barriers to care for PLHIV. Participants reported increased mental health challenges, loss of personal relationships with their HIV care providers, and limited opportunities to connect with peers socially. Qualitative research with First Nations PLHIV in Manitoba also found increased mental health concerns and experiences of discrimination leaving many isolated during the pandemic [52]. As healthcare systems move out of pandemic restrictions, it is important to consider how the pandemic exacerbated disparities in underserved communities [6,52–56] to enable reconnections to care.

The participants shared various experiences of internalized stigma, which has been linked with a lower retention in HIV care in adolescent girls and boys [26]. Our findings showed that participants experienced intersectional stigma (i.e., a compounding of stigma and experiences of discrimination based on more than one intersecting identity) [57] by primary healthcare providers and social networks because of HIV status, unstable housing, or substance use. This led to participants feeling angry and disappointed with providers who should deliver care safely and respectfully, leading to distrust and reluctance to return to places where they had experienced discrimination. Intersectional stigma has been described across HIV syndemic research as being a key factor influencing HIV transmission, mental health, substance use, and barriers to HIV care [57]. Our findings build on a growing body of work in the literature calling for more comprehensive interventions to address the HIV intersectional stigma to reduce negative health outcomes and better connect people with care [58,59]. Other studies have shown the promising results of decreasing HIV stigma and discrimination in primary healthcare settings by using targeted educational campaigns which could be explored in settings that are mandated to provide healthcare for all Manitobans [27].

Social and structural factors interacted with health conditions to hinder HIV care in this study. Two-thirds of participants were living below the official Canadian poverty line

(CAD 25,471/year [60]). Poverty affects every aspect of a person's life, and for people experiencing houselessness, the negative impact on linkage and retention in HIV care cannot be overstated [61,62]. The findings from this study show that PLHIV who are experiencing houselessness have other competing priorities before HIV care. Houselessness and poverty led many participants to find ways to support themselves, such as stealing, which placed them at higher risk of criminalization and victimization. Likewise, theft of belongings made it hard for people experiencing houselessness to adhere to their medication and treatment, since besides "trying to survive", they must spend time obtaining new medications. These participants felt worried and anxious about their viral load increasing to a transmissible level due to missed doses. These worries are not unfounded as at an individual level non-adherence to antiretroviral therapy can lead to increased HIV replication [63] and reduced CD4 cell counts [64], and at a population level it can lead to higher rates of HIV transmission, healthcare utilization [65,66] and increased mortality [67,68].

According to participants, current responses to these problems are insufficient as they remarked on a lack of preventative strategies, such as outreach and street-based nursing for PLHIV experiencing houselessness, that could engage people at risk. Similarly, participants shared frustration over the lack of universal coverage of HIV medicine in Manitoba (approved in 2024, after completion of this study) as some people without coverage cannot afford to pay their annual Pharmacare deductible, adding the financial consideration of cost of managing comorbidities to the choice of HIV care. We call on decision makers to prioritize evidence-based [62], accessible, permanent, and emergency housing options for PLHIV, which would support increased access to and retention in HIV care [69].

The findings in this study also suggest facilitators that enable participants' engagement in HIV care, such as caring service providers and welcoming healthcare environments. The emotion with which many participants described their HIV care providers, and a welcoming environment highlights the enormous work providers have done to create trust and safety. For many participants, HIV clinics were among the few safe spaces in their lives. These experiences align with past qualitative research that has emphasized how providers who embody care, compassion, empathy, and empowerment in their patient interactions serve as facilitators in engaging PLHIV with care [25,70–76]. Funding to retain and support these services is critical, given the body of evidence on the importance of these patient interactions in facilitating people into HIV care.

The main limitations of this study include the required time commitment for data collection sessions. Not all PLHIV in Manitoba may have had time to commit to this study, and we may have missed some perspectives. However, our research design allowed for low-barrier and flexible data collection methods to include participants experiencing complex situations, providing confidence that our findings represent diverse populations. Additionally, we may have missed PLHIV in communities outside Winnipeg and Brandon who have different barriers to their care. To address this, we engaged with community partner organizations, enabling the participation of PLHIV who have received care while living outside of the two largest cities in Manitoba. An additional limitation is that we did not measure the biological factors that may serve the basis of social–biological interaction. This is a complex task that was beyond the scope of the current project.

5. Conclusions

Manitoba is the province with the second-highest number of new HIV diagnoses in Canada. Women, men, and non-binary people face barriers to HIV care including individual, healthcare, and social and structural factors intersecting and challenging the achievement of UNAIDS 95-95-95 goals [1]. Using syndemic theory, our findings add to the literature on how specific biological (e.g., substance use, mental health) and socioeconomic (e.g., poverty, social seclusion) create adverse effects in PLHIV's engagement with HIV care [11,33]. These findings shed light on the interacting diseases and inequalities that further marginalize the health of underserved populations. In addition, our findings emphasize the need to move beyond siloed interventions and, instead, focus on holistic person-centered care options that address the interconnected root causes such as poverty, houselessness, and stigma and discrimination contributing to the rising HIV diagnoses in Manitoba. While managing all the conditions PLHIV are experiencing (Figure 3) might seem organizationally complex, there are integrated interventions (i.e., addressing multiple problems) such as offering education for HIV, individualized and group mental health supports, housing assistance, supervised injection programs within HIV and primary care facilities, and collaborations between academic, civic, and community organizations, that show encouraging results in contexts similar to Manitoba [69,77–79]. Future research should assess the feasibility of implementing such interventions as part of the HIV care model in Manitoba and the effects such interventions have on immune activation as a surrogate measure of converging risks.

Supplementary Materials: The following supporting information can be downloaded at: https://www.mdpi.com/article/10.3390/tropicalmed9120287/s1, Supplementary File S1: Operational Definitions; Supplementary File S2: Participant Survey: Demographics & Life Circumstances. References [80–85] are cited in the Supplementary Materials.

Author Contributions: Conceptualization, Z.V.R., M.H-B., Y.K., K.M., K.K., L.J.M. and L.I.; methodology, E.V.-A., C.S., K.M., M.L., C.D. (Chantal Daniels), H.P., J.B., N.D., R.M., R.R., C.D. (Clara Dan), F.W., S.C., L.P., M.S., K.D., M.H.-B., Y.K. and Z.V.R.; software, E.V.-A.; validation, E.V.-A., C.S. and K.M.; formal analysis, E.V.-A., C.S., K.M. and Z.V.R.; investigation, E.V.-A., C.S., K.M., H.P., J.B., N.D., R.M., R.R., C.D. (Clara Dan), F.W., S.C., L.P., M.S., M.P. and K.T.; data curation, E.V.-A., C.S. and K.M.; writing—original draft preparation, E.V.-A.; writing—review and editing, E.V.-A., C.S., K.M., M.L., C.D. (Chantal Daniels), H.P., J.B., N.D., R.M., R.R., C.D. (Clara Dan)., F.W., S.C., L.P., M.S., M.P., K.K., L.J.M., L.I., K.T., K.D., M.H.-B., Y.K. and Z.V.R.; visualization, E.V.-A. and Z.V.R.; supervision, Z.V.R., M.H-B., K.M. and Y.K.; project administration, Z.V.R.; funding acquisition, Z.V.R., M.H.-B. and Y.K. All authors have read and agreed to the published version of the manuscript.

Funding: This research was funded by the Canadian Institutes of Health Research (grant number EG5-179453), and The Manitoba Medical Service Foundation (grant number: 2021-13. This research was also supported, in part, by the Canada Research Chairs Program for ZVR (Award # 950-232963). Production of this manuscript has been made possible in part through a financial contribution of the Public Health Agency of Canada (PHAC) to the National Collaborating Centre for Infectious Diseases. Disclaimer for PHAC: the views expressed here do not necessarily represent the views of the Agency.

Institutional Review Board Statement: This study was approved by the University of Manitoba Health Ethics Research Board (HS25572; H2022:218, 22 June 2022), the First Nations Health and Social Secretariat of Manitoba, Nine Circles Community Health Centre, Shared Health Manitoba (SH2022:194, 21 October 2022), and the 7th Street Health Access Centre.

Informed Consent Statement: Informed consent was obtained from all subjects involved in this study.

Data Availability Statement: Individual qualitative participant data will not be available since it contains potential and sensible identifiable information. Data dictionaries, qualitative codebooks, and quantitative data will be available upon request on a case-by-case basis.

Acknowledgments: We are grateful for all the participants, physicians, clinicians, program managers, social workers, health educators, and all stakeholders who dedicatedly collaborated to bring this project together. We thank Mariana Echeverri, Allison Chalmers-Justl, Kelly Merkeley-Paulsen, Deanne Baker, Kaylee Crepeele, Chris Trimble, Jody Jollimore, Jacqueline Gahagan, Neora Pick, Tara Faye Myran, Veda Koncan, and Adrienne Meyers.

Conflicts of Interest: The authors declare no conflicts of interest. The funders had no role in the design of this study; in the collection, analyses, or interpretation of data; in the writing of the manuscript; or in the decision to publish the results.

References

1. UNAIDS Global HIV & AIDS Statistics 2023. Available online: https://www.unaids.org/en/resources/fact-sheet (accessed on 1 September 2023).
2. Public Health Agency of Canada Estimates of HIV Incidence, Prevalence and Canada's Progress on Meeting the 90-90-90 HIV Targets. 2020. Available online: https://www.canada.ca/en/public-health/services/publications/diseases-conditions/estimates-hiv-incidence-prevalence-canada-meeting-90-90-90-targets-2020.html (accessed on 10 August 2023).
3. Manitoba HIV Program Manitoba HIV Program Report 2018–2021. 2022. Available online: https://mbhiv.ca/wp-content/uploads/2022/11/Report-MB-HIV-Program-FINAL-Nov-30-2022-Reduced-size.pdf (accessed on 1 August 2023).
4. Sharp, A.; Sorokopud-Jones, M.; Haworth-Brockman, M.; Kasper, K.; MacKenzie, L.; Ireland, L.; Gawlik, K.; Lopez, L.; Vanegas, J.M.; Bullard, J.; et al. Sex Differences in Houselessness, Injection Drug Use, and Mental Health Conditions among People Newly Diagnosed with HIV in Manitoba, Canada from 2018 to 2021: A Retrospective Cohort Study. *Lancet Reg. Health–Am.* **2024**, *36*, 100805. [CrossRef] [PubMed]
5. Sorokopud-Jones, M.; Sharp, A.; Haworth-Brockman, M.; Kasper, K.; MacKenzie, L.; Ireland, L.; Gawlik, K.; Lopez, L.; Vanegas, J.M.; Bullard, J.; et al. Sexually Transmitted and Blood-Borne Infections by Sex, Methamphetamine Use, and Houselessness before, at, and after HIV Diagnosis in Manitoba, Canada. *IJID Reg.* **2024**, *13*, 100433. [CrossRef] [PubMed]
6. Shiau, S.; Krause, K.; Valera, P.; Swaminathan, S.; Halkitis, P. The Burden of COVID-19 in People Living with HIV: A Syndemic Perspective. *AIDS Behav.* **2020**, *24*, 2244–2249. [CrossRef] [PubMed]
7. Statistics Canada Focus on Geography Series, 2016 Census. Available online: https://www12.statcan.gc.ca/census-recensement/2016/as-sa/fogs-spg/Facts-PR-Eng.cfm?TOPIC=9&LANG=Eng&GK=PR&GC=46 (accessed on 27 July 2022).
8. Brandon, J. The Winnipeg Street Census 2022: Final Report 2022. Available online: https://endhomelessnesswinnipeg.ca/street-census/ (accessed on 2 October 2023).
9. Gabel, C.; Powell, A. The Future of Indigenous Healthcare in Manitoba: Moving Beyond Soft Reconciliation in Health. *Int. Indig. Policy J.* **2023**, *14*, 1–18. [CrossRef]
10. Bromberg, D.J.; Mayer, K.H.; Altice, F.L. Identifying and Managing Infectious Disease Syndemics in Patients with HIV. *Curr. Opin. HIV AIDS* **2020**, *15*, 232. [CrossRef] [PubMed]
11. Singer, M. A Dose of Drugs, a Touch of Violence, a Case of AIDS: Conceptualizing the Sava Syndemic. *Free Inq. Creat. Sociol.* **1996**, *28*, 13–24.
12. Jain, J.P.; Strathdee, S.A.; Patterson, T.L.; Semple, S.J.; Harvey-Vera, A.; Magis-Rodríguez, C.; Martinez, G.; Pines, H.A. Perceived Barriers to Pre-Exposure Prophylaxis Use and the Role of Syndemic Factors among Female Sex Workers in the Mexico-United States Border Region: A Latent Class Analysis. *AIDS Care* **2020**, *32*, 557–566. [CrossRef]
13. Rhodes, T.; Singer, M.; Bourgois, P.; Friedman, S.R.; Strathdee, S.A. The Social Structural Production of HIV Risk among Injecting Drug Users. *Soc. Sci. Med.* **2005**, *61*, 1026–1044. [CrossRef]
14. Tyagi, M.; Bukrinsky, M.; Simon, G.L. Mechanisms of HIV Transcriptional Regulation by Drugs of Abuse. *Curr. HIV Res.* **2016**, *14*, 442–454. [CrossRef]
15. Wang, L.-B.; Xu, L.-L.; Chen, L.-J.; Zhang, K.-K.; Zhang, Q.-Y.; Chen, Y.-K.; Li, J.-H.; Liu, J.-L.; Wang, Q.; Xie, X.-L. Methamphetamine Induces Intestinal Injury by Altering Gut Microbiota and Promoting Inflammation in Mice. *Toxicol. Appl. Pharmacol.* **2022**, *443*, 116011. [CrossRef]
16. Li, Y.; Kong, D.; Bi, K.; Luo, H. Related Effects of Methamphetamine on the Intestinal Barrier via Cytokines, and Potential Mechanisms by Which Methamphetamine May Occur on the Brain-Gut Axis. *Front. Med.* **2022**, *9*, 783121. [CrossRef]
17. Fulcher, J.A.; Shoptaw, S.; Makgoeng, S.B.; Elliott, J.; Ibarrondo, F.J.; Ragsdale, A.; Brookmeyer, R.; Anton, P.A.; Gorbach, P.M. Brief Report: Recent Methamphetamine Use Is Associated With Increased Rectal Mucosal Inflammatory Cytokines, Regardless of HIV-1 Serostatus. *J. Acquir. Immune Defic. Syndr.* **2018**, *78*, 119–123. [CrossRef] [PubMed]
18. Stevenson, M.; Stanwick, T.L.; Dempsey, M.P.; Lamonica, C.A. HIV-1 Replication Is Controlled at the Level of T Cell Activation and Proviral Integration. *EMBO J.* **1990**, *9*, 1551–1560. [CrossRef] [PubMed]
19. Carrico, A.W.; Flentje, A.; Kober, K.; Lee, S.; Hunt, P.; Riley, E.D.; Shoptaw, S.; Flowers, E.; Dilworth, S.E.; Pahwa, S.; et al. Recent Stimulant Use and Leukocyte Gene Expression In Methamphetamine Users with Treated HIV Infection. *Brain Behav. Immun.* **2018**, *71*, 108. [CrossRef] [PubMed]
20. Massanella, M.; Gianella, S.; Schrier, R.; Dan, J.M.; Pérez-Santiago, J.; Oliveira, M.F.; Richman, D.D.; Little, S.J.; Benson, C.A.; Daar, E.S.; et al. Methamphetamine Use in HIV-Infected Individuals Affects T-Cell Function and Viral Outcome during Suppressive Antiretroviral Therapy. *Sci. Rep.* **2015**, *5*, 13179. [CrossRef] [PubMed]
21. Walter, T.J.; Iudicello, J.; Cookson, D.R.; Franklin, D.; Tang, B.; Young, J.W.; Perry, W.; Ellis, R.; Heaton, R.K.; Grant, I.; et al. The Relationships between HIV-1 Infection, History of Methamphetamine Use Disorder, and Soluble Biomarkers in Blood and Cerebrospinal Fluid. *Viruses* **2021**, *13*, 1287. [CrossRef]
22. Hobkirk, A.L.; Towe, S.L.; Lion, R.; Meade, C.S. Primary and Secondary HIV Prevention among Persons with Severe Mental Illness: Recent Findings. *Curr. HIV/AIDS Rep.* **2015**, *12*, 406–412. [CrossRef]
23. Arranz, L.; de Vicente, A.; Muñoz, M.; De la Fuente, M. Impaired Immune Function in a Homeless Population with Stress-Related Disorders. *Neuroimmunomodulation* **2009**, *16*, 251–260. [CrossRef]

24. Currie, L.B.; Patterson, M.L.; Moniruzzaman, A.; McCandless, L.C.; Somers, J.M. Examining the Relationship between Health-Related Need and the Receipt of Care by Participants Experiencing Homelessness and Mental Illness. *BMC Health Serv. Res.* **2014**, *14*, 404. [CrossRef]
25. Holtzman, C.W.; Shea, J.A.; Glanz, K.; Jacobs, L.M.; Gross, R.; Hines, J.; Mounzer, K.; Samuel, R.; Metlay, J.P.; Yehia, B.R. Mapping Patient–Identified Barriers and Facilitators to Retention in HIV Care and Antiretroviral Therapy Adherence to Andersen's Behavioral Model. *AIDS Care* **2015**, *27*, 817–828. [CrossRef]
26. Pantelic, M.; Casale, M.; Cluver, L.; Toska, E.; Moshabela, M. Multiple Forms of Discrimination and Internalized Stigma Compromise Retention in HIV Care among Adolescents: Findings from a South African Cohort. *J. Int. AIDS Soc.* **2020**, *23*, e25488. [CrossRef] [PubMed]
27. Yuvaraj, A.; Mahendra, V.S.; Chakrapani, V.; Yunihastuti, E.; Santella, A.J.; Ranauta, A.; Doughty, J. HIV and Stigma in the Healthcare Setting. *Oral Dis.* **2020**, *26*, 103–111. [CrossRef] [PubMed]
28. Laprise, C.; Bolster-Foucault, C. Understanding Barriers and Facilitators to HIV Testing in Canada from 2009-2019: A Systematic Mixed Studies Review. *Can. Commun. Dis. Rep. Releve Mal. Transm. Au Can.* **2021**, *47*, 105–125. [CrossRef] [PubMed]
29. Gahagan, J.C.; Fuller, J.L.; Proctor-Simms, E.M.; Hatchette, T.F.; Baxter, L.N. Barriers to Gender-Equitable HIV Testing: Going beyond Routine Screening for Pregnant Women in Nova Scotia, Canada. *Int. J. Equity Health* **2011**, *10*, 18. [CrossRef]
30. Khan, M.; MacEntee, K.; Kiptui, R.; Van Berkum, A.; Oudshoorn, A.; Ayuku, D.O.; Apondi, E.; Lee, E.O.J.; Abramovich, A.; MacDonald, S.-A.; et al. Barriers to and Facilitators of Accessing HIV Services for Street-Involved Youth in Canada and Kenya. *BMC Public Health* **2022**, *22*, 1901. [CrossRef]
31. Liboro, R.M.; Bell, S.; Ranuschio, B.; Barnes, L.; Despres, J.; Sedere, A.; Puno, T.; Shuper, P.A. Barriers and Facilitators to Promoting Resilience to HIV/AIDS: A Qualitative Study on the Lived Experiences of HIV-Positive, Racial and Ethnic Minority, Middle-Aged and Older Men Who Have Sex with Men from Ontario, Canada. *Int. J. Environ. Res. Public Health* **2021**, *18*, 8084. [CrossRef]
32. Rueda, Z.V.; Haworth-Brockman, M.; Sobie, C.; Villacis, E.; Larcombe, L.; Maier, K.; Deering, K.; Sanguins, J.; Templeton, K.; MacKenzie, L.; et al. Social and Structural Barriers and Facilitators to HIV Healthcare and Harm Reduction Services for People Experiencing Syndemics in Manitoba: Study Protocol. *BMJ Open* **2023**, *13*, e067813. [CrossRef]
33. Singer, M.; Bulled, N.; Ostrach, B.; Mendenhall, E. Syndemics and the Biosocial Conception of Health. *Lancet* **2017**, *389*, 941–950. [CrossRef]
34. Mendenhall, E.; Singer, M. What Constitutes a Syndemic? Methods, Contexts, and Framing from 2019. *Curr. Opin. HIV AIDS* **2020**, *15*, 213. [CrossRef]
35. Mendenhall, E. Beyond Co-Morbidity: A Critical Anthropological Perspective of Syndemic Depression and Diabetes in Cross-Cultural Contexts. *Med. Anthropol. Q.* **2015**, *30*, 462. [CrossRef]
36. Government of Canada, S.C. Focus on Geography Series, 2021 Census—Manitoba. Available online: https://www12.statcan.gc.ca/census-recensement/2021/as-sa/fogs-spg/Page.cfm?lang=E&topic=1&dguid=2021A000246 (accessed on 14 September 2024).
37. Bernstein, D.; Stein, J.; Newcomb, M.; Walker, E.; Pogge, D.; Ahluvalia, T.; Stokes, J.; Handelsman, L.; Medrano, M.; Desmond, D.; et al. Development and Validation of a Brief Screening Version of the Childhood Trauma Questionnaire. *Child Abus. Negl.* **2003**, *27*, 169–190. [CrossRef] [PubMed]
38. Rogers, E.S.; Ralph, R.O.; Salzer, M.S. Validating the Empowerment Scale with a Multisite Sample of Consumers of Mental Health Services. *Psychiatr. Serv. Wash. DC* **2010**, *61*, 933–936. [CrossRef] [PubMed]
39. World Health Organization. *A Conceptual Framework for Action on the Social Determinants of Health*; World Health Organization: Geneva, Switzerland, 2010.
40. Braun, V.; Clarke, V. Using Thematic Analysis in Psychology. *Qual. Res. Psychol.* **2006**, *3*, 77–101. [CrossRef]
41. Braun, V.; Clarke, V. Reflecting on Reflexive Thematic Analysis. *Qual. Res. Sport Exerc. Health* **2019**, *11*, 589–597. [CrossRef]
42. Kohrt, B.A.; Worthman, C.M.; Adhikari, R.P.; Luitel, N.P.; Arevalo, J.M.G.; Ma, J.; McCreath, H.; Seeman, T.E.; Crimmins, E.M.; Cole, S.W. Psychological Resilience and the Gene Regulatory Impact of Posttraumatic Stress in Nepali Child Soldiers. *Proc. Natl. Acad. Sci. USA* **2016**, *113*, 8156–8161. [CrossRef]
43. Cole, S.W.; Levine, M.E.; Arevalo, J.M.G.; Ma, J.; Weir, D.R.; Crimmins, E.M. Loneliness, Eudaimonia, and the Human Conserved Transcriptional Response to Adversity. *Psychoneuroendocrinology* **2015**, *62*, 11–17. [CrossRef]
44. Seedat, S. Interventions to Improve Psychological Functioning and Health Outcomes of HIV-Infected Individuals with a History of Trauma or PTSD. *Curr. HIV/AIDS Rep.* **2012**, *9*, 344–350. [CrossRef]
45. Leserman, J. Role of Depression, Stress, and Trauma in HIV Disease Progression. *Psychosom. Med.* **2008**, *70*, 539–545. [CrossRef]
46. Remien, R.H.; Stirratt, M.J.; Nguyen, N.; Robbins, R.N.; Pala, A.N.; Mellins, C.A. Mental Health and HIV/AIDS: The Need for an Integrated Response. *AIDS* **2019**, *33*, 1411–1420. [CrossRef]
47. Gilbert, L.; Raj, A.; Hien, D.; Stockman, J.; Terlikbayeva, A.; Wyatt, G. Targeting the SAVA (Substance Abuse, Violence and AIDS) Syndemic among Women and Girls: A Global Review of Epidemiology and Integrated Interventions. *J. Acquir. Immune Defic. Syndr.* **2015**, *69*, S118. [CrossRef]
48. *Trauma and Substance Abuse: Causes, Consequences, and Treatment of Comorbid Disorders*; American Psychological Association: Washington, DC, USA, 2014; ISBN 978-1-4338-1523-2.
49. Carrico, A.W. Substance Use and HIV Disease Progression in the HAART Era: Implications for the Primary Prevention of HIV. *Life Sci.* **2011**, *88*, 940–947. [CrossRef] [PubMed]

50. Berg, R.C.; Page, S.; Øgård-Repål, A. The Effectiveness of Peer-Support for People Living with HIV: A Systematic Review and Meta-Analysis. *PLoS ONE* **2021**, *16*, e0252623. [CrossRef] [PubMed]
51. Brezing, C.; Ferrara, M.; Freudenreich, O. The Syndemic Illness of HIV and Trauma: Implications for a Trauma-Informed Model of Care. *Psychosomatics* **2015**, *56*, 107–118. [CrossRef] [PubMed]
52. Larcombe, L.; Ringaert, L.; Restall, G.; McLeod, A.; Hydesmith, E.; Favel, A.; Morris, M.; Payne, M.; Souleymanov, R.; Keynan, Y.; et al. "Because of COVID...": The Impacts of COVID-19 on First Nation People Accessing the HIV Cascade of Care in Manitoba, Canada. *PLoS ONE* **2023**, *18*, e0288984. [CrossRef] [PubMed]
53. Bonn, M.; Palayew, A.; Bartlett, S.; Brothers, T.D.; Touesnard, N.; Tyndall, M. Addressing the Syndemic of HIV, Hepatitis C, Overdose, and COVID-19 Among People Who Use Drugs: The Potential Roles for Decriminalization and Safe Supply. *J. Stud. Alcohol Drugs* **2020**, *81*, 556–560. [CrossRef]
54. Public Health Agency of Canada Survey of the Impact of COVID-19 on Access to STBBI-Related Health Services Including Harm Reduction Services Among People Who Use Drugs or Alcohol in Canada. Available online: https://health-infobase.canada.ca/datalab/covid-19-stbbi-services.html (accessed on 22 July 2022).
55. McLinden, T.; Stover, S.; Hogg, R.S. HIV and Food Insecurity: A Syndemic Amid the COVID-19 Pandemic. *AIDS Behav.* **2020**, *24*, 2766–2769. [CrossRef]
56. Spinelli, M.A.; Hickey, M.D.; Glidden, D.V.; Nguyen, J.Q.; Oskarsson, J.J.; Havlir, D.; Gandhi, M. Viral Suppression Rates in a Safety-Net HIV Clinic in San Francisco Destabilized during COVID-19. *AIDS* **2020**, *34*, 2328–2331. [CrossRef]
57. Viswasam, N.; Schwartz, S.; Baral, S. Characterizing the Role of Intersecting Stigmas and Sustained Inequities in Driving HIV Syndemics Across Low- and Middle-Income Settings. *Curr. Opin. HIV AIDS* **2020**, *15*, 243. [CrossRef]
58. Operario, D.; Sun, S.; Bermudez, A.N.; Masa, R.; Shangani, S.; van der Elst, E.; Sanders, E. Integrating HIV and Mental Health Interventions to Address a Global Syndemic among Men Who Have Sex with Men. *Lancet HIV* **2022**, *9*, e574–e584. [CrossRef]
59. Smith, L.R.; Patel, V.V.; Tsai, A.C.; Mittal, M.L.; Quinn, K.; Earnshaw, V.A.; Poteat, T. Integrating Intersectional and Syndemic Frameworks for Ending the US HIV Epidemic. *Am. J. Public Health* **2022**, *112*, S340. [CrossRef]
60. Laidley, J.; Tabbara, M. Welfare in Canada, 2022. *Récupéré le* **2023**, *30*.
61. Saha, R.; Miller, A.P.; Parriott, A.; Horvath, H.; Kahn, J.G.; Malekinejad, M. Viral Blood-Borne Infections Testing and Linkage to Care Cascade among Persons Who Experience Homelessness in the United States: A Systematic Review and Meta-Analysis. *BMC Public Health* **2022**, *22*, 1421. [CrossRef] [PubMed]
62. Riley, E.D.; Hickey, M.D.; Imbert, E.; Clemenzi-Allen, A.A.; Gandhi, M. Coronavirus Disease 2019 (COVID-19) and HIV Spotlight the United States Imperative for Permanent Affordable Housing. *Clin. Infect. Dis.* **2021**, *72*, 2042–2043. [CrossRef] [PubMed]
63. Maggiolo, F.; Di Filippo, E.; Comi, L.; Callegaro, A.; Colombo, G.L.; Di Matteo, S.; Valsecchi, D.; Rizzi, M. Reduced Adherence to Antiretroviral Therapy Is Associated with Residual Low-Level Viremia. *Pragmatic Obs. Res.* **2017**, *8*, 91–97. [CrossRef] [PubMed]
64. Wood, E.; Hogg, R.S.; Yip, B.; Harrigan, P.R.; O'Shaughnessy, M.V.; Montaner, J.S.G. The Impact of Adherence on CD4 Cell Count Responses among HIV-Infected Patients. *J. Acquir. Immune Defic. Syndr. 1999* **2004**, *35*, 261–268. [CrossRef] [PubMed]
65. Abara, W.E.; Adekeye, O.A.; Xu, J.; Rust, G. Adherence to Combination Antiretroviral Treatment and Clinical Outcomes in a Medicaid Sample of Older HIV-Infected Adults. *AIDS Care* **2017**, *29*, 441–448. [CrossRef]
66. Fielden, S.J.; Rusch, M.L.A.; Yip, B.; Wood, E.; Shannon, K.; Levy, A.R.; Montaner, J.S.G.; Hogg, R.S. Nonadherence Increases the Risk of Hospitalization among HIV-Infected Antiretroviral Naive Patients Started on HAART. *J. Int. Assoc. Physicians AIDS Care* **2008**, *7*, 238–244. [CrossRef]
67. Castillo-Mancilla, J.R.; Cavassini, M.; Schneider, M.P.; Furrer, H.; Calmy, A.; Battegay, M.; Scanferla, G.; Bernasconi, E.; Günthard, H.F.; Glass, T.R.; et al. Association of Incomplete Adherence to Antiretroviral Therapy With Cardiovascular Events and Mortality in Virologically Suppressed Persons With HIV: The Swiss HIV Cohort Study. *Open Forum Infect. Dis.* **2021**, *8*, ofab032. [CrossRef]
68. Glass, T.R.; Sterne, J.A.C.; Schneider, M.-P.; De Geest, S.; Nicca, D.; Furrer, H.; Günthard, H.F.; Bernasconi, E.; Calmy, A.; Rickenbach, M.; et al. Self-Reported Nonadherence to Antiretroviral Therapy as a Predictor of Viral Failure and Mortality. *AIDS* **2015**, *29*, 2195–2200. [CrossRef]
69. Rajabiun, S.; Tryon, J.; Feaster, M.; Pan, A.; McKeithan, L.; Fortu, K.; Cabral, H.J.; Borne, D.; Altice, F.L. The Influence of Housing Status on the HIV Continuum of Care: Results From a Multisite Study of Patient Navigation Models to Build a Medical Home for People Living With HIV Experiencing Homelessness. *Am. J. Public Health* **2018**, *108*, S539–S545. [CrossRef]
70. Padilla, M.; Carter, B.; Gutierrez, M.; Fagan, J. The Boundary of HIV Care: Barriers and Facilitators to Care Engagement Among People with HIV in the United States. *AIDS Patient Care STDs* **2022**, *36*, 321. [CrossRef]
71. Kuchinad, K.E.; Hutton, H.E.; Monroe, A.K.; Anderson, G.; Moore, R.D.; Chander, G. A Qualitative Study of Barriers to and Facilitators of Optimal Engagement in Care among PLWH and Substance Use/Misuse. *BMC Res. Notes* **2016**, *9*, 229. [CrossRef] [PubMed]
72. Yehia, B.R.; Stewart, L.; Momplaisir, F.; Mody, A.; Holtzman, C.W.; Jacobs, L.M.; Hines, J.; Mounzer, K.; Glanz, K.; Metlay, J.P.; et al. Barriers and Facilitators to Patient Retention in HIV Care. *BMC Infect. Dis.* **2015**, *15*, 246. [CrossRef] [PubMed]
73. Carey, J.W.; Carnes, N.; Schoua-Glusberg, A.; Kenward, K.; Gelaude, D.; Denson, D.; Gall, E.; Randall, L.A.; Frew, P.M. Barriers and Facilitators for Clinical Care Engagement Among HIV-Positive African American and Latino Men Who Have Sex with Men. *AIDS Patient Care STDs* **2018**, *32*, 191–201. [CrossRef] [PubMed]

74. Taylor, B.S.; Fornos, L.; Tarbutton, J.; Muñoz, J.; Saber, J.A.; Bullock, D.; Villarreal, R.; Nijhawan, A.E. Improving HIV Care Engagement in the South from the Patient and Provider Perspective: The Role of Stigma, Social Support, and Shared Decision-Making. *AIDS Patient Care STDs* **2018**, *32*, 368–378. [CrossRef] [PubMed]
75. Beima-Sofie, K.; Begnel, E.R.; Golden, M.R.; Moore, A.; Ramchandani, M.; Dombrowski, J.C. "It's Me as a Person, Not Me the Disease": Patient Perceptions of an HIV Care Model Designed to Engage Persons with Complex Needs. *AIDS Patient Care STDs* **2020**, *34*, 267–274. [CrossRef]
76. Davoust, M.; Drainoni, M.-L.; Baughman, A.; Campos Rojo, M.; Estes, T.; Rajabiun, S.; Ross-Davis, K.; McCann, K.; Sullivan, M.; Todd, L.; et al. "He Gave Me Spirit and Hope": Client Experiences with the Implementation of Community Health Worker Programs in HIV Care. *AIDS Patient Care STDs* **2021**, *35*, 318–326. [CrossRef]
77. Buchbinder, S.P.; Havlir, D.V. Getting to Zero San Francisco: A Collective Impact Approach. *J. Acquir. Immune Defic. Syndr.* **2019**, *82*, S176–S182. [CrossRef]
78. Crepaz, N.; Baack, B.N.; Higa, D.H.; Mullins, M.M. Effects of Integrated Interventions on Transmission Risk and Care Continuum Outcomes in Persons Living with HIV: Meta-Analysis, 1996–2014. *AIDS* **2015**, *29*, 2371–2383. [CrossRef]
79. Krüsi, A.; Small, W.; Wood, E.; Kerr, T. An Integrated Supervised Injecting Program within a Care Facility for HIV-Positive Individuals: A Qualitative Evaluation. *AIDS Care* **2009**, *21*, 638–644. [CrossRef]
80. Canada, H. Health Portfolio Sex and Gender-Based Analysis Policy. 2017. Available online: https://www.canada.ca/en/health-canada/corporate/transparency/heath-portfolio-sex-gender-based-analysis-policy.html (accessed on 5 December 2023).
81. Scandurra, C.; Mezza, F.; Maldonato, N.M.; Bottone, M.; Bochicchio, V.; Valerio, P.; Vitelli, R. Health of Non-binary and Genderqueer People: A Systematic Review. *Front. Psychol.* **2019**, *10*, 1453. [CrossRef]
82. Canadian Institutes of Health Research. Meet the Methods Series: "What and Who Is Two-Spirit?" in Health Research—CIHR. 2020. Available online: https://cihr-irsc.gc.ca/e/52214.html (accessed on 11 December 2023).
83. Feyissa, G.T.; Woldie, M.; Munn, Z.; Lockwood, C. Exploration of facilitators and barriers to the implementation of a guideline to reduce HIV-related stigma and discrimination in the Ethiopian healthcare settings: A descriptive qualitative study. *PLoS ONE* **2019**, *14*, e0216887. [CrossRef] [PubMed]
84. Gulliford, M.; Figueroa-Munoz, J.; Morgan, M.; Hughes, D.; Gibson, B.; Beech, R.; Hudson, M. What does "access to health care" mean? *J. Health Serv. Res. Policy* **2002**, *7*, 186–188. [CrossRef] [PubMed]
85. Homeless Hub. Canadian Definition of Homelessness | The Homeless Hub. Available online: https://www.homelesshub.ca/resource/canadian-definition-homelessness (accessed on 5 December 2023).

Tropical Medicine and Infectious Disease

MDPI

Article

Occupational Syndemics in Farmworkers in the Cape Winelands, South Africa

Nicola Bulled

Institute for Collaboration on Health, Intervention, and Policy (InCHIP), University of Connecticut, 2006 Hillside Road, Storrs, CT 06269, USA; nicola.bulled@uconn.edu

Abstract: Occupational exposures in the agricultural industry globally have been associated with heightened risk for several diseases. Reports written in South Africa in the last decade have raised awareness of the harsh occupational conditions and human rights abuses suffered by farmworker communities in the wine industry. Despite receiving "fair trade" labels upon reentry into the global market in the 1990s, the working conditions on wine farms in South Africa have remained unchanged and exploitative for centuries. Farmworkers remain dependent on substandard farm housing, have insecure land tenure rights, are exposed to toxic pesticides, are denied access to benefits and unionization, and endure long working hours in harsh environmental conditions with low pay. These occupational conditions are linked to interacting disease clusters: metabolic syndrome, problematic drinking, and communicable diseases including tuberculosis, HIV, and COVID-19. This milieu of interacting diseases with deleterious outcomes is an under-considered occupational syndemic that will likely worsen given both the lasting impacts of COVID-19 and more recent shifts in global public health funding.

Keywords: occupational health; HIV; tuberculosis; syndemics; wine farms; South Africa

1. Introduction

Agriculture is the single largest form of employment in the world, playing a role in the economies of most countries and in the lives of local populations [1,2]. Agriculture is also a hazardous occupation, with one of the highest occupational fatality, non-fatal injury, and occupational illness rates [3,4]. Over 25 years ago, a review of the links between agriculture and health by Lipton & De Kadt [5] highlighted the direct link between agriculture, disease, death via malnutrition, and chronic and infectious diseases.

Farming as a means of employment entails unique characteristics including settings, organizational structure, policies, and oversight. Farmworkers are exposed to several health hazards as a result of their professional activities, including ultraviolet radiation; inhalation of organic dust from spores and minerals; exposure to microorganisms such as viruses, bacteria, and infectious parasites, and their toxic products; and exposure to pesticides [2,4,6–8]. Hazards extend beyond the workplace to include limited protections in housing [9], lack of access to clean water and sanitation facilities [10,11], and inaccessible healthcare.

A number of studies have suggested a unique pattern of disease among farmers when compared to other populations [3]. A study by Davila et al. [12] established that farmworkers in the US have an increased prevalence of metabolic syndrome. Studies from around the world have documented significantly higher rates of depression, anxiety, and suicide among farmers than the general population [13–19]. The prevalence of chronic kidney disease of unknown etiology has been steadily increasing in agricultural communities globally [20]. Occupational and environmental exposures in agricultural settings are also known to elicit lung inflammatory responses and increase risk for numerous lung diseases including asthma, COPD, and COVID-19 [21,22].

In this paper, I present a syndemic examination of farmworkers in South Africa's Cape Winelands, arguing that the confluence of social and biological forces that support a milieu of interacting chronic, infectious, and mental health conditions is an occupational syndemic. First, I present how the syndemic framework offers a way to comprehensively consider the increased health risks presented by occupational settings. Second, I consider historic and current labor practices and their impact on comorbid disease clusters in the Cape Winelands. Third, I argue how these labor practices support an occupational syndemic consisting of a clustering of interacting diseases (tuberculosis [TB], HIV, metabolic syndrome [MetS], problematic drinking) in socially, economically, and politically marginalized farmworkers. In so doing, I use a syndemic lens to draw attention to the complex occupational health crisis endured by vulnerable workers globally and the need for comprehensive global health and occupational reforms. Data for this paper are drawn from a variety of sources including published scientific literature, country, industry, and global health organization reports, and grey and periodical literature.

2. Applying the Syndemics Framework to Understand Occupational Risks

Syndemics theory has gained traction in medical and public health applications, with a tenfold rise in related published scientific output in the past decade [23,24]. It offers a comprehensive and contextualized understanding of adverse disease clusters in marginalized populations [25]. The concept has informed policy and programming on numerous disease epidemics including most recently MPOX [26], COVID-19 [27], and Ebola [28]. Understanding the biological and social elements of a syndemic can inform a comprehensive response to address individual disease elements, relationships between disease conditions, and the social determinants of health [29–31].

Syndemics theory provides a critical alternative to the concepts of comorbidities and social determinants of health by recognizing two detrimental elements simultaneously: (1) the driving effects of unequal and unjust social and structural determinants resulting in disease clusters, and (2) the interaction of coexisting diseases resulting in excess health burden beyond comorbidity. In this, the objective of the syndemic framework is to understand the whole health picture and the alignment of its constituent biological and social/structural elements. In the investigation of these issues, the syndemics approach addresses three primary questions: (1) How do diseases interact in ways that enhance harm? (2) How do social and structural conditions promote disease clustering and disease interaction? (3) How can we prevent and mitigate syndemics?

Scholars have recently applied the syndemic framework to address disease clusters in specific occupational settings, driven by observations of excess COVID-19 burden. For example, Lemke et al. [32,33] presented an argument for COVID-19-related syndemics in long-haul truck drivers in the US. Truck drivers experience higher rates of COVID-19 infection, morbidity, and mortality, overlapping with already disproportionate health burdens of cardiometabolic and respiratory comorbidities, including obesity, hypertension, diabetes, bronchitis, emphysema, and lung cancer. The COVID-19 syndemics in this population are shaped by the unique occupational configurations of long-haul trucking, including harmful work organization characteristics, toxic workplace environments, and structural factors. Long periods of time away from home, excessive time pressures, shift work, and non-working hours in worksite environments encourage detrimental lifestyle and behavioral patterns such as poor diet, lack of physical activity, poor sleep health, and high rates of cigarette smoking. Workplace environments expose truck drivers to noxious air pollutants such as carbon monoxide, nitrogen oxides, and particulate matter, including road dust. Compounding the health ramifications of these occupational factors is limited healthcare access, reflected in both poor insurance coverage and lack of available medical services, leading to failures in screening, diagnosis, and treatment for acute and chronic conditions.

Studies of Mexican migrant farm laborers in the US indicated a two-to-three-times-higher rate of COVID-19 infection, morbidity, and mortality among farmworkers than the general population, a population already heavily burdened by high rates of food insecurity, stress, depression, anxiety, obesity, high blood pressure, and diabetes. Singer and Cook [34] linked these disproportionate health burdens to occupational exposures, as the employment sector was deemed "essential" during the early years of the COVID-19 pandemic when preventive measures such as vaccines were not available. In addition, the nature of agricultural labor and related communal living increases airborne disease transmission through close contact and confined shared spaces. Furthermore, structural factors include the historical exclusion of farmworkers from health and labor protections, low wages, limited access to healthcare due to travel distances related to the rural nature of farmwork; the cost of healthcare, with few farm contracts including healthcare insurance; and the fear of engaging with healthcare institutions given the lack of legal documentation or ill-defined temporary work permits.

Singer [35] presented an empirical argument for the syndemic nature of comorbid disease conditions experienced by commercial fishers. He argued that the occupational characteristics of commercial fishing contribute directly to excess health burdens including substance abuse, violence, mental health disorders, injuries, and chronic pain, as well as COVID-19 infection, morbidity, and mortality. The physically demanding and dangerous working conditions of commercial fishing and crowded working sites, as well as the monotony of the work, the social isolation, sleep deprivation, fatigue, and economic uncertainty, promote detrimental behavior such as poor diets, alcohol, tobacco, and drug use as well as increase exposure to airborne disease.

The historical labor policies of the mining sector in South Africa, including short-term migratory labor contracts, low wages, crowded and unsanitary communal housing, limited family accommodations, and risky working conditions, are driving features of high levels of adversely interacting disease comorbidities of TB, HIV, silicosis, and COVID-19, argue Bulled and Singer [30]. The dangerous working conditions and limited worker protections increase risk for lung diseases such as silicosis, as well as communal diseases such as TB and COVID-19, among mine laborers. While reforms have been made in the industry to address the HIV epidemic, with HIV rates high among mine laborers, the industry has not undergone comprehensive occupational reforms, failing to meet social and labor plan targets, with workers continuing to have limited access to secure job contracts, acceptable housing, and robust healthcare.

The literature on occupational syndemics to date affirms the conclusion of Abrams [36] that "if we are to understand the history of occupational health, it must be viewed in the context of the labor-capital relationship: work-related disease is socially produced and is, therefore, preventable." However, as noted by Merrill Singer, the developer of the syndemics framework, "Despite promising initial efforts, as yet the full potential of a syndemics framework for deconstructing the complexities of occupational health under neoliberal capitalism remains unrealized" [37]. With this paper, I aim to contribute to further evidencing the application of the syndemics framework in occupational settings in which disease burdens are compounded.

3. Working on Cape Wine Farms

Out of South Africa's nine provinces, the greatest number of farmworkers live in the wealthy and fertile Western Cape. South Africa's wine industry contributed 0.9% of the national GDP, 1.8% of national employment, and ZAR 18.85 billion in household income in 2024 [38]. Its links to other industries in its value chain generates greater multiplier effects than the average South African industry, making it particularly important to the national and individual economies. Consequently, the wine industry has a greater contribution to GDP (ZAR 1.57 vs. 1.3 million) and employment (7.51 vs. 6.58 jobs) for every ZAR 1 million in output relative to the average South African industry.

In reports published in 2003, 2008, and 2011, the South African Human Rights Commission documented clear abuses of wine farmworkers and labor law violations [39]. To varying degrees, farmworkers are subject to exploitative conditions and abusive practices, perpetrated by farm owners or managers. Wine farm work is physically demanding, involving long hours in harsh weather conditions, with workers exposed to toxic pesticides that are sprayed on crops. Inadequate safety equipment, limited to only overalls and rubber gloves, in contravention of health and safety regulations, exposes farmworkers to toxic pesticides. Farmworkers report covering their faces with their caps or with ineffective dust masks in an attempt to block the spray of chemicals as they have no access to respirators [39]. Workers who work with chemicals report having no appropriate cleaning facilities to use, consequently exposing others including family members to toxic chemicals. Workers report often having no access to hand washing facilities, toilets, or drinking water, as required by labor regulations [39]. Transportation of workers on the back of trucks, a contentious but common and legal practice in South Africa, also presents a risk. In addition to accidents involving workers being flung from the backs of trucks [40], the close proximity of workers to one another in the truck bed increases the likelihood of airborne disease transmission.

Farmworkers earn among the lowest wages in South Africa and are often denied benefits to which they are legally entitled [39]. Under Sectorial Determination 13 (SD13), passed by the Department of Labor in 2003 in an effort to protect workers, employers are required to pay sick leave, annual leave, and maternity leave [39]. SD13 also requires employers to pay at least the minimum wage, limits the amount of deductions that employers can make from wages for food and accommodation, and regulates the hours worked. However, under SD13, employers are only required to pay sick leave if workers have accrued sufficient sick leave, accruing sick leave at a ratio of 1 day of sick leave for every 26 days worked [41]. Paid leave and family responsibility leave only have to be granted to fixed-term workers if their contracts are for more than four months [41]. To limit their obligations under SD13, employers opt to employ workers on short-term contracts, and when farmworkers are ill or injured, they are often denied sick leave or are required to present a medical certificate [39,41].

Farmworkers also struggle to obtain timely or affordable healthcare given their remote location, limited transportation options, and low wages [39]. A study conducted in 2003 pointed to the impact of significant health budget cuts and the centralization of healthcare delivery, reducing mobile clinic visits to farms by 64% between 1997 and 2000 [42]. The changes resulted in public clinics operating in fixed facilities or on centrally situated farms up to 5 km away and operating only on weekdays during office hours. These findings are consistent with a more recent study conducted in Limpopo, with the majority of farmworkers reporting walking 2–5 km to the nearest public health clinic, with a third living beyond a 5 km radius [43].

Farm owners are not responsible for providing housing, although many have historically done so. Moreover, there are no specific regulations governing the conditions of on-farm housing. This gap in legislation means that housing for farmworkers often is substandard [39]. Human Rights Watch reported on Isaak, a farmworker who had lived for 10 years in a former pig stall with no electricity, water, or ability to provide adequate shelter from the elements [39]. In hostels, primarily maintained for seasonal workers, conditions are often overcrowded and unclean, with reports of as many as 17 sharing a single room [41].

Farm owners have no incentive to maintain housing in good condition, as the Extension of Security and Tenure Act (no.62 in 1997) stipulates that any farm dweller, even those whose employment has been terminated, may only be evicted from on-farm housing if the farmer obtains a court order and if suitable alternative housing is available. To avoid the ESTA's strictures, farmers appoint workers on short fixed-term rather than permanent contracts and accommodate them in on-farm hostels or not at all [41]. Farmworkers endure this housing because moving elsewhere is often not financially feasible due to both their low wages and the transportation costs of getting to work. The skewed land-holding patterns in South Africa mean that poor people in rural areas have very few options for affordable and decent housing near remote farms. In recent years, overcrowded, unsafe, and unsanitary informal settlements have been growing outside wine-producing towns [44].

Despite these evident occupational hazards, farmworkers have limited avenues to report grievances. Most workers keep quiet, fearing that if they complain they will lose their jobs or get deported if they are foreign migrant workers [41]. A study of citrus workers in the Western Cape found that about a third of workers were represented by a worker committee to which they lodged their grievances [41]. Farmers have actively attempted to block union formation on farms [39]. In the Western Cape region, unionization of farmworkers is low at 5–8%, compared to a national average of 25% [39].

4. Wine Farms as Disease Hotspots

There is currently limited to no literature or data available on the prevalence of diseases among farmworkers in South Africa, and even less that detail the health conditions of farmworkers in the Cape Winelands. One study in the Cape Winelands District Municipality, formerly known as the Boland District Municipality, found a high prevalence of MetS among farmworkers [45]. MetS is a cluster of risk factors including high blood pressure, elevated fasting blood glucose, increased waist circumference, and high cholesterol, that are mostly associated with people living with obesity and diabetes. Research has also shown that the wine farmworker population is chronically malnourished, despite a large portion of their income being spent on food [42]. Another study among farmworkers in the Cape Winelands District found the incidence of TB to be exceptionally high, with a reported new smear-positive TB incidence rate of 1685 per 10,000 population [46], three times the provincial rate and almost five times the national level [47,48]. Although there is a dearth of studies on TB incidence and prevalence among farmworkers in South Africa, it has been reported that there is an increased risk of TB for agricultural workers globally when compared to workers in other occupations [49,50]. According to the National Occupational Mortality Surveillance South Africa (NOMS-SA), of the 114,706 deaths due to TB reported between 2013 and 2015, agriculture constituted the largest share of TB-related deaths at 20% [51]. The odds of dying from TB are 58% higher among agricultural laborers compared to those in other occupations with odds increasing among workers exposed to silica dust [52].

High levels of exposure to silica in the agricultural industry has been reported in South Africa [53]. As noted elsewhere [30], the lung damage resulting from silica exposure likely contributed to increased COVID-19 infectivity in certain occupations in South Africa. High levels of pesticide and other chemical exposure are common on farms, known to increase asthma and other lung conditions. The limited pesticide-protective equipment and overcrowded living and transportation conditions further supports a likely higher burden of COVID-19 among South African farmworkers, as present elsewhere [22,54,55]. It is not possible to gauge whether the area's morbidity and mortality from COVID-19 was more or less than the national, as population statistics were based on 2011 census data and not representative of current area population and, as elsewhere, statistics were probably an undercount [41].

In 2010, farmworkers were reported to have a higher burden of HIV (35–42% vs. 18%) [56,57] relative to the general South Africa population [58]. In 2001, the HIV prevalence among pregnant women attending public health antenatal facilities in Cape Winelands Municipality District was 8.3% [59]. Farmworkers have an increased HIV risk due to several factors, most notably the link between farm work and migration [60]. Migration is described as the single greatest predictor of HIV risk and prevalence in Sub-Saharan Africa [61]. In South Africa, farmworkers who are migrants (internal and foreign) and their partners have a higher burden of HIV compared with non-migrants and their partners [62–64].

Finally, harmful alcohol consumption and its negative impact has been identified as particularly high among farming communities in the Western Cape [65–68]. Rates of fetal alcohol syndrome or partial fetal alcohol syndrome in the province are among the highest in the world [69,70], and alcohol-related interpersonal violence and child neglect has been highlighted as serious problems [65,69,71,72]. A study on alcohol use in wine farms in Stellenbosch/Franschoek and Vredendal in the Western Cape, demonstrated a high prevalence of both current drinking (69%) and, among current drinkers, symptoms of problem drinking (73%), with the drinking scores surpassing provincial estimates by 2 for men and 3.5 times for women [68]. Farmworkers in the Cape Winelands describe their community as "characterized by excessive drinking", with intergenerational problematic drinking, drinking-related interpersonal violence, physical violence and injury, and sexual infidelity considered norms [73]. Rather than viewing excessive drinking as problematic, wine farmworkers view drinking as serving important functions, including as a facilitator of pleasure, recreation, stress release, and social connection [73].

5. Occupational Syndemic of Farmworkers in the Cape Winelands

Two elements constitute a syndemic: (1) negative disease interactions within a specified population; and (2) inequitable structural relationships driving disease interaction and increased health burden. In the case of occupational syndemics, structural factors and anthropogenic environments are expressed in unsafe work and living conditions and ineffective labor policies. For South Africa's wine industry, occupational syndemics include a high burden of MetS, TB, HIV, and problem drinking driven by high levels of exposure to pesticides damaging lung tissue, crowded and unsanitary living conditions increasing airborne disease transmission, and a historical legacy of the "dop" system supporting intergenerational excess drinking which contributes to risky sexual practices and interpersonal violence; see Figure 1. Moreover, labor policies that perpetuate low wages and substandard housing and limit workers' ability to take sick leave, and centralized healthcare systems that limit access to health facilities, further support disease transmission and increase disease morbidity.

Addressing the first element of the syndemic—the interaction of diseases resulting in deleterious health outcomes—South African wine farmworkers experience a high prevalence of four deadly diseases (MetS, TB, HIV, problematic drinking) and these diseases are known to adversely interact. Interaction exists if the joint effect is significantly larger than the sum of the individual effects. In diseases, this can occur across multiple pathways and mechanisms, including (1) diseases/conditions that weaken the effectiveness of components of the body's immune system; (2) diseases that damage organs and tissues, facilitating the onset of other diseases/conditions; and (3) diseases that disrupt body cellular signaling, causing a downgrading of cell functioning, increasing vulnerability to and the impact of other diseases.

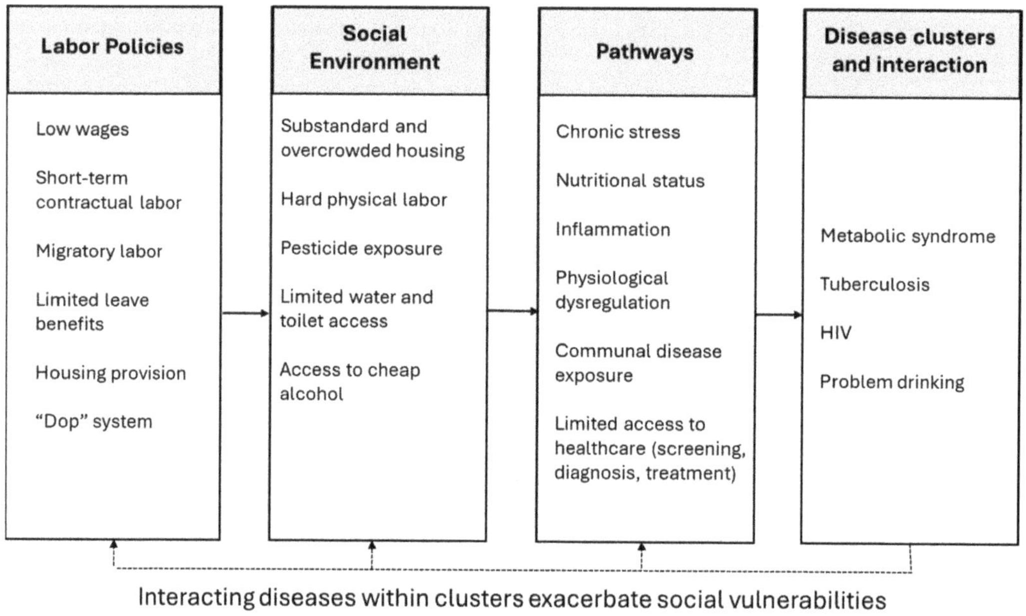

Figure 1. Occupational syndemic model of wine farmworkers in South Africa.

In South Africa, high TB/HIV co-infection rates are an important contributory factor to increased TB risk in farmworkers. Population TB risk is elevated an additional 25% by HIV [74,75]. In 2020, Africa was reported as the region with the highest cases of HIV/TB co-infection, with South Africa contributing to an astounding 50% of these [76]. HIV was directly responsible for 55% (4.8 million) of the TB cases and 69% (1.4 million) of TB deaths [77].

As described elsewhere [30], HIV infection alters the general immune system as well as specifically attacking *M. tuberculosis*-specific T cells, rendering individuals highly susceptible to developing active TB. Conversely, *M. tuberculosis* infection has a negative impact on the immune system's response to HIV, increasing the likelihood of HIV infection and accelerating the progression from HIV infection to AIDS [78]. HIV and TB infections have also been found to impact the morbidity and mortality of other diseases, including COVID-19. A cohort study of the South African active hospital surveillance system for COVID-19 hospital admissions found that the odds of COVID-19 in-hospital mortality were higher in people with current or past TB infections (AOR 1.48, 95% CI 1.32–1.67) and for those with HIV (1.34, 1.27–1.43) [79].

HIV-related inflammation, toxicity of treatments, and increasing longevity of people living with HIV increases vulnerability to chronic communicable diseases, including MetS [80]. Modern HIV treatments are known to result in an increase in body weight [81–83]. Excess body weight has consequential spillover effects on other metabolic outcomes, including increased risks for diabetes and hypertension [84,85]. Poorly managed HIV, including detectable and/or fluctuating viral load levels, has been shown to be associated with higher comorbid rates with hypertension, diabetes, and cardiovascular diseases [80,85,86].

Alcohol use is a risk factor for TB, HIV, and MetS. A meta-analysis determined that alcohol use is associated with a 35% higher risk of TB compared to no alcohol use, which increased to 56% in high-TB burden countries [87]. Furthermore, TB risk rises as ethanol intake increases, with ethanol intake of more than 60 g per day associated with a 68% higher risk of tuberculosis compared to no alcohol use [87]. Problem drinking increases HIV exposure through increased likelihood of sexual violence, and reduced engagement with condom use [88,89]. Finally, a meta-analysis of prospective studies found that problem drinkers had a 84% higher risk of MetS than non-drinkers [90].

HIV, TB, and MetS can all be aggravated by high levels of pesticide exposure. Aside from acute poisonings that can occur, persistent pesticide exposure can disrupt immune system function by inhibiting lymphocytes and monocyte proliferation, affecting the production of cytokines and immunoglobulins, altering the cell's phagocytic activity, and inducing apoptosis, thereby increasing infectivity and worsening progression of HIV and TB [91,92]. Long-term exposure to pesticides has the potential to induce energy metabolic disorders by disturbing the physical process of energy absorption in the intestine and energy storage in the liver, adipose tissue, and skeletal muscle, as well as energy regulation by the pancreas and immune cells [93]. These pesticide-induced disruptions ultimately cause abnormal levels of blood glucose and lipids, which in turn induce the development of related metabolic diseases, including overweight, underweight, and diabetes [94]. Pesticide exposure can also increase risk for chronic respiratory illnesses, malnutrition, depression, and problem drinking [95–99].

The second aspect of a syndemic—structural factors creating unsafe occupational conditions that drive disease—is also evident on farms in the Cape Winelands. Many argue that occupational health hazards in the Western Cape are related partly to the legacy of institutionalized distribution of alcohol by means of the "dop" (tot) system, a form of remuneration practiced during the colonial and apartheid eras whereby farmworkers were part-paid with low-quality wine supplied throughout the day [100–103]. This practice was a means to control and maintain farmworkers as a cheap source of labor and was not restricted to workers involved in the wine industry. The "dop" system and its legacy of inexpensive and readily available alcohol reflects the wider dispersion of a culture of alcohol consumption in rural communities in the region today [68].

Current labor policies further contribute to compounding disease burden among wine farmworkers. As noted previously, the ESTA, aiming to protect workers from housing evictions, has resulted in worse housing conditions, or no housing, as employers are unable to evict terminated employees, resulting in less housing availability. Employers are not required to provide housing, and under SD13, are not allowed to deduct housing costs from wages. SD13 also requires employers to provide benefits, such as paid sick leave, as described previously. To reduce this cost, employers offer only limited-term contracts that are not subject to the same benefit and labor regulation requirements. Furthermore, union formation for wine farmworkers has been blocked and there is limited labor policy compliance oversight (see "Efforts to address occupational syndemics in Cape Winelands"). In addition, the centralization of healthcare services limits access to rural farm dwellers with limited access to transportation.

Singer termed these conditions of employment a form of "occupational violence" [37]. Over time this produces chronic occupational stress experienced both physiologically and emotionally as constant fatigue, anxiety, feelings of hopelessness, and the sense of being a disposable commodity [41]. Chronic stress induces enduring exposure to stress-related hormones (e.g., corticotrophin-releasing hormone, cortisol, catecholamines, and thyroid hormone). Prolonged exposure to these chemical messengers, which places the body in a constant state of alertness, weakens the immune system, affects muscle and cognitive function, and promotes mental health issues [104], increasing the risk for multiple interacting health conditions and the development of occupational syndemics.

6. Efforts to Address Occupational Syndemics in Cape Winelands

Efforts to improve conditions on farms in the Cape Winelands have been made by various private actors, including farmers' associations, industry bodies, and retailers [39]. In 2001, Agri Wes-Cape, the largest farmers' association in the province and the provincial affiliate of Agri SA, the largest agricultural organization in South Africa, adopted a comprehensive Code of Conduct for its members. In 2002, the wine industry created the Wine Industry Ethical Trade Association (WIETA), a multi-stakeholder initiative that audits members. In 2008, the fruit industry began an ethical trade program. Some international retailers have imposed their own audit requirements and supported other programs within their supply chains.

During the COVID-19 pandemic, the WIETA collaborated with government institutions and industry bodies to obtain information and guidance on how to mitigate the pandemic. In response to the pandemic, in 2022, 24 farmworkers were trained as community health workers, a Western Cape Government Health initiative in collaboration with non-profit and agricultural industry partners [105]. The Aurum Institute in Malmesbury, Western Cape, implemented the USAID-funded TB Local Organizations Network (LON) project in 2022 to support organizations to implement locally generated solutions to improve TB diagnosis, treatment, and prevention services [106].

These initiatives have had varying degrees of reach and impact, but have so far failed to substantially alter conditions across all farms in the Western Cape, both because the state's lack of enforcement of farmworkers' rights [107,108] and recent shifts in global health and development funding. In 2013, the ratio of labor inspectors to workers in the Western Cape was 1:16,090, exceeding the International Labor Organization's recommended ratio of 1:10,000. At the time, Inspection and Enforcement Services in the Department of Labor had only 56 inspectors in the Western Cape, of which just 6 were Occupational Health Safety inspectors. Given that these 56 inspectors had to inspect all workplaces in the province, they only managed to conduct 23% of inspections in the Agriculture, Forestry and Fishing sector [109]. In addition, an agreement between the Department of Labor, AgriSA, and other parties requires that labor inspectors give farmers prior notice of inspections, undermining inspectors' capacity to identify violations [39].

The COVID-19 pandemic further challenged efforts to improve occupational conditions. With an influx of COVID-19 patients admitted to medical facilities, South Africa observed a 50% reduction in the number of TB tests performed and in the collection of HIV and TB medication during pandemic years [110,111]. As facilities and resources were reallocated to treat COVID-19 patients, other patients with major diseases, like HIV or TB, were at risk of not being treated or of developing complications [112,113]. Similar disruptions in HIV testing, positive HIV tests, and initiation of antiretroviral therapy were reported as an impact of COVID-19 [114]. Models project that this will dramatically increase incidence of both HIV and TB for years to come [115].

In January 2025, the USAID issued blanket stop-orders to pause the implementation of USAID-funded activities, and in February terminated all USAID-funded programs in South Africa. In South Africa, PEPFAR and USAID make up 14% of the national TB budget. The reduction in funding has impacted linkage to TB care, prevention, screening, testing, treatment and follow-up, community-based services, and TB-HIV integration, threatening progress in reducing TB incidence and mortality, and undermining the significant progress made in South Africa in addressing both HIV and TB over the past decade [116].

7. Conclusions

The syndemics lens affords insights into the sociobiological dynamics of health as codetermined by interacting biological and social forces. This examination of wine farmworkers in South Africa indicates that these forces include physically demanding and dangerous working conditions, labor policies which support substandard and unsanitary living environments, labor migration, precarious working contracts, minimal benefits and low pay, and a centralized healthcare system that limits access to robust healthcare. In addition, farmworkers in the Western Cape region are still impacted by the historical practice of the "dop" system, which created a culture of problem alcohol use. These conditions of occupational violence increase the susceptibility of wine farmworkers to high levels of chronic stress, which increases susceptibility to communicable and non-communicable diseases that present as an occupational syndemic. The syndemics framework offers an important tool to understand the impact of national and global social and structural relationships and their impact on worker health and can be used to inform public health and clinical responses and comprehensive labor reforms.

Funding: This research received no external funding.

Institutional Review Board Statement: Not applicable.

Informed Consent Statement: Not applicable.

Conflicts of Interest: The author declares no conflict of interest.

References

1. de-Assis, M.P.; Barcella, R.C.; Padilha, J.C.; Pohl, H.H.; Krug, S.B.F. Health problems in agricultural workers occupationally exposed to pesticides. *Rev. Bras. Med. Trab.* **2021**, *18*, 352–363. [CrossRef]
2. Ghafari, M.; Cheraghi, Z.; Doosti-Irani, A. Occupational risk factors among Iranian farmworkers: A review of the available evidence. *Epidemiol. Health* **2017**, *39*, e2017027. [CrossRef] [PubMed]
3. Donham, K.J.; Thelin, A. *Agricultural Medicine: Occupational and Environmental Health for the Health Professions*; Blackwell Pub.: Hoboken, NJ, USA, 2006.
4. Lessenger, J.E. *Agricultural Medicine*; Springer: Berlin/Heidelberg, Germany, 2006.
5. Lipton, M.; de Kadt, E. *Agriculture–Health Linkages*; World Health Organization: Geneva, Switzerland, 1988.
6. Lemarchand, C.; Tual, S.; Levêque-Morlais, N.; Perrier, S.; Belot, A.; Velten, M.; Guizard, A.-V.; Marcotullio, E.; Monnereau, A.; Clin, B. Cancer incidence in the AGRICAN cohort study (2005–2011). *Cancer Epidemiol.* **2017**, *49*, 175–185. [CrossRef]
7. Arcury, T.; Quandt, S. (Eds.) *Latinx Farmworkers in the Eastern United States: Health, Safety, and Justice*, 2nd ed.; Springer: Berlin/Heidelberg, Germany, 2020.
8. Quandt, S.A.; Wiggins, M.F.; Chen, H.; Bischoff, W.E.; Arcury, T.A. Heat index in migrant farmworker housing: Implications for rest and recovery from work-related heat stress. *Am. J. Public Health* **2013**, *103*, e24–e26. [CrossRef]
9. Arcury, T.A.; Weir, M.; Chen, H.; Summers, P.; Pelletier, L.E.; Galván, L.; Bischoff, W.E.; Mirabelli, M.C.; Quandt, S.A. Migrant farmworker housing regulation violations in North Carolina. *Am. J. Ind. Med.* **2012**, *55*, 191–204. [CrossRef]
10. Arcury, T.A.; Weir, M.M.; Summers, P.; Chen, H.; Bailey, M.; Wiggins, M.F.; Bischoff, W.E.; Quandt, S.A. Safety, security, hygiene and privacy in migrant farmworker housing. *New Solut. A J. Environ. Occup. Health Policy* **2012**, *22*, 153–173. [CrossRef] [PubMed]
11. Quandt, S.A.; Summers, P.; Bischoff, W.E.; Chen, H.; Wiggins, M.F.; Spears, C.R.; Arcury, T.A. Cooking and eating facilities in migrant farmworker housing in North Carolina. *Am. J. Public Health* **2013**, *103*, e78–e84. [CrossRef]
12. Davila, E.P.; Florez, H.; Fleming, L.E.; Lee, D.J.; Goodman, E.; LeBlanc, W.G.; Caban-Martinez, A.J.; Arheart, K.L.; McCollister, K.E.; Christ, S.L.; et al. Prevalence of the metabolic syndrome among U.S. workers. *Diabetes Care* **2010**, *33*, 2390–2395. [CrossRef] [PubMed]
13. Belyea, M.J.; Lobao, L.M. Psychosocial consequences of agricultural transformation: The farm crisis and depression 1. *Rural Sociol.* **1990**, *55*, 58–75. [CrossRef]
14. Elliott, M.; Heaney, C.; Wilkins, J., III; Mitchell, G.; Bean, T. Depression and perceived stress among cash grain farmers in Ohio. *J. Agric. Saf. Health* **1995**, *1*, 177–184. [CrossRef]

15. Jones-Bitton, A.; Best, C.; MacTavish, J.; Fleming, S.; Hoy, S. Stress, anxiety, depression, and resilience in Canadian farmers. *Soc. Psychiatry Psychiatr. Epidemiol.* **2020**, *55*, 229–236. [CrossRef] [PubMed]
16. Linn, J.G.; Husaini, B.A. Determinants of psychological depression and coping behaviors of Tennessee farm residents. *J. Community Psychol.* **1987**, *15*, 503–512. [CrossRef]
17. Onwuameze, O.E.; Paradiso, S.; Peek-Asa, C.; Donham, K.J.; Rautiainen, R.H. Modifiable risk factors for depressed mood among farmers. *Ann. Clin. Psychiatry* **2013**, *25*, 83–90. [PubMed]
18. Rudolphi, J.M.; Berg, R.L.; Parsaik, A. Depression, anxiety and stress among young farmers and ranchers: A pilot study. *Community Ment. Health J.* **2020**, *56*, 126–134. [CrossRef]
19. Younker, T.; Radunovich, H.L. Farmer mental health interventions: A systematic review. *Int. J. Environ. Res. Public Health* **2021**, *19*, 244. [CrossRef]
20. Johnson, R.J.; Wesseling, C.; Newman, L.S. Chronic kidney disease of unknown cause in agricultural communities. *N. Engl. J. Med.* **2019**, *380*, 1843–1852. [CrossRef]
21. Nordgren, T.M.; Charavaryamath, C. Agriculture occupational exposures and factors affecting health effects. *Curr. Allergy Asthma Rep.* **2018**, *18*, 65. [CrossRef]
22. Chicas, R.; Xiuhtecutli, N.; Houser, M.; Glastra, S.; Elon, L.; Sands, J.M.; McCauley, L.; Hertzberg, V. COVID-19 and agricultural workers: A descriptive study. *J. Immigr. Minor. Health* **2022**, *24*, 58–64. [CrossRef]
23. Singer, M.; Bulled, N.; Ostrach, B. Whither syndemics?: Trends in syndemics research, a review 2015–2019. *Glob. Public Health* **2020**, *15*, 943–955. [CrossRef]
24. Mendenhall, E.; Newfield, T.; Tsai, A.C. Syndemic theory, methods, and data. *Soc. Sci. Med.* **2022**, *295*, 114656. [CrossRef]
25. Singer, M.; Bulled, N.; Ostrach, B.; Mendenhall, E. Syndemics and the biosocial conception of health. *Lancet* **2017**, *389*, 941–950. [CrossRef] [PubMed]
26. McQuiston, J.; Braden, C.; Bowen, M.; McCollum, A.; McDonald, R.; Carnes, N.; Carter, R.; Christie, A.; Doty, J.; Ellington, S.; et al. The CDC Domestic Mpox Response—United States, 2022–2023. *MMWR Morb. Mortal. Wkly. Rep.* **2023**, *72*, 547–552. [CrossRef]
27. Horton, R. Offline: COVID-19 is not a pandemic. *Lancet* **2020**, *396*, 874. [CrossRef] [PubMed]
28. Delphin, K.; Remco Van De, P.; Thierno Oumar, F.; Alexandre, D.; Willem Van De, P.; Wim Van, D. Guinea's response to syndemic hotspots. *BMJ Glob. Health* **2021**, *6*, e006550. [CrossRef]
29. Singer, M.; Bulled, N.; Ostrach, B.; Lerman Ginzburg, S. Syndemics: A cross-disciplinary approach to complex epidemic events like COVID-19. *Annu. Rev. Anthropol.* **2021**, *50*, 41–58. [CrossRef]
30. Bulled, N.; Singer, M. The occupational syndemics of miners in South Africa. *Discov. Soc. Sci. Health* **2024**, *4*, 36. [CrossRef]
31. Singer, M.; Bulled, N.; Ostrach, B. Syndemics and human health: Implications for prevention and intervention. *Ann. Anthropol. Pract.* **2012**, *36*, 205–211. [CrossRef]
32. Lemke, M.K.; Apostolopoulos, Y.; Sönmez, S. Syndemic frameworks to understand the effects of COVID-19 on commercial driver stress, health, and safety. *J. Transp. Health* **2020**, *18*, 100877. [CrossRef]
33. Lemke, M.K.; Apostolopoulos, Y.; Sönmez, S. A novel COVID-19 based truck driver syndemic? Implications for public health, safety, and vital supply chains. *Am. J. Ind. Med.* **2020**, *63*, 659–662. [CrossRef]
34. Singer, M.; Cook, J. Deadly Companions: The Diabetes/COVID-19 (DiaCOVID-19) Syndemic in Mexico and the U.S. Mexican Diaspora. In *COVID-19 Syndemics and the Global South: A World Divided*; Routledge: Oxfordshire, UK, 2024.
35. Singer, M. Syndemics of the sea: Adverse disease interactions and the stressors of fisher livelihoods. *Fish Fish.* **2023**, *25*, 205–217. [CrossRef]
36. Abrams, H. A Short History of Occupational Health. *J. Public Health Policy* **2001**, *22*, 34–80. [CrossRef] [PubMed]
37. Singer, M. Occupational Syndemics & the Anthropology of Work. *Exertions*. 2024. Available online: https://saw.americananthro.org/pub/pxfx0pnr/release/1 (accessed on 2 June 2025).
38. FTI Consulting, Inc. *Overview of the South African Wine Industry*; FTI Consulting, Inc.: Washington, DC, USA, 2025. Available online: https://www.fticonsulting.com/-/media/files/insights/reports/2025/feb/overview-south-african-wine-industry.pdf (accessed on 2 June 2025).
39. Human Rights Watch. *Ripe with Abuse: Human Rights Conditions in South Africa's Fruit and Wine Industries*; Human Rights Watch: New York, NY, USA, 2011. Available online: https://www.hrw.org/report/2011/08/23/ripe-abuse/human-rights-conditions-south-africas-fruit-and-wine-industries (accessed on 23 August 2011).
40. Ngcakani, N. Transportation: Your Farm Workers Aren't Cattle. *Foodformzansicoza*. 2021. Available online: https://www.foodformzansi.co.za/transportation-farmworkers/ (accessed on 2 June 2025).
41. Visser, M. *The Impact of COVID-19 on South African Migrant Wage Workers and the Self-Employed*; Working Paper; International Labor Organization: Geneva, Switzerland, 2022. Available online: https://webapps.ilo.org/static/english/intserv/working-papers/wp088/index.html#ID0E1DAG (accessed on 2 June 2025).
42. Clarke, M.; Dick, J.; van Zyl, H.; Johansson, E. Farmers' perceptions of the lay health worker on farms in the Western Cape, South Africa. *Agrekon* **2004**, *43*, 465–483. [CrossRef]

43. Mlangeni, N.; Malotle, M.; Made, F.; Ramodike, J.; Sikweyiya, Y.; Du Preez, C.; Thompson, N.S.; Zungu, M. Factors associated with TB screening among agricultural workers in Limpopo Province, South Africa. *Glob. Health Action* **2023**, *16*, 2162227. [CrossRef]
44. Pannenbecker, J. Labour Conditions in South African Wine Industry Remain Appalling. *SOMO 2020*. Available online: https://www.somo.nl/labour-conditions-in-south-african-wine-industry-remain-appalling/ (accessed on 28 January 2020).
45. Kruger, M.J.; Nell, T.A. The prevalence of the metabolic syndrome in a farm worker community in the Boland district, South Africa. *BMC Public Health* **2017**, *17*, 61. [CrossRef]
46. Clarke, M.; Dick, J.; Zwarenstein, M.; Diwan, V. DOTS for temporary workers in the agricultural sector. An exploratory study in tuberculosis case detection. *Curationis* **2003**, *26*, 66–71. [CrossRef]
47. Boland District Municipality. *Tuberculosis Information: Areas 614*; Boland District Municipality: Paarl, South Africa, 2003.
48. South African National Tuberculosis Control Programme. *Tuberculosis Report on Tuberculosis Recording and Reporting*; Department of Health: Pretoria, South Africa, 2003.
49. Ciesielski, S.D.; Seed, J.R.; Esposito, D.H.; Hunter, N. The epidemiology of tuberculosis among North Carolina migrant farm workers. *JAMA* **1991**, *265*, 1715–1719. [CrossRef]
50. Semilan, H.M.; Abugad, H.A.; Mashat, H.M.; Abdel Wahab, M.M. Epidemiology of tuberculosis among different occupational groups in Makkah region, Saudi Arabia. *Sci. Rep.* **2021**, *11*, 12764. [CrossRef]
51. National Institute for Occupational Health. *Occupation and Mortality: Tuberculosis-Related Mortality in South Africa, 2013–2015*; National Institute for Occupational Health: Braamfontein, South Africa, 2021. Available online: https://www.nioh.ac.za/wp-content/uploads/2021/04/TB_NOMS_report_31_March_2021.pdf (accessed on 2 June 2025).
52. Kootbodien, T.; Wilson, K.; Tlotleng, N.; Ntlebi, V.; Made, F.; Rees, D.; Naicker, N. Tuberculosis Mortality by Occupation in South Africa, 2011–2015. *Int. J. Environ. Res. Public Health* **2018**, *15*, 2756. [CrossRef]
53. Swanepoel, A.; Rees, D.; Renton, K.; Kromhout, H. Exposure to respirable crystalline silica in south african farm workers. *J. Phys. Conf. Ser.* **2009**, *151*, 012005. [CrossRef]
54. Liebman, A.K.; Seda, C.H.; Galván, A.R. Farmworkers and COVID-19: Community-Based Partnerships to Address Health and Safety. *Am. J. Public Health* **2021**, *111*, 1456–1458. [CrossRef]
55. Lusk, J.L.; Chandra, R. Farmer and farm worker illnesses and deaths from COVID-19 and impacts on agricultural output. *PLoS ONE* **2021**, *16*, e0250621. [CrossRef] [PubMed]
56. Colvin, M. *Integrated Biological and Behavioural Surveillance Survey (IBBSS) in the Commercial Agricultural Sector in South Africa*; International Organization for Migration: Geneva, Switzerland, 2010. Available online: https://reliefweb.int/sites/reliefweb.int/files/resources/E3AEF43DCC2CFA1F492577E70021F885-Full_Report.pdf (accessed on 2 June 2025).
57. Klaas, N.E.; Thupayagale-Tshweneagae, G.; Makua, T.P. The role of gender in the spread of HIV and AIDS among farmworkers in South Africa. *Afr. J. Prim. Health Care Fam. Med.* **2018**, *10*, e1–e8. [CrossRef]
58. National Department of Health. *The 2010 National Antenatal Sentinel HIV & Syphilis Prevalence Survey in South Africa*; South African NDoH: Pretoria, South Africa, 2010. Available online: https://www.hst.org.za/publications/NonHST%20Publications/hiv_aids_survey.pdf (accessed on 2 June 2025).
59. Western Cape Department of Health. *The Provincial and District HIV Antenatal Survey*; Provincial Department of Health: Cape Town, South Africa, 2001.
60. International Organization for Migration. *HIV/AIDS, Population Mobility and Migration in Southern Africa: Defining a Research and Policy Agenda*; International Organization for Migration: Geneva, Switzerland, 2005. Available online: http://www.iom.int (accessed on 2 June 2025).
61. Nicholas, P.K.; Mfono, N.; Corless, I.B.; Davis, S.M.; O'Brien, E.; Padua, J.; Ahmed, S.; Sheldon, L.K.; Oas, K.; Sadler, L.; et al. HIV vulnerability in migrant populations in southern Africa: Sociological, cultural, health-related, and human-rights perspectives. *Int. J. Afr. Nurs. Sci.* **2016**, *5*, 1–8. [CrossRef]
62. Coffee, M.; Lurie, M.N.; Garnett, G.P. Modelling the impact of migration on the HIV epidemic in South Africa. *AIDS* **2007**, *21*, 343–350. [CrossRef]
63. Lurie, M.; Harrison, A.; Wilkinson, D.; Karim, S.A. Circular Migration and Sexual Networking in Rural KwaZulu/Natal: Implications for the Spread of HIV and Other Sexually Transmitted Diseases. *Health Transit. Rev.* **1997**, *7*, 17–27. Available online: http://www.jstor.org/stable/40608686 (accessed on 2 June 2025).
64. Lurie, M.N.; Williams, B.G.; Zuma, K.; Mkaya-Mwamburi, D.; Garnett, G.; Sturm, A.W.; Sweat, M.D.; Gittelsohn, J.; Abdool Karim, S.S. The impact of migration on HIV-1 transmission in South Africa: A study of migrant and nonmigrant men and their partners. *Sex. Transm. Dis.* **2003**, *30*, 149–156. [CrossRef] [PubMed]
65. Gossage, J.; Snell, C.; Parry, C.; Marais, A.; Barnard, R.; De Vries, M.; Blankenship, J.; Seedat, S.; Hasken, J.; May, P. Alcohol Use, Working Conditions, Job Benefits, and the Legacy of the "Dop" System among Farm Workers in the Western Cape Province, South Africa: Hope Despite High Levels of Risky Drinking. *Int. J. Environ. Res. Public Health* **2014**, *11*, 7406–7424. [CrossRef]
66. Holtman, Z.; Shelmerdine, S.; London, L.; Flisher, A. Suicide in a poor rural community in the Western Cape, South Africa: Experiences of five suicide attempters and their families. *S. Afr. J. Psychol.* **2011**, *41*, 300–309. [CrossRef]

67. Ojo, O.A.; Louwagie, G.; Morojele, N.; Rendall-Mkosi, K.; London, L.; Olorunju, S.; Davids, A. Factors associated with female high-risk drinking in a rural and urban South African site. *S. Afr. Med. J.* **2010**, *100*, 180–182. [CrossRef]
68. McLoughlin, J.-A.; Little, F.; Mazok, C.; Parry, C.; London, L. Prevalence of and Associations With Papsak Wine Consumption Among Farm Workers in the Western Cape Province, South Africa. *J. Stud. Alcohol Drugs* **2013**, *74*, 879–888. [CrossRef]
69. May, P.; Gossage, J.; Marais, A.; Adnams, C.; Hoyme, H.; Jones, K.; Robinson, L.; Khaole, N.; Snell, C.; Kalberg, W.; et al. The epidemiology of fetal alcohol syndrome and partial FAS in a South African community. *Drug Alcohol Depend.* **2007**, *88*, 259–271. [CrossRef] [PubMed]
70. May, P.A.; Blankenship, J.; Marais, A.S.; Gossage, J.P.; Kalberg, W.O.; Barnard, R.; De Vries, M.; Robinson, L.K.; Adnams, C.M.; Buckley, D. Approaching the Prevalence of the Full Spectrum of Fetal Alcohol Spectrum Disorders in a South African Population-Based Study. *Alcohol Clin. Exp. Res.* **2013**, *37*, 818–830. [CrossRef] [PubMed]
71. Parry, C.; Gossage, J.; Marais, A.; Barnard, R.; de Vries, M.; Blankenship, J.; Seedat, S.; May, P. Comparison of baseline drinking practices, knowledge, and attitudes of adult s residing in communities taking part in the FAS prevention study in South Africa. *Afr. J. Drug Alcohol Stud.* **2012**, *11*.
72. Parenzee, P.; Smythe, D. *Domestic Violence and Development: Looking at the Farming Context*; Institute of Criminology, University of Cape Town Cape Town: Cape Town, South Africa, 2003.
73. Lesch, E.; Adams, A.R. Couples living with and around alcohol abuse: A study of a farmworker community in the Cape Winelands, South Africa. *Soc. Sci. Med.* **2016**, *156*, 167–174. [CrossRef]
74. Park, H.H.; Girdler-Brown, B.V.; Churchyard, G.J.; White, N.W.; Ehrlich, R.I. Incidence of tuberculosis and HIV and progression of silicosis and lung function impairment among former Basotho gold miners. *Am. J. Ind. Med.* **2009**, *52*, 901–908. [CrossRef] [PubMed]
75. Corbett, E.L.; Charalambous, S.; Moloi, V.M.; Fielding, K.; Grant, A.D.; Dye, C.; De Cock, K.M.; Hayes, R.J.; Williams, B.G.; Churchyard, G.J. Human immunodeficiency virus and the prevalence of undiagnosed tuberculosis in African gold miners. *Am. J. Respir. Crit. Care Med.* **2004**, *170*, 673–679. [CrossRef]
76. World Health Organization. *Global Tuberculosis Report 2013*; 9241564652; World Health Organization: Geneva, Switzerland, 2013.
77. Kubjane, M.; Osman, M.; Boulle, A.; Johnson, L.F. The impact of HIV and tuberculosis interventions on South African adult tuberculosis trends, 1990–2019: A mathematical modeling analysis. *Int. J. Infect. Dis.* **2022**, *122*, 811–819. [CrossRef]
78. Bruchfeld, J.; Correia-Neves, M.; Källenius, G. Tuberculosis and HIV Coinfection. *Cold Spring Harb. Perspect. Med.* **2015**, *5*, a017871. [CrossRef]
79. Jassat, W.; Cohen, C.; Tempia, S.; Masha, M.; Goldstein, S.; Kufa, T.; Murangandi, P.; Savulescu, D.; Walaza, S.; Bam, J.-L.; et al. Risk factors for COVID-19-related in-hospital mortality in a high HIV and tuberculosis prevalence setting in South Africa: A cohort study. *Lancet HIV* **2021**, *8*, e554–e567. [CrossRef]
80. Dominick, L.; Midgley, N.; Swart, L.M.; Sprake, D.; Deshpande, G.; Laher, I.; Joseph, D.; Teer, E.; Essop, M.F. HIV-related cardiovascular diseases: The search for a unifying hypothesis. *Am. J. Physiol. Heart Circ. Physiol.* **2020**, *318*, H731–H746. [CrossRef]
81. Venter, W.D.F.; Moorhouse, M.; Sokhela, S.; Fairlie, L.; Mashabane, N.; Masenya, M.; Serenata, C.; Akpomiemie, G.; Qavi, A.; Chandiwana, N.; et al. Dolutegravir plus Two Different Prodrugs of Tenofovir to Treat HIV. *N. Engl. J. Med.* **2019**, *381*, 803–815. [CrossRef] [PubMed]
82. Vos, A.G.; Barth, R.E.; Klipstein-Grobusch, K.; Tempelman, H.A.; Devillé, W.L.J.; Dodd, C.; Coutinho, R.A.; Grobbee, D.E. Cardiovascular Disease Burden in Rural Africa: Does HIV and Antiretroviral Treatment Play a Role?: Baseline Analysis of the Ndlovu Cohort Study. *J. Am. Heart Assoc.* **2020**, *9*, e013466. [CrossRef]
83. McCann, K.; Shah, S.; Hindley, L.; Hill, A.; Qavi, A.; Simmons, B.; Serenata, C.; Sokhela, S.; Venter, W.D.F. Implications of weight gain with newer anti-retrovirals: 10-year predictions of cardiovascular disease and diabetes. *AIDS* **2021**, *35*, 1657–1665. [CrossRef]
84. Thienemann, F.; Ntusi, N.A.B.; Battegay, E.; Mueller, B.U.; Cheetham, M. Multimorbidity and cardiovascular disease: A perspective on low- and middle-income countries. *Cardiovasc. Diagn. Ther.* **2020**, *10*, 376–385. [CrossRef]
85. Magodoro, I.M.; Okello, S.; Dungeni, M.; Castle, A.C.; Mureyani, S.; Danaei, G. Association between HIV and Prevalent Hypertension and Diabetes Mellitus in South Africa: Analysis of a Nationally Representative Cross-Sectional Survey. *Int. J. Infect. Dis.* **2022**, *121*, 217–225. [CrossRef] [PubMed]
86. Shah, A.S.V.; Stelzle, D.; Lee, K.K.; Beck, E.J.; Alam, S.; Clifford, S.; Longenecker, C.T.; Strachan, F.; Bagchi, S.; Whiteley, W.; et al. Global Burden of Atherosclerotic Cardiovascular Disease in People Living with HIV: Systematic Review and Meta-Analysis. *Circulation* **2018**, *138*, 1100–1112. [CrossRef]
87. Imtiaz, S.; Shield, K.D.; Roerecke, M.; Samokhvalov, A.V.; Lönnroth, K.; Rehm, J. Alcohol consumption as a risk factor for tuberculosis: Meta-analyses and burden of disease. *Eur. Respir. J.* **2017**, *50*, 1700216. [CrossRef] [PubMed]
88. Fisher, J.C.; Bang, H.; Kapiga, S.H. The Association Between HIV Infection and Alcohol Use: A Systematic Review and Meta-Analysis of African Studies. *Sex. Transm. Dis.* **2007**, *34*, 856–863. [CrossRef]
89. Fisher, J.C.; Cook, P.A.; Kapiga, S.H. Alcohol use before sex and HIV risk: Situational characteristics of protected and unprotected encounters among high-risk African women. *Sex. Transm. Dis.* **2010**, *37*, 571–578. [CrossRef]

90. Sun, K.; Ren, M.; Liu, D.; Wang, C.; Yang, C.; Yan, L. Alcohol consumption and risk of metabolic syndrome: A meta-analysis of prospective studies. *Clin. Nutr.* **2014**, *33*, 596–602. [CrossRef]
91. Lopez, L.; Kogut, K.; Rauch, S.; Gunier, R.B.; Wong, M.P.; Harris, E.; Deardorff, J.; Eskenazi, B.; Harley, K.G. Organophosphate pesticide exposure and risk of SARS-CoV-2 infection. *Environ. Res.* **2024**, *255*, 119214. [CrossRef] [PubMed]
92. Fagundes, T.R.; Kawassaki, A.C.B.; Concato, V.M.; Assolini, J.P.; Silva, T.F.; Gonçalves, M.D.; da Silva Siqueira, E.; Sahd, C.S.; Inoue, F.S.R.; da Silva, T.P.; et al. Impact of Pesticides on Immune-Endocrine Disorders and Its Relationship to Cancer Development. In *Handbook of Cancer and Immunology*; Rezaei, N., Ed.; Springer International Publishing: Cham, Switzerland, 2022; pp. 1–30.
93. He, B.; Ni, Y.; Jin, Y.; Fu, Z. Pesticides-induced energy metabolic disorders. *Sci. Total Environ.* **2020**, *729*, 139033. [CrossRef] [PubMed]
94. Kahn, L.G.; Philippat, C.; Nakayama, S.F.; Slama, R.; Trasande, L. Endocrine-disrupting chemicals: Implications for human health. *Lancet Diabetes Endocrinol.* **2020**, *8*, 703–718. [CrossRef]
95. London, L. Human rights and health: Opportunities to advance rural occupational health. *Int. J. Occup. Environ. Health* **2011**, *17*, 80–92. [CrossRef] [PubMed]
96. Surplus People Project. Pesticide Health Risks for South African Emerging Farmers. 2011. Available online: https://www.spp.org.za/wp-content/uploads/2016/07/pesticide_booklet.pdf (accessed on 2 June 2025).
97. Curl, C.L.; Spivak, M.; Phinney, R.; Montrose, L. Synthetic Pesticides and Health in Vulnerable Populations: Agricultural Workers. *Curr. Environ. Health Rep.* **2020**, *7*, 13–29. [CrossRef]
98. Cancino, J.; Soto, K.; Tapia, J.; Muñoz-Quezada, M.T.; Lucero, B.; Contreras, C.; Moreno, J. Occupational exposure to pesticides and symptoms of depression in agricultural workers. A systematic review. *Environ. Res.* **2023**, *231*, 116190. [CrossRef]
99. Mamane, A.; Baldi, I.; Tessier, J.F.; Raherison, C.; Bouvier, G. Occupational exposure to pesticides and respiratory health. *Eur. Respir. Rev.* **2015**, *24*, 306–319. [CrossRef]
100. London, L. The 'dop' system, alcohol abuse and social control amongst farm workers in South Africa: A public health challenge. *Soc. Sci. Med.* **1999**, *48*, 1407–1414. [CrossRef]
101. Te Water Naude, J.; London, L.; Pitt, B.; Mahomed, C. The 'dop' system around Stellenbosch--results of a farm survey. *S. Afr. Med. J. Suid-Afr. Tydskr. Vir Geneeskd.* **1998**, *88*, 1102–1105.
102. London, L. Alcohol consumption amongst South African farm workers: A challenge for post-apartheid health sector transformation. *Drug Alcohol Depend.* **2000**, *59*, 199–206. [CrossRef]
103. Mager, A. 'White liquor hits black livers': Meanings of excessive liquor consumption in South Africa in the second half of the twentieth century. *Soc. Sci. Med.* **2004**, *59*, 735–751. [CrossRef] [PubMed]
104. Geronimus, A. *Weathering: The Extraordinary Stress of Ordinary Life in an Unjust Society*; Little Brown: Boston, MA, USA, 2023.
105. Democratic, A. Farm Worker Project for Better Health is Progressing Swiftly. *Where We Govern.* 2022. Available online: https://www.da.org.za/government/where-we-govern/2022/08/farm-worker-project-for-better-health-is-progressing-swiftly (accessed on 2 June 2025).
106. The Aurum Institute. Aurum Tackles TB in Western Cape farmlands. 2022. Available online: https://www.auruminstitute.org/component/content/article/28-blog/aurum-news/668-aurum-tackles-tb-in-western-cape-farmlands?Itemid=101 (accessed on 2 June 2025).
107. Barrientos, S.; Visser, M. South African horticulture: Opportunities and challenges for economic and social upgrading in value chains. *SSRN* **2013**, *2209718*. [CrossRef]
108. Visser, M.; Ferrer, S. *Farm Workers' Living and Working Conditions in South Africa: Key Trends, Emergent Issues, and Underlying and Structural Problems*; International Labour Organization: Pretoria, South Africa, 2015.
109. Department of Labour. *Adequacy of Resources for Effective Inspections to be Conducted Within the South African Labour Market*; Department of Labour: Cape Town, South African, 2017.
110. Hogan, A.B.; Jewell, B.L.; Sherrard-Smith, E.; Vesga, J.F.; Watson, O.J.; Whittaker, C.; Hamlet, A.; Smith, J.A.; Winskill, P.; Verity, R. Potential impact of the COVID-19 pandemic on HIV, tuberculosis, and malaria in low-income and middle-income countries: A modelling study. *Lancet Glob. Health* **2020**, *8*, e1132–e1141. [CrossRef] [PubMed]
111. National Department of Health. *COVID-19 South African Coronavirus News and Information Portal*; National Department of Health: Pretoria, South Africa, 2021. Available online: https://sacoronavirus.co.za/ (accessed on 2 June 2025).
112. Alene, K.A.; Wangdi, K.; Clements, A.C.A. Impact of the COVID-19 Pandemic on Tuberculosis Control: An Overview. *Trop. Med. Infect. Dis.* **2020**, *5*, 123. [CrossRef]
113. Eike, D.; Hogrebe, M.; Kifle, D.; Tregilgas, M.; Uppal, A.; Calmy, A. How the COVID-19 Pandemic Alters the Landscapes of the HIV and Tuberculosis Epidemics in South Africa: A Case Study and Future Directions. *Epidemiologia* **2022**, *3*, 297–313. [CrossRef]
114. Jardim, C.G.R.; Zamani, R.; Akrami, M. Evaluating the Impact of the COVID-19 Pandemic on Accessing HIV Services in South Africa: A Systematic Review. *Int. J. Environ. Res. Public Health* **2022**, *19*, 11899. [CrossRef]

115. StopTB Partnership. *The Potential Impact of the COVID-19 Response on Tuberculosis in High-Burden Countries: A Modelling Analysis*. 2020. Available online: https://stoptb.org/assets/documents/news/Modeling%20Report_1%20May%202020_FINAL.pdf (accessed on 2 June 2025).
116. Ndjeka, N.; Kubjane, M.; Abdullah, F.; Mohr-Holland, E.; Subrayen, P.; Loveday, M.; Dube, M.; Boffa, J. Impact of US funding cuts and stop work orders on TB services and research in South Africa. *IJTLD Open* **2025**, *2*, 241–243. [CrossRef]

MDPI AG
Grosspeteranlage 5
4052 Basel
Switzerland
Tel.: +41 61 683 77 34

Tropical Medicine and Infectious Disease Editorial Office
E-mail: tropicalmed@mdpi.com
www.mdpi.com/journal/tropicalmed

www.ingramcontent.com/pod-product-compliance
Lightning Source LLC
Chambersburg PA
CBHW061628210926
51850CB00009B/2478
9783725846436